Language Learning and
Communication Disorders in Children

Language Learning an

GERTRUD L. WYATT

Communication Disorders in Children

THE FREE PRESS, NEW YORK · COLLIER-MACMILLAN LIMITED, LONDON

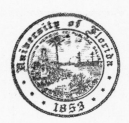

For Cornelia

Contents

Foreword

This volume is indeed a gold mine of dynamic interdisciplinary information about the whole child. It will be of great value not only to the speech therapist but also to the child psychologist, the child psychiatrist, the school psychologist, the pediatrician, and the psychiatric social worker. It will be of value, also, to school administrators, the key people who can make possible the flexible team approach in the application of research findings to the remediation of the many problems in language and communication confronting educators today.

The opening chapter presents a model of adult–child verbal interaction necessary for the child's learning of language in the phonetic, semantic, and grammatical dimensions. The verbal model, the author maintains, must be a good one, and it must be continuous. Not only must the model be correct for the mother tongue in the above characteristics; to be effective, it must also be appropriate to the child's level of intellectual and verbal development and it must be presented in an emotional atmosphere of affection and warmth. To the usually recognized linguistic, physiological, and acoustic levels of language development the author adds the psychological level. This, she holds, is essential in enabling the child to acquire the necessary internal feedback system that allows him to progress from the dualistic form of communication with the mother or other language model to a pluralistic system of communicating with a variety of persons.

Two fascinating case studies, presented in carefully objectified, anecdotal style, vividly illustrate the basis for the author's emphasis on the quality and continuity of the mother's interaction with the child in the acquisition of speech. One is of an institutionalized child in transition to a foster home; the other, of a young stutterer who is followed longitudinally in diary fashion.

The author's rich background in the Viennese school of speech therapy and early contact with outstanding psychoanalysts and developmental psychologists was followed by scientific training in clinical psychology in the United States, where her developmental crisis theory of stuttering was the subject of her doctoral research (summarized in Chapter 6).

Descriptions of subsequent applications of her diagnostic techniques and therapies in a school setting—where she has unusual opportunities to work with other professionals from a variety of other disciplines and where she has enjoyed continued support for research—make this book essentially the author's professional autobiography. Personal experiences and scientific objectivity are skillfully woven together in an easy, readable style, without belaboring either case material or statistical data, so that the whole work has a ring of sincerity and integrity. The author is quick to point out where her initial ideas required modification in the light of scientific inquiry and to call attention to areas needing further research.

Although the syndrome of the stuttering child is a primary focus of the book, the author's broad conception of language and communication leads her to secondary chapters on the diagnosis and treatment of children with other types of language disturbances whom she encounters in her work. There are helpful discussions of children with articulatory defects (both with and without stuttering) as well as of children whose language and communication difficulties seem to be associated with neurological signs and perceptual-motor impairments.

The detailed appendixes—providing descriptions of diagnostic aids, tests, and check-lists employed in the studies described—make this a most helpful manual. The bibliography of approximately 500 pertinent titles, deftly referred to in the text, is multilingual and thoroughly up-to-date. The description of applications of the author's insightful and demonstrably successful techniques to disadvantaged children in compensatory educational programs, as described in Chapter 15, should do much to overcome current educational lags.

The book is indeed timely, and it is one of very few works presenting practical solutions to clinical problems arrived at on the basis of solidly grounded research.

Fordham University, New York   DOROTHEA MCCARTHY

Preface and Acknowledgments

The aims of this book are (1) to present clinical observations of children's language behavior and (2) to report in detail the results of a series of original research studies carried out during the last ten years by myself and my collaborators, at the Wellesley Public Schools, Wellesley, Massachusetts. An attempt has been made to explore the processes of language teaching and language learning occurring during a child's early years within the framework of adult-child relationships. I perceived the acquisition of language by the child as an ongoing process, depending at all times upon the stage of maturation and the physiological functioning of the organism, but also upon the sociocultural setting in which the child finds himself and upon the kind and frequency of verbal stimulation he experiences within a given network of interpersonal relationships.

The observations reported here were made partly in Central European and partly in North American settings. The cultures concerned were of the kind in which the mother—or her substitute—has the primary responsibility for the care and upbringing of the young child, thus serving as the primary love object and the primary speech model for him. The thesis is put forward that, within such cultural settings, *certain forms of mother-child interaction tend to facilitate language development in the child and others tend to inhibit it or interfere with it.*

I believe with Heinz Werner and Bernard Kaplan that "there are multiple approaches to the problems of language . . . each of which probes into these problems with its own presuppositions, its specific concerns, its own techniques and modes of analysis . . . Each approach yields some information on the complex and many-sided problems and none can claim reasonably to be the only avenue to truth."[1]

---

1. Werner and Kaplan (1963), p. v.

My early training in the observation of children's language and behavior was guided by some of the outstanding teachers under whom I had the privilege of studying: Professor Emil Froeschels, then head of the Voice and Speech Clinic at the Vienna General Hospital, University of Vienna; Miss Anna Freud, then director of the training program for educators at the Vienna Psychoanalytic Institute; and the late Dr. Susan Isaacs, of London University, who introduced me to the study of child development.

The conceptual framework of the studies described here was derived from genetic psychology, in particular from the work of Heinz Werner and Jean Piaget; from the psychology of language and communication; and from psychoanalytic ego-psychology. Research findings were considered in the areas of language development, psycholinguistics, speech pathology, psychotherapy, and remedial education.

As most of our original research studies were carried out within a school setting, a developmental approach to the problems of language behavior was found most fruitful. Within this framework correlations between teaching and learning and the identification of orderly sequences of behavior over time provided the essential coordinates against which each child's linguistic development or deviations could be plotted. A field theory of language behavior was adopted in which the unit of analysis was no longer the individual child. Observations were focused upon the *process of interaction* between speaker and listener and the characteristic *patterns* of these interactions, changing with the age and the developmental stage of the child and differing between settings and between interacting speech partners.

Moral and financial support for most of these studies came from the Wellesley School Department and from the U.S. Department of Health, Education, and Welfare, the National Institute of Mental Health. The latter supported our work from 1958 to 1959, through Small Grant M-2667-A, and from 1961 to 1964, through Research Grant MH-4643.

My collaborators and I appreciate the support we received from various persons connected with the Wellesley Public School System. We are deeply grateful to Mr. John B. Chaffee, Superintendent of Schools; to Mr. Roger Woodbury and Mr. Wilbert Rook, Assistant Superintendents; to the members of the Wellesley School Committee; and to the principals of the eleven elementary schools for their active sympathy with our projects and interests and for the constructive help given in our professional interactions with teachers, parents, and children. All members of the research staff benefitted immeasurably from our continuous contact with the well-trained and highly motivated teachers of the Wellesley Public School System. Our diagnostic skills and therapeutic ingenuity were challenged constantly by our ongoing work with the children and parents of Wellesley. In addition, we received much professional encouragement and scientific stimulation from the pediatricians practicing in the Wellesley area and from the staff of the Wellesley Human Relations Service, Incorporated.

In spite of my lifelong interest in children's language behavior, however, my work would never have come to fruition without the contributions made by my collaborators in the research project, Treating Children with Non-Organic Language Disorders. From 1961 to 1964 it was my great good fortune to be associated with the following persons: the sponsor of the project, Mr. John B. Chaffee; our research assistant, Mrs. Harriet M. Stanton; therapists and parent counselors Mrs. Louise S. Brown (who participated in the project from 1961 to 1964), Dr. Ronald P. Dutton (1961 to 1964), Mrs. Jacqueline Harmon (1961 to 1963), Mrs. Marilyn Prentice (1962 to 1964), Miss Dorothy A. Savre (1963 to 1964), Mrs. Lois L. Scott (1961 to 1964), and Mr. John Stout (1961 to 1962); consultants Drs. Austin W. Berkeley, John K. Brines, and Helen M. Herzan, data analysts Mrs. Marion Kagan, Dr. Newton von Sander, and Miss Cornelia K. Wyatt; and our executive secretary, Mrs. Doris B. Adams. The integrity and ingenuity of all members of the team was matched only by the unselfish generosity with which they contributed their time and skills.

One member of the team must be mentioned with particular appreciation: Dr. Helen M. Herzan, the consultant in psychiatry. The methods of therapy used in working with stuttering children and parents were developed in constant collaboration with her, and our team might have functioned less harmoniously without the wisdom of her advice and the unfailing tact and kindness which prompted her supervisory work with our therapists and parent counselors.

I am grateful also to Mrs. Lois Scott and Miss Jean Taylor for contributing some of the observations of children in Head Start programs, mentioned in Chapter 15.

I am much indebted to a number of friends and associates for critical reading of sections of this book. Mrs. Harriet Stanton and Dr. Newton von Sander, my fellow psychologists at the Wellesley Public Schools, as well as Dr. Frederick Wyatt, Chief of the Psychological Clinic at the University of Michigan, have read and reflected upon much of the manuscript. Individual chapters have been read and suggestions for improvement have been made by Mr. John Chaffee, Dr. Helen Herzan, Mrs. Barbara Johnson, Dr. Lewis Klebanoff, Mrs. Katherine Morrill, Mrs. Roberta Perlin, Mr. Alton Reynolds, Mrs. Lois Scott, and Dr. Leonard Weiner. Miss Cornelia Wyatt has given me much help in matters of style and organization.

Mrs. Doris B. Adams, our devoted secretary, not only typed and retyped the many forms and reports needed during our research, she also prepared the subsequent drafts of this volume—for all of which I am most grateful to her.

I also wish to acknowledge the patience of The Free Press for waiting several years for this book in the making, and I appreciate the assistance given me by various persons there.

Furthermore, I am deeply grateful to the John Simon Guggenheim Memorial Foundation, whose generous support, awarded to me in 1965, made it possible for me to devote time to the preparation of this volume.

I close this preface with the hope that this book will be of help to the many people dedicated to the study, care, and education of young children: psychologists, speech therapists, physicians, educators, social workers, public health nurses, and—last, not least—interested parents. The book is meant as a form of communication through which we may share our therapeutic experiences with the reader and bring to his attention patterns of adult-child interaction which have not been comprehended sufficiently in the past.

GERTRUD L. WYATT

Introduction: The Plan of the Book

The plan of the book is as follows: Part I contains examples of interaction between adults and children, followed by the history of two children with deviations in language development. In Part II a number of interrelated research studies in the area of communication disorders are described and their results discussed.

Part I is devoted mainly to examples of adult-child interaction patterns and of children's language behavior in everyday life situations as well as under unusual circumstances. It is hoped that the examination of these "raw" transcripts of children's speech will sharpen the reader's perception of some of the specific features to be observed in adult-child interaction and will prepare him for the hypotheses tested and the techniques adopted in the formal research studies contained in Part II.

In addition to these examples, Part I also contains the description and analysis of the language behavior of two children: Debby (Chapter 2) and Nana (Chapters 3 and 4). Debby's language deficit was observed during a truly traumatic episode occurring in the third year of her unusual life history. In contrast to the limited observation of Debby, Nana's language development was followed from birth through adolescence. The appearance of stuttering in Nana's speech during the third year of her life was totally unexpected. Thus I had the unique opportunity of watching the development of her symptoms from day to day, of realizing the mother's distress in reaction to Nana's difficulties, of observing the gradual disappearance of Nana's symptoms, and, finally, of witnessing her mastery of speech and language in later years. Samples of these observations have been presented in Chapters 3 and 4, together with a theoretical discussion of the behavior observed.

I knew Debby in 1938, and I have known Nana since her birth in 1942. By necessity, my reports about these two children had to be anecdotal and impressionistic in style. I do believe, however, that no similar descriptions exist in the literature on language development and that the rarity of the observations justifies their publication. I am grateful particularly to the late Professor Heinz Werner, who encouraged me to continue my recording of Nana's language development.

The information gained from the first four chapters is summarized in Chapter 5. A number of hypotheses concerning the interpersonal aspects of language learning in childhood are presented, and the role of imitation, repetition, and corrective feedback in language development is discussed.

Research studies to test these hypotheses were carried out between 1958 and 1964, and their results are reported in Part II. In Chapters 6 to 14 three different groups of children with developmental speech and language disorders are described, and problems of differential diagnosis, therapy, and work with teachers and parents are discussed in detail. Most of the information concerning these children was gained through a series of original studies carried out at the Wellesley Public Schools. Two of these studies were partly supported by the National Institute of Mental Health. Some of our research findings were presented previously in reports to the National Institute of Mental Health (Wyatt 1959 and 1964). However, while these earlier reports were technical in nature and statistically oriented, the emphasis in the present volume is clinical. In order to illuminate the treatment process, detailed case studies and verbatim excerpts from children's test responses and from therapists' reports have been included in Chapters 6 to 13.

In 1965 some members of our group had the opportunity of observing children and consulting teachers and parents connected with two Head Start programs carried out in the Greater Boston area. In this way we learned how to adapt our treatment techniques to the needs of educationally deprived young chidren and their mothers. Our experiences with this group and our recommendations for compensatory language training of children are presented in Chapter 15.

Finally, in Chapter 16, the problems of primary and secondary prevention of communication disorders in children are discussed and ways are suggested to organize educational and therapeutic programs for children with developmental language disorders.

Oh Sprache, beschreibende, selber unbeschreibliche,
sucherische, hindraengend zum Unbeschreibbaren.
Kein Wort wuerde leben, waere es nicht durchzittert von
  dem fremden Klang aus anderm Tal,
dem Hauchklang von dort, der das Beschreibbare ins
  Unbeschreibliche hebt.

—HERMANN BROCH *

Oh language, describing, itself indescribable, searching,
pressing towards the indescribable.
No word would live unless a-tremble with the strange sound
from the valley beyond,
the spirit-sound from beyond, lifting the describable
  into the indescribable.

Language is the most significant and colossal work that the human spirit has evolved—nothing short of a finished form of expression for all communicable experience. This form may be endlessly varied by the individual without thereby losing its distinctive contours; and it is constantly reshaping itself as is all art. Language is the most massive and inclusive art we know, a mountainous and anonymous work of unconscious generations.

—EDWARD SAPIR

---

* By permission of Suhrkamp Verlag, Frankfurt, Germany
Copyright 1953 by Rhein-Verlag A G Zuerich

PART I

Patterns of Interaction Between Adults and Children

CHAPTER ONE

A Model for the Study of Adult-Child Interaction

A clinical study of developmental language disorders in children must begin with an understanding of the conditions and the structure of normal developmental processes. In order to understand deviations or deficiencies in children's language development, we must be able to determine under what conditions, in what manner, and at what point in the child's development the process of language learning was disrupted or delayed and language development began to deteriorate.

Since the appearance of Clara and William Stern's famous work *Die Kinder-sprache* (1907), research in children's language development has expanded greatly. Necessarily, studies in language development carried out earlier in the century were mostly normative, focusing upon the number of different sounds and words mastered by the majority of children at a given age. The most comprehensive survey of the literature was presented by Dorothea McCarthy in the *Manual of Child Psychology* (1954). The bibliography following her review extends over 17 pages, covering approximately 700 publications culled from both American and European publications.

The paramount importance of the preschool years for language development has been established in many studies (McCarthy, 1954, 1959 and 1960). McCarthy (1954) referred to the "amazingly rapid acquisition of an extremely complex system of symbolic habits by young children," while Penfield and Roberts (1959) stressed the "biological time table for language learning," assuming that the most intensive learning occurs between two and four years of age.

Edward Sapir, the anthropologist, in his classical study of language was among the first to stress the sociocultural determinants of language behavior in man in contrast to the merely physiological aspects of the act of speaking. He wrote:

The process of acquiring speech is, in sober fact, an utterly different sort of thing from the process of learning to walk. In the case of the latter function, culture, in other words,

the traditional body of social usage, is not seriously brought into play. The child is individually equipped, by the complex set of factors that we term biological heredity, to make all
the needed muscular and nervous adjustments that result in walking. . . . In a very real
sense the normal human being is predestined to walk, not because his elders will assist him to
learn the art, but because . . . walking is an inherent, biological function of man.

Not so language. It is of course true that in a certain sense the individual is predestined
to talk, but that is due entirely to the circumstance that he is born not merely in nature, but
in the lap of a society that is reasonably certain to lead him to its traditions. . . . Walking is
an organic, an instinctive function (not, of course, itself an instinct); speech is a non-instinctive, acquired, "cultural function."[1]

Language is a purely human and non-instinctive method of communicating ideas,
emotions and desires by means of a system of voluntarily produced symbols. . . . We must
not be misled by the term "the organs of speech." There are, properly speaking, no organs
of speech, there are only organs that are incidentally useful in the production of speech
sounds. . . . Physiologically, speech is an overlaid function, or, to be more precise, a group
of overlaid functions. . . . We cannot define it as an entity in psychophysical terms alone,
however much the psycho-physical basis is essential to its functioning in the individual. . . .
Our study of language is not to be one of the genesis and operation of a concrete mechanism;
it is, rather, to be an inquiry into the function and form of the arbitrary systems of symbolism
that we term languages.[2]

Sapir's emphasis upon interpersonal variables, however, has been overlooked
almost completely in the field of speech pathology and therapy, where the medical
model prevails. A wealth of information concerning the physiology and pathology
of speech and hearing has been accumulated, but the focus of investigation is
still primarily upon the child as an isolated individual. As a rule the child is perceived as speech defective, or speech handicapped; in the German literature, for
instance, the expression *das sprach-kranke Kind* is found frequently.

Sapir's appeal has found considerable response in the psychology of language
and communication. In the past few years much attention has been paid to the
social context within which the child's language learning occurs (Bullowa, Jones,
and Bever, 1961; Bullowa, Jones, and Duckert, 1964; Slobin, 1964a and 1964b;
Brown and Cazden, 1965). Most recently, sociologists, psychologists, and educators
engaged in developing compensatory programs for culturally deprived children
have been particularly concerned with environmental stimulation or deprivation
and its effect upon children's language learning and cognitive development
(Bernstein, 1961; C. P. Deutsch, 1964; John and Goldstein, 1964; Olim, Hess, and
Shipman, 1965, and others).

In our own research we have been particularly interested in the process of
verbal interaction between child and mother, its importance for language learning,
and its relation to language deviations in the child.

My interest concerning the effect of maternal stimulation upon children's

---

1. Edward Sapir, *Language: An introduction to the study of speech* (New York: Harcourt, Brace &
World, Inc., 1921), pp. 1-2. Reprinted by permission of Harcourt, Brace & World, Inc., and Rupert
Hart-Davis Ltd.
2. Sapir, pp. 7-10.

language development goes back to the early 1950s. When I looked through the literature for descriptions of verbal interaction patterns between adult and child, I found almost none. Outside of Piaget's (1951) studies of sensory-motor learning through imitation of a model, hardly any systematic observations of interaction between adults and children existed. I did find, finally, a vivid description of verbal interaction between adults and children in Margaret Mead's anthropological study of life in New Guinea:

> Children are taught to talk through the men's and older boys' love of playing with children. There is no belief that it is necessary to give a child formal teaching, rather chance adult play devices are enlisted. One of these is the delight in repetition. Melanesian languages very frequently use repetition to give an intensity to speech. To go far is expressed by "go go go," to be very large by "big big big." . . . A crowd also has a tendency to pick up a phrase and repeat it or turn it into a low monotonous song.
>
> This random affection for repetitiousness makes an excellent atmosphere in which the child acquires facility in speech. There is no adult boredom with the few faulty words of babyhood. Instead these very groping words form an excellent excuse for indulging their own passion for repetition. So the baby says "me," and the adult says "me." The baby says "me" and the adult says "me," on and on in the same tone of voice. I have counted sixty repetitions of the same monosyllabic word, either a true word or a nonsense syllable. And at the end of the sixtieth repetition, neither baby nor adult was bored.
>
> What is true of speech is equally true of gesture. Adults play games of imitative gesture with children. . . .
>
> So in this atmosphere of delight in repetition and imitation, a new language is taught painlessly by one age group to another.[3]

In comparing Mead's description of Manus patterns of communication between adults and children with the interaction between experimenter and child described by Piaget (1951), we find that both authors mention *games of mutual imitation* between partners who are imitating each other's gestures, words, and phrases. We are all familiar with the growing child's passion for *repetition*, an aspect of human development which seems to guarantee the necessary overlearning which is essential for the eventual mastery of speech and language. Furthermore, the *adults' delight* in the children's imitations and repetitions should be noted.

In recent years my collaborators, my students, and I have have collected our own samples of adult-child interaction. We made our observations generally with the permission of the parents concerned; occasionally without it. Sitting in a train, in a physician's waiting room, or in any other public place, one often has the opportunity to observe verbal interaction between parent and child. With some practice it is possible to take notes discreetly. During a casual conversation with the parent following the observation, one usually can learn the age of the child observed. Anybody interested in the development of language should turn into an observer and collector of parent-child conversations. Indeed, it is an enlightening and enchanting pastime.

---

3. Mead, 1953, pp. 30–33.

In addition to such casual observations, systematic notes were taken whenever a preschool child was referred to our research project for a diagnostic evaluation. As part of the evaluation procedure we made it a practice to visit at the child's home, often during mealtime. Such visits offer an excellent opportunity for observing the interaction process in a normal life situation between the child, his mother, and often his brothers and sisters.

EXAMPLES OF ADULT-CHILD INTERACTION

Let us now look at some of these examples of mother-child interaction.

Observation 1

I made the following observation on a hot summer day at a crowded beach. The child observed was Ricky, a 17-months-old boy. With him at the beach were his mother and grandmother.

Ricky was running around rather aimlessly, and his mother said to him:
"Come on . . . dig . . . dig in the sand . . . come on . . . there is your spoon . . . dig in the sand . . . don't cry . . . we will build a house . . . there is your spoon . . . dig in the sand. . . ."

A few minutes later Ricky began to run around again, and his mother said: "Want to go in the water? . . . all right . . . we go in the water . . . all right . . . come on, we go in the water . . . see the water . . ."

Holding hands, mother and son ran toward the water, while the mother said: "See the water . . . see the water . . . the water. . . ."

Ricky echoed: "Water! Water!"

Mother: "See the water . . . see the water . . . there is the water . . . there we go . . . there we go . . . see the water!"

Both waded into the water and soon they were out of my range of hearing. A few minutes later they both returned, Ricky riding on his mother's shoulders, screaming with delight.

Both sat down next to the grandmother, who remarked: "The water is too cold."

Their conversation continued. Mother (to grandmother): "I washed his pants off, the water is too cold." (To Ricky): "Now put your robe on . . . you need your robe, here is your robe."

The mother wrapped Ricky in a little white bathrobe. Ricky yelled happily and skipped around in his bathrobe.

Mother: "You show-off! You show-off! Oh, you do look pretty, you look pretty, oh boy! Want to go for a walk? Go for a walk?"

Ricky: "Go . . . go!"

Mother: "This way" (laughing), "this way!"

Ricky laughed and ran away from his mother. She ran after him, and held his hand as both walked off again toward the water.

Several features of this observation are of interest to us. The interaction between mother and child was as much nonverbal as it was verbal. The mother followed Ricky with her eyes almost continuously; she played with him; she cuddled him, carried him, directed and protected him. Mother and child obviously were close to each other, both physically and emotionally. This young mother, from her appearance a lower-middle-class woman, was an excellent speech model for her small son. She spoke to him in short simple sentences, using a limited vocabulary that most probably he was able to comprehend. Her short phrases and sentences were gramatically correct, and she articulated clearly. Watching her play with Ricky, one could sense her delight in the child. During the time of the observation she talked much more with her son than with her mother. Most striking in her speech with the child were the frequent repetitions she used. Altogether, she used language not on an elaborate adult level but approximately on the level of a 2-year-old child, thus matching her own speech production very closely with the child's level of maturation. Such a match is possible only if the mother permits herself a "positive regression" to a kind of behavior and speech which she must have enjoyed earlier in her own life. It was evident that this particular mother felt comfortable in using this simple form of language.

Observation 2

The second observation was made during a recent taxi ride in London.

Travelling from one station to another, I shared a taxi with a small family: a grandmother and a young mother with two children, a girl of 7 months and a boy of 2 years. During the brief trip the grandmother talked a good deal to the little boy, who was standing at the window, while the mother was occupied with the baby girl, whom she held on her lap. The grandmother explained to the boy that they were riding in a taxi; she referred to the driver as *the taximan.*While the mother and the grandmother exchanged remarks about the trip, the little boy uttered the word *taximan* from time to time. Each time, the grandmother responded immediately, repeating the word two or three times: "Yes, a taximan, taximan, taximan!" When we drove across Trafalgar Square with its fountains, the grandmother said to the little boy: "Look, see the water, see the water!" Turning to the mother she said: 'He wouldn't know what a fountain is.' The little boy repeated: "Water . . . taximan,' and the grandmother reiterated: "Yes, a taximan. And see the water, see the water." The little girl, who was only half awake, began to babble "oohahwooah . . ." and the grandmother echoed back "oohahwooah."

In this situation the mother primarily communicated nonverbally with her younger child, cuddling and rocking her, while the grandmother served as language teacher for the older boy. Both women appeared to belong to the working class or the lower-middle class. In providing her little grandson with labels for his experiences, the grandmother demonstrated a high degree of empathy (*Einfuehlung*) with the child's developmental level. She purposely used simple terms such as *taximan* for *taxidriver* and *water* for *fountain*. It was particularly striking to observe that in talking to the little boy, the grandmother repeated her words and phrases much more frequently than the boy did. All that he could handle at his stage of development were two basic words—*taximan* and *water*—which he repeated from time to time.

My observations made in this case agree with Slobin's (1954a). In analyzing the language development of two children 18 and 27 months old, Slobin found that their mothers repeated the children's words much more frequently—about three times more often—than the children imitated their mothers' words.

Observation 3

The next observation was made by a graduate student who was a trained nursery school teacher. Like myself, the student chose the beach for observing a 2-year-old boy and his family:

The mother I observed had three children: Cathy who was 4 years old, Bobby who was 2, and an infant in a baby carriage. Prior to this observation, the mother had been trying to keep the two older children off the blanket on which she and another young mother were sunning themselves. She wanted the children to play by themselves at the water's edge.

Bobby came up from the water's edge bringing a stone, which he silently offered to his mother. The mother took the stone, said "Okay," and put the stone down on the sand. Bobby walked away without saying anything, but returned immediately with another stone, which he again held out to his mother. With some annoyance, she said: "Okay, okay, go down by the water." Bobby picked up this second stone, which his mother had put down on the sand near the first one, and seemed about to throw it. Mother said: 'Don't throw it, don't throw it!" Bobby put down the stone and walked toward the water. He soon stopped to pick up a branch which was lying on the ground. His mother called: "Leave it, leave it"; and Bobby left it.

Bobby finally reached the water. He seemed attracted to a plastic boat which an older boy was sailing and said to a teenage girl who happened to be walking by: "Lookadat." The girl did not answer him.

Bobby stood at the water's edge for a brief moment. He then picked up some sand, turned around, and began to move toward his mother. The mother saw him coming. She pointed to the water and called out to him: "Get down by the water!" Bobby turned around and again approached the water's edge. He went over to the boy with the plastic boat and tried to grab it from him. He seemed about to burst into tears, when he suddenly caught sight of his sister Cathy, who was running toward the mother. He ran after her, smiling and pointing at his mother.

Cathy flopped down in the sand near the mother and said to her: "Will you help me to make a castle?" The mother and Cathy were already building in the sand when Bobby reached them. He looked at the sand structure and said excitedly: "Whatisit, Mommy?" The mother took a tissue and began to wipe his runny nose. She did not answer his question.

After his nose was wiped, Bobby suddenly smashed the castle with his foot. Cathy cried out and Mother said angrily to Bobby: "Why did you do that?" Bobby answered something that sounded like: "Howdoser." Cathy moved away and said to the other mother on the blanket: "You put the radio on?" The other mother replied: "Yes, I did." Bobby said "Whadisit?" Mother said to Bobby: "Go down by the water now." Bobby made no move to go. His mother picked him up by the arms and pushed him toward the water. Bobby turned around and came back to her. Mother said: "Bobby, go down there with Cathy!" Bobby moved away toward the other woman and said: "Dat's a boat, is it? Dat's a boat, is it? Dat's a boat, is it?" The woman didn't hear him because his voice was drowned out by the sound of the radio.

The mother was continually rejecting Bobby. She did not answer any of his requests for information; she disregarded all his offerings; she seemed to take no pleasure in the child at all. She never matched her words with those of the child, and her tone of voice was always angry.

The child showed his anger and frustration in many ways, all of them nonverbal. The most noticeable of these was the smashing of his sister's castle. The mother had been playing with the sister but had excluded Bobby from the project, even to the point of not responding to his question about what they were making. Bobby's retaliation had been to smash the product.

In this particular 10-minute observation the mother was certainly a poor speech model and an inadequate teacher of language for Bobby. However, later the same afternoon I had the opportunity of observing a different type of interaction between the same mother and her little boy. They were in the water together. The mother was telling Bobby to kick his feet. She showed him how, and then helped him do it. Bobby was smiling and laughing. He heard the sound of a motorboat and said: "Boat!" An airplane was passing at the same moment and the mother said: "No, plane!" Then she saw the boat and added: "Oh yes, there is a boat!" Bobby saw the plane and said: "Plane"; and his mother said: "The boat goes in the water, the plane goes in the sky."

During this second period of conversation the mother's attitude to the child had changed completely She was listening to him; smiling at him; helping him to learn a new skill, kicking; and teaching him new words and their meaning.

The mother's diction and articulation of sounds were clear at all times. When her feelings for the child were positive, she acted as a good speech model for him.

During the first observation, I was interested in seeing that when his mother failed him, Bobby called out to other females. He told the teenage girl to look at the boat, and he repeated to the other woman on the blanket: "Dat's a boat, is it? Dat's a boat, is it?" Unfortunately for Bobby, neither of these females responded to him either.

Bobby's articulation was somewhat poor for a 2-year-old child. I wondered how often his mother felt inclined to spend time with him alone, adapting her way of speaking to his age and his needs.

The difference in this mother's communicating style during the two observations is most interesting. When the mother was alone with Bobby and felt friendly toward him, she had no difficulty keeping in tune with his interests. She shared his perceptions of the world around him and taught him the appropriate words and phrases to verbalize his experiences. But when the mother was preoccupied with other people and activities, a situation of disturbed communication developed between her and Bobby. Ruesch (1957), in his study of the genesis of disturbed communication, states that for a child's healthy psychological development to be assured, his messages have to be replied to appropriately and at the right moment. By disregarding Bobby's verbal and nonverbal messages and by shifting the communication from his questions and appeals to her commands, Bobby's mother gave him what Ruesch would call "a tangential reply." Ruesch explains: "In replying tangentially, the receiver deprives the sender of the pleasure of being understood; at the same time, he makes a bid for control by launching another statement which he expects to be acknowledged" (1957, p. 55). This form of inappropriate response evokes in the child feelings of confusion, frustration, and eventually rage. At his age, unable to express his feelings in verbal language, Bobby had no other choice but to express them through action language.

The following three examples will illustrate patterns of communication between mothers and their four-year-old children.

Observation 4

The following observation was made by another graduate student, an experienced school teacher. She observed Lisa, a 4-year-old girl, and her mother, a middle-class woman. Lisa was her mother's only child.

(*Lisa sits in a small rocking chair showing a book to her mother.*)
Lisa (*holding up the book*). This is my cat.
Mother (*leaning over to look*). Where is the cat?
Lisa. Up a tree. He wouldn't come down for his supper. The daddy cat wasn't home.
Mother. He wasn't home?
Lisa. No, he runned up a tree—oh—my toe! (*She grabs her foot.*)
Mother. What happened to your toe? Did you rock on it?
Lisa. No, I bent it. (*Examines her toe.*)
Mother (*rubbing Lisa's foot*). Is it all right now?
Lisa (*finding another picture in her book*). Yes. Look at the man. He's writing on the thing.
Mother. That's a typewriter. He's writing on the typewriter.
Lisa (*rocking back and forth*). See the fence. He can't climb over.
Mother. No, the fence is too high.
Lisa. A hangaroo could jump over the fence. See me jump. (*Laughs and jumps twice.*)
Mother (*laughs*). You'd make a good kangaroo.
Lisa (*returns to her chair, looks at the book quietly for several seconds*). See the boys. They're playing. I'm hot. (*Puts the book on the floor.*)
Mother. Put the book away if you're through reading.
Lisa. Over here? (*Walks across the room. Points to the bookcase.*)
Mother. Yes. (*Points.*) Put it on the middle shelf.
Lisa. This one? (*Touches the middle shelf.*)
Mother. That's right. You're a good girl. Come and give me a kiss.
(*Lisa laughs and runs to her mother. Climbs onto the couch and hugs her. Mother hugs and kisses Lisa.*)
Mother. You are hot. We'll all go swimming in the pool after lunch.
Lisa (*skips out to the hall, chanting*). Swimming, swimming, swimming. I'm going swimming in my swimming pool!

I do not hesitate to call this an ideal teaching-learning situation. The mother is an excellent speech model for the child. She speaks with clear articulation, she uses short, simple sentences that are appropriate for the child's age and state of development, she matches her words and phrases closely with those of the child, she teaches the child new words, she teaches differentiation among similar objects and concepts, she provides the child with immediate and specific verbal feedback, and she teaches casually in a setting of mutual delight in each other. In fact, her way of matching words with the child makes her the ideal speech model. Her form of communication—which, of course, she used quite spontaneously—can be seen as a model for "therapeutic communication," which we will discuss later.

Observation 5

Next follows an example of a very different type of mother-child interaction. Like Lisa, Nicky was 4 years old. One of our therapists described this scene.

I was successful in observing Nicky alone with his mother for only a few minutes. Because there are five children in this family, both older and younger than Nicky, it is almost impossible to observe him alone with his mother.

Nicky came into the house to get something to eat. First he asked: "Tan I have some tooties?"

Mother: "Yes. Get down. I will get them. You can have two."

Nicky: "Tis many?"

Mother: "No—two."

Nicky: "Tis many?"

Mother: "Yes."

Nicky: "Tan I have some choc'lat milt?"

Mother: "Yes, I will fix it."

Nicky wanted to put the chocolate syrup into the milk, but his mother insisted on doing it: "You will make a mess."

Mrs. B. fixed the milk, while Nicky continued to insist that he could do it.

Mother: "The thing is broken, you can't do it. I have to take the top off."

The top of the jar of chocolate had a spout that could be depressed so that the syrup would pump easily. This spout was broken. Nicky became furious and threw himself to the floor in a temper tantrum, screaming: "I wanta do it!"

His mother continued to fix the milk as Nicky screamed.

Mother: "Look, it's broken, it does not work."

Nicky refused to drink the milk, screaming: "I hate you! You dumb!"

The mother remained calm, but firm: "Are you going to drink that?"

Nicky yelled: "No!"

Mrs. B. told him that she would save it and someone else would drink it. Nicky went into the next room and continued to fuss for a few minutes. Then he came back into the kitchen and said: "You going to buy a new thing, huh?"

His mother answered: "Yes."

Nicky drank the milk and announced that he was going out.

The name of the object under discussion was used only once by each person. Thereafter it was "thing," "it," "some," and so forth. The word spout was not used at all. There was little word matching.

Mrs. B. was pleasant and willing to assist Nicky. His temper tantrums did not cause her to be angry. She simply explained the situation and let him decide what to do. When Nicky shouted "I hate you! You dumb," Mrs. L. looked at me and winked as though to say, "Isn't he a character?"

Obviously, here we have a communication pattern quite different from the first one. This mother provided little, if any, corrective feedback. As mentioned in the report, there was little word matching. The mother did not teach names for objects, and she did not teach the child to differentiate among similar objects. The child's speech was immature in articulation, vocabulary, and sentence structure. Because of the large number of small children in the family the mother was frequently unavailable to Nicky, a circumstance that contributed significantly to his language deficit.[4]

However, the example should remind us that we must not confuse the concepts mother–child interaction pattern and mother–child relationship. Nicky and

---

4. The prevalence of language deficits in families with many small children was demonstrated in our research studies (see Chapter 14).

his mother had a basically good relationship, although the mother was neither an ideal provider of specific *verbal* feedback nor a good speech model. In comparing the two examples, one might assume that Lisa's mother considered the teaching of speech and language as an important aspect of her maternal role and that Nicky's mother was not aware of this responsibility.

Observation 6

As our final example, we will observe another mother of five children with her youngest child, Ann, a 4-year-old. Ann's brothers and sisters were already in junior or senior high school. Ann's mother was of upper-middle-class background.

Ann's mother had been referred to me by her pediatrician because of Ann's severely defective articulation. Ann's hearing had been tested and found normal, but her spontaneous speech was almost incomprehensible to a stranger. As usual, I made a home visit to observe the setting and the interaction between child and mother.

Ann and her mother received me in a very formal manner in the living room of their home. Ann, a pretty child, was wearing a party dress and black patent leather pumps. After having exchanged some words of greeting with the mother and the child, I followed my usual procedure and asked both of them to sit down on a couch and to look at a picture book together.

Mother and child were looking at a picture of the seashore, with water, boats, birds, sea animals, a little boy standing at the beach with a bucket and shovel, and a lighthouse in the background. This is what I observed.

The mother said: "Look at that, isn't that a nice picture! You remember, that's just like Cape Cod, isn't it? Now look at the sailboats and the steamboat and the birds and all the animals, the crabs, the seagulls, the lizard. Now look at this animal here. What's that? Do you remember what that is? You know—you must remember it—the kind of animal that Daddy and I like to eat, and you don't like to eat it, remember that? Don't you remember it? We go down to the Harbor House to eat it—you must know the name: a lobster!"

Ann replied: "O ye—I know—I wemember—a wobser, I wemember it."

The mother continued: "And look what's there. Now what is that in the back there? Remember that? You saw that on the Cape too. You remember the lighthouse? You know what a lighthouse is for? A lighthouse has a light shining all night to protect the ships so they won't get off their course and run into a rock."

Ann responded with a relatively long sentence which was so poorly articulated that it was impossible for me to understand it or to write it down.

Ann's mother had flooded the child with an overabundance of information, pointing out many details in the picture before her. At the same time the mother neglected to give the child specific corrective feedback with regard to her articulation of speech sounds. The mother talked at a great rate of speed, with a somewhat blurred articulation, using advanced vocabulary and elaborate sentence structure.

In our research we have labeled this type of maternal stimulation "overloading the system." Apparently Ann comprehended the meaning of her mother's speech well enough, but it was impossible for her to perceive and to filter out the configuration of single sounds and of sequences of sounds occurring in single words.

After having observed Ann and her mother for a while, I asked the mother to observe Ann and me looking at pictures together. We were looking at the picture of a farm, and I said slowly and distinctly: "A barn—a barn—a big red barn." Ann spontaneously repeated: "A barn."
Therapist: "A cow!"
Ann: "A cow."
Therapist: "A hor-se, a white hor-se, a white hor-se in the barn."
Ann: "A horse, a white horse."
Therapist: "Another horse, here is another horse."
Ann: "Anover horse, a boy, a tat."
Therapist: "A cat, a cat on the roof," and so forth.

Thus I provided Ann with specific corrective feedback, with the emphasis upon clear articulation of speech sounds. I also used short phrases and sentences, avoiding "overexpansion" of sentences. We call this technique *lessening the linguistic load*.

During my visit I made the following observation: Ann, obviously a healthy child of normal intelligence, quickly switched her style of verbal response from her mother to me, adapting to the style of the adult talking to her. Ann's mother, in talking to the child, had focused upon intellectual explanations, while my emphasis was on the teaching of auditory discrimination of speech sounds.

Evidently, an adult's conscious or unconscious emphasis upon certain part aspects of communication determines his style of talking with a child. The child in his turn, in a one-to-one speaking situation with a trusted adult, tries to match his verbal response closely with the formal speech characteristics of the adult— even if the adult's speech pattern should be deficient, overly complex, or otherwise inappropriate as a model for the child. If the adult's language style is completely beyond the child's ability of adaptation, the child will either withdraw into silence or become inattentive and restless. This discovery is of great significance for our understanding of the process of language therapy and, beyond that, of the processes of teaching and learning in general.

J. McVicker Hunt, in a paper on the psychological basis for preschool enrichment (1964), discussed in detail the concept of the match between the incoming information and that already stored within the listener (the child). He pointed to the discrepancy that often exists between the level of complexity encountered in the language of parents and teachers, and the level of complexity a child's organism can handle comfortably and effectively.

In Ann's case we observed how the child—the less developed organism— tried to match her performance with that of her mother—the more developed organism—attempting to communicate in a style that obviously was too complex for her. We propose that all good teaching, or good therapy, requires two inter-

related modes of communication: First, the adult, through listening and observation, must ascertain what information the child has already stored and understood
and what skills he already commands; second, it must be the adult, the more
developed organism, who consciously matches his style of communication with
that of the child, the less developed one.

TYPES AND QUALITIES OF CORRECTIVE FEEDBACK

In acting as speech model for a child, the interested adult frequently will improve upon the child's speech performance. When Lisa (observation 4) talked about
a "hangaroo," her mother replied that Lisa would make a good "kangaroo," thus
providing the child with a corrective feedback in the area of articulation or phonics.
When Lisa talked about the "thing" on which the man typed, her mother gave
her a semantic feedback, calling the "thing" a typewriter. When Ricky (observation 1) called out "go . . . go," his mother expanded his statement into "let's
go," thus giving him a corrective grammatical feedback. Slobin in his studies of
children's acquisition of syntax (1964a) found that such *expansions* were among the
most important teaching devices used by adults.

Thus the concept of corrective feedback must be further refined in accordance
with the multiple aspects of language. The child has to learn sounds and sequences
of sounds. He must learn names for objects and experiences and differentiation
between the names for similar objects and experiences. Finally, he has to learn
the patterns of grammar and syntax characteristic for a given language. To accomplish all this, he needs *phonetic, semantic,* and *grammatical feedback.* Looking back
at our six examples of adult-child interaction, we find that not all adults did
provide feedback on all levels. Ann's mother (observation 6) provided semantic
and grammatical but no phonetic feedback. Nicky's mother (observation 5)
provided little corrective feedback on any level, and Nicky's speech was deficient
in articulation, vocabulary, and grammar.

Lisa's mother (observation 3) provided feedback on all levels of speech and
language. Taking her clues from the child and matching her own sentences
closely with the child's level of language skill, she frequently improved upon the
child's performance. By being always just a little bit ahead of the child, this mother
used the technique of small steps in teaching her child to speak.

Judson S. Brown (1949) suggested that there are at least three different types
of feedback: informational, rewarding, and motivating feedback. Lisa's mother
(observation 4) provided all three types. In addition her feedback was immediate
and continuous, and it was at all times appropriate for the age of the child and for
her stage of development.

If the child's mother—or another interested adult significant in the child's
life—continuously and habitually provides the child during his early years with
verbal and nonverbal feedback, the child develops a set of *trustworthy expectancies*
(Roger Brown, 1958). If the child's feedback expectancies are not fulfilled, if the
mother provides verbal feedback in certain situations but withholds it in others,

the child reacts to the absence of customary and expected feedback with bewilderment, frustration, and, eventually, aggression. Thus discontinuous feedback can provoke a disturbance in the mother-child relationship, similar to that illustrated in our third example.

In analyzing patterns of communication between adults and children, both content and emotional quality must be considered. We will have to discern whether the feedback provided by the adult encompasses all levels of linguistic complexity —phonetic, semantic, and grammatical; whether it is rewarding or punishing, continuous or discontinuous; and whether it is appropriate or inappropriate for the child's developmental stage. Beyond this, we will be interested in the general feeling tone or the emotional atmosphere prevailing during the interaction process. The emotional quality of adult-child interaction can range from mutual delight to mutual indifference or irritation or open conflict. It will be expressed in both verbal and nonverbal modes of communication: choice of words, tone of voice, expressive gestures, and overt behavior acts. Examples can be found in the bodily closeness, the stroking and kissing between Lisa and her mother, on the one hand, and in Nicky's temper tantrum and running out of the room on the other hand.

THE MODEL OF THE "SPEECH CHAIN"

Having analyzed various examples of adult-child interactions occurring in everyday situations, we are now ready to seek a theoretical model that will represent the basic structure of all possible patterns of adult-child interaction, regardless of the degree of satisfaction or frustration the partners experience during the act of communicating. P. B. Denes and E. N. Pinson have presented a model of person-to-person communication which—with certain modifications—will be useful for our purpose.

The authors start from the situation of two people in conversation. One of them, the speaker, is transmitting information to the other, the listener. The speaker has to arrange his thoughts, decide what he wants to say, and put his message into linguistic form "by selecting the right words and phrases to express its meaning, and by placing these words in the correct order required by the grammatical rules of language (Denes and Pinson, 1963, p. 3). This is the *linguistic level* of communication. This process in turn is "associated with activity in the speaker's brain, and it is in the brain that the proper instructions, in the form of impulses along the motor nerves, are sent to the muscles of the vocal organs, the lips and the vocal cords" (the *physiological level*). The nerve impulses will set the vocal muscles into movement, producing sound waves, which travel through the air between speaker and listener (the *acoustic level*). Pressure changes at the listener's ear activate his hearing mechanism and produce nerve impulses that travel along the acoustic nerve to the listener's brain. In the listener's brain a considerable amount of nerve activity is already taking place, and this activity is modified by the nerve impulses arriving from the ear. "This modification of brain activity, in ways which we do not fully understand, brings about recognition of the speaker's message" (1963, p. 5). Denes and Pinson conclude: "We see, therefore, that speech communication consists of a chain of events linking the speaker's brain with the listener's brain. We shall call this chain of events *the speech chain.*"

In addition there is internal feedback. The speaker not only speaks but constantly also listens to his own voice while speaking. He continuously compares the quality of the sounds he produces with the sound qualities he intended to produce, making adjustments in his linguistic performance if necessary.

As Denes and Pinson show, the speech chain involves activity on at least three different levels—the linguistic, physiological, and physical—first on the speaker's and then, in reverse, on the listener's end. During this process "the speaker's linguistic code of words and sentences is transformed into physiological and physical codes before being reconverted into a linguistic code at the listener's end" (1963, p. 6).

In applying this model to communication between adult and child, some modifications are necessary.

1. In actual life situations speaker and listener invariably participate in some form of interpersonal relationship in which the respective mood of the speech partners, their feelings, their expectancies of each other, their degree of strangeness or familiarity, in short, a number of psychological variables, will affect the form and manifestation of the speech chain. It therefore seems justified to add the *psychological level* to the physiological, linguistic, and physical levels.

2. In putting a message into linguistic form, the speaker must not only select from his memory storage the right words and phrases to express his meaning and place them into correct grammatical order; he must also select the correct sounds or phonemes necessary for the pronunciation of each word. Thus on the linguistic level the process of *encoding* demands a rapid structuring of the intended message—from the conceptual and feeling level to naming or word finding, articulation and proper sequential ordering of sounds, and syntactical and grammatical ordering of words. The listener, in turn, goes through a similar process of recognition in receiving and *decoding* the message (Fry, 1963).

3. In adult-child communication enormous differences exist between the levels of linguistic accomplishment of the speech partners. The adult has at his command a highly developed linguistic system functioning at a high rate of speed. The child, depending on his age, commands a more-or-less rudimentary and primitive linguistic system, correlated with an immature, still-developing neurophysiological organism. Denes and Pinson's model of the speech chain is based upon the assumption of equipotentiality between speech partners. A model for adult-child interaction must, however, include recognition of the basic neurophysiological and linguistic *inequality* between them.

In particular, the adult's well-developed and continuously effective feedback system permits him the constant monitoring of his speech performance, comparing the speech he produces with the speech he intended to produce. In innumerable experiments with delayed feedback, in which the speaker's voice was recorded on tape and played back to him through earphones a fraction of a second later, it was demonstrated that the speaker's performance deteriorated rapidly. Stammering or slurring speech appeared as soon as the speaker missed, even briefly, the self-corrective effect of the feedback link. A similar example is the gradual deterioration of speech in persons suffering from prolonged deafness (Yates, 1963).

Richard A. Chase (1963) investigated the role of sensory feedback in the control of ongoing speech motor activities. He assumed that in order to make possible the correct organization and patterning of speech motor activity, there must occur at all times a process of matching or mismatching of the ongoing motor activities with a central representation of the desired form of that activity. These operations constitute error detection, and error detection requires the existence of some standard against which the sensory feedback can be checked. Chase further assumed that the development of such a standard for error detection would depend upon the incorporation of organized acoustical information from the environment, as well as on progressive shaping of the inflow of sensory feedback associated with the imitation of complex acoustical inputs from the environment.[5]

However, the young child in the process of primary learning does not yet possess an internalized standard against which to compare the results of his motor activities. It is our assumption that the child only gradually develops an internal verbal feedback system. While acquiring such a dependable system, the child needs constant and consistent external corrective feedback from significant adults to monitor his speech and other motor productions. He needs the mother—or a mother substitute, such as the father or a teacher—as a dependable source of corrective feedback in order to learn language in all its forms: speaking, listening, reading, writing. Figure 1 presents a schema of speech transmission between adult and child.

THE ROLE OF THE MOTHER IN THE CHILD'S LANGUAGE DEVELOPMENT

In the reality of life and development it is the mother—or her substitute—who first brings the language of her social group to her child, serving as a temporary interpreter for a permanent medium (Wyatt, 1949). Thus the learning of the "mother tongue" is an intensely emotional experience for the young child; and like all emotional learning, it is achieved through the processes of conscious imitation and unconscious identification (Freud and Burlingham, 1944). Learning to speak, like all primary learning, is influenced, therefore, by the child's relationship to the mother.

As Sapir (1921) suggested, language development cannot be fully understood if studied exclusively within a framework of biological growth and maturation.

---

5. For further information concerning the work of Chase and his collaborators see *Annual Report, 1967,* listed in the Bibliography.

One would like to say with D. McCarthy (1955): "We have continued to worship too long at the shrine of maturation." The acquisition of language by the child, though dependent upon maturation by the organism, is essentially a process of learning through imitation of a model. In this learning process it is the mother— as a rule—who serves as the primary model for the child's groping attempts at imitation of sounds and words and as a guide for the child's experimentation with word meanings and sentence structure.

The most detailed study so far of the infant's learning of sensory-motor skills through imitation of a model has come from Jean Piaget (1951). He describes the stages by which imitative learning is accomplished. He also hints at the possibility that the nature of the psychological relationship between the child and his model may affect the learning process.

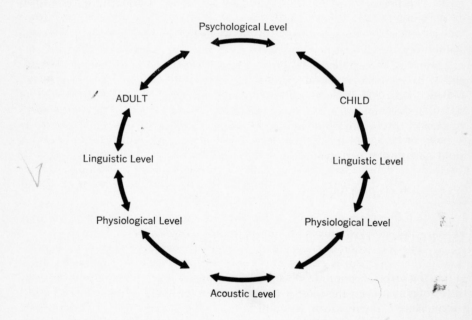

FIGURE 1.   SPEECH TRANSMISSION BETWEEN ADULT AND CHILD*

PSYCHOLOGICAL LEVEL. *The feelings of speech partners for each other, their relationship, their mutual expectancies, and the respective levels of maturation, which determine the choice of words by the speaker and the interpretation of their meaning by the listener.*

LINGUISTIC LEVEL. *Process of word finding; selecting the correct sounds and putting them into correct sequences; putting words into correct grammatical order to form sentences.*

PHYSIOLOGICAL LEVEL. *Neural activities affecting the speaker's perceptual and motor mechanisms and activating the hearing mechanisms of speaker and listener.*

ACOUSTIC LEVEL. *Sound waves traveling through the air between speaker and listener.*

  * (Reproduced by permission of *Pediatrics* [Wyatt, 1965].)

Apparent confirmation of the crucial role that the relationship between mother and child plays in the acquisition of language has come from a number of studies of children reared in orphanages or foundling homes. In these studies the severe retardation of language development was attributed in the majority of the children to the loss of the child's natural mother, prolonged separation from the mother early in the child's life, or unavailability of a permanent mother figure.[6]

Unmistakable confirmation of the mother's role as speech model and provider of corrective feedback has come from a painstaking experimental study carried out by Margaret Bullowa and her collaborators at the Massachusetts Mental Health Center and at Harvard University (Bullowa, Jones, and Duckert, 1964). This longitudinal study of normal first language acquisition is being conducted by a group of researchers that includes psychiatrists and linguists. Film and high fidelity tape recordings are used for the observation of infants and their mothers in their own homes. In their paper "The acquisition of a word," a child's learning of the word *shoe* has been documented. Together with other items in her rapidly growing vocabulary, the child acquired phonetic control and semantic use of the word *shoe* in a sequence of stages extending over a period of time from the age of 9 months and 12 days to 22 months and 15 days. The authors describe in detail the mother's interest in the child's language development, her frequent verbal stimulation of the child, the naming games mother and child played with each other, the mother's correction of the child's utterances, her encouragement of the child in order to keep her trying, and finally her pleased acceptance of the child's word *shoe* as a valid imitation of her own word.

BASIC ASSUMPTIONS

The following assumptions will provide the basis for our study of language learning and of developmental language disorders in children.

1. The acquisition of language by the child, though dependent upon maturation of the organism, is essentially a learning process occurring within an interpersonal matrix of reciprocal feedback between adult and child. During the early stages of this process the mother (or her substitute) serves as the primary model for the child's attempts at imitation of the language patterns specific for the given culture.

2. The optimum condition for successful language learning in early childhood is a continuous, undisrupted, and affectionate relationship between mother and child, manifested in frequent and appropriate communication, both nonverbal and verbal. Such communication is appropriate for the child if the mother takes her cues from the child's behavior and verbalizations and provides the child with a corrective feedback.

3. Language learning goes through a series of interrelated stages. Each new

---

6. A summary and critical review of these studies was presented by Bowlby (1951). His conclusions, in turn, were critically evaluated by Casler (1961), Yarrow (1961), and Ainsworth *et al.* (1962).

TABLE 1—SCHEMA OF LANGUAGE DEVELOPMENT**

	Child's Language Development	Mother's* Role
Birth to 1 Year	Presymbolic Stage Preverbal communication with mother through crying, smiling, comfort and discomfort sounds, babbling.	Dualistic Speech Relationship Mother is child's primary love-object and primary speech model; mother communicates preverbally with child through touch, tone of voice, facial expression, mothering, finger-games, and so forth.
1 to 2 Years	Early Symbolic Stage Naming, learning of words; beginning of auditory discrimination between speech sounds.	Mutual adaptation and imitation between mother and child; word matching; development of reciprocal identification. Mother provides corrective feedback for child.
2 to 3 Years	Early Relational Stage Beginnings of grammatical speech, phrases, and short sentences; learning of words and of sound patterns continues.	Mutual imitation and reciprocal feedback continues; matching of phrases and sentences.

Child Changes Gradually from Dualistic to Pluralistic Speech Relationships

	Child's Language Development	Mother's* Role
3 to 6 Years	Early relational stage continues. Learning of additional words; experimentation with word meanings; further learning of sound patterns, syntax, and sentence structure.	Child's early speech patterns gradually become internalized. Thus child gradually becomes independent of mother and can learn speech and language from other models (other familiar people).
6 to 7 Years	Beginning of formal instruction (school entrance). Sound patterns in most children mastered by age 7.	Teachers, peers, radio, TV, finally books become partners in communication and models for speech and language usage.
7 to 10 Years	Advanced Relational Stage Emergence of complex sentence structures. Learning of *visual* symbols: reading and writing.	
Pre-adolescence and Adolescence	Language learning continues in all areas: speaking, listening, reading, writing. Gradual acquisition of adult language structure.	

* *Note*: M. = Mother, or mother substitute.

** Reproduced by permission of *Pediatrics* (Wyatt, 1965).

and higher stage of development represents fundamentally an innovation, not merely an addition of certain characteristics to those of the previous level (Werner, 1957). The child's relationship to the original model is of particular importance during the practicing stage of a new function or activity, when the child is learning new patterns of a more complex nature, prior to the attainment of efficient performance. In individual children and under specific circumstances, shifting from a less differentiated to a more differentiated stage may produce a crisis in language learning. This may be expressed in the form of a total or partial arrest (fixation) or regression in language development (Hendrick, 1942; Buxbaum, 1947).

4. Increasing mastery of language permits the child to sustain the relationship with the mother at a greater and greater distance in place and time. Once the child has reached the stage of internalizing the basic linguistic patterns of the model, he can reproduce them even if the model has been absent for some time (Mowrer, 1950; Piaget, 1951; Shands, 1954). Eventually, autonomy of function will be reached when the child can dispense with the original model. He will then be able increasingly to modify the linguistic patterns at will, and he will turn to a variety of different models (people) for additional learning. Thus the child's interpersonal network of communication changes gradually from a dualistic to a pluralistic one. Together with the genetic endowment of each child, the vicissitudes—satisfactions and frustrations—of the primary dualistic speech relationship will affect the child's rate of learning to speak, the degree of skill he achieves at a given time, his expectancies concerning future speech partners, and thus his behavior in later speech situations.

In Table 1 a schematic summary of the child's language development from birth to adolescence is presented, together with the mother's contributions to this development. The time spans printed on the left side of the table should be read as averages only.

CHAPTER TWO

Debby: A Case of "Hospitalism"

Having explored the mother's role in the child's language development, let us consider now the language behavior of a child growing up without a mother or a continuous mother substitute. This was the case with Debby, who grew up in a hospital.

The negative effects of lack of maternal care upon children growing up in institutions have been reported by a number of investigators (Durfee and Wolf, 1933; Lowrey, 1940; Freud and Burlingham, 1943; Goldfarb, 1945; Spitz, 1945; Roudinesco and Appell, 1950; Bowlby, 1951; Rheingold, 1956; Brodbeck and Irwin, 1964). All observers agreed that the majority of the children in this category were retarded in their development and that language was the area most affected. Severely delayed language development and persistent speech disabilities were mentioned as the outstanding deficiency of children reared in institutions. Most children were more handicapped in expressive speech than in their understanding of language. Freud and Burlingham mentioned that some children with retarded language development showed marked and rapid improvement while they were away from the war-time nursery for several weeks, visiting in their own homes. Spitz, in his well-known study of children growing up in a foundling home, used the term *hospitalism* in referring to the morbid consequences of prolonged confinement to a hospital and, beyond that, to the evil effects of institutional care on infants placed in institutions at an early age.

The case of Debby, which will be presented here, should be of particular interest to students of child development. Not only was Debby in the extraordinary situation of being a *healthy* child living within the confines of a hospital; in addition, when she was finally transferred from the hospital to a foster family, she had to forget her first language, German, and had to learn a new language, English.

OBSERVATIONS

I encountered Debby in Austria in February 1938, shortly before the country was overrun by the Nazis. Because of the special circumstances and political upheaval of those days, my observations of the child had to be rather casual. Many questions concerning details of her early development and training had to remain unanswered. However, the fact that I saw Debby repeatedly and traveled with her from Vienna to London in June 1938 made it possible for me to notice some significant aspects of her behavior and language development.

My observations of Debby coincided with a crisis in my own life. Leaving Austria, entering England as a political refugee, and later emigrating to the United States, I was unable to preserve the detailed records of my observations. The following account has been taken almost verbatim from a report I presented in the fall of 1938 at a seminar conducted at London University by the late Susan Isaacs.

I first met Debby in the toddler's ward of a children's hospital in Vienna. The well-equipped hospital was surrounded by a large park and was beautifully situated in the Vienna Woods. A major purpose of the institution was the care of premature infants, and one wing was used exclusively for this. Each premature infant was kept in a separate glass-partitioned cubicle. Rooms for nursing mothers were located in the same building. In addition to maintaining the division for premature babies, the institution functioned as a regular children's hospital, offering medical and surgical treatment for children up to 14 years of age. The hospital also served as training center for pediatric nurses.

During the winter of 1937–38 I attempted to organize at the hospital a child guidance clinic, which would serve children with behavior as well as speech problems. My work at the hospital consisted of administering psychological and speech tests to children, counseling parents, and providing speech therapy for children between 3 and 6 years of age who were brought to my attention by the resident physicians.

Soon after I began my part-time work at the hospital, I became aware of a lively 3-year-old girl who lived in one of the large wards on the ground floor. The child showed no sign of physical illness or malfunction. Her English name, Deborah or Debby, sounded unfamiliar among all the Viennese Mitzies, Lieserls, and Greterls in the wards. Debby was a vigorous, plump, and pretty little girl with very fair hair, blue eyes, and a light complexion. Playing with other children on the ward, she was extremely active and quite unrestrained in the expression of her moods and feelings. She either dominated her playmates—who were convalescent children—or played in a self-absorbed way without any consideration for the other children in the room. All the physicians and nurses knew her well, and she seemed to be the pet child of staff members and helpers. Her general behavior gave the impression that she was of normal intelligence. However, her speech and language were strikingly poor in vocabulary and grammar, and her articulation of words was severely defective.

My inquiries evoked the following case history. Debby was the illegitimate child of a British mother, who had come to Austria to give birth to the child away from her home. Mother and child had entered the hospital a few days after Debby's birth. A few weeks later the mother returned to England, leaving the child in the care of the hospital. Thus Debby had spent practically all her life at the children's hospital. The mother had made regular payments towards the child's maintenance, but she had never been able to visit her child. When Debby was 2 years old, the hospital had suggested to the mother that she be placed in a foster home; but the mother preferred having Debby stay in the hospital because "she was there under medical supervision." Debby lived at first in the hospital's neo-natal department; later she was transferred to the toddlers' division and, finally, to the 2- to 6-year-old group, where I first met her.

As the primary aim of the hospital was the treatment and care of children who were acutely and often dangerously ill, physicians and nurses had neither the time nor the inclination to devote themselves to Debby's education. No child psychiatrist or psychiatric social worker was on the hospital staff at that time. Though Debby was a healthy child, she was included automatically in all daily hospital routines necessary for the care of the sick. For example, all through her life in the hospital her temperature was taken three times a day. As no physician or nurse was allowed to enter the infants' cubicles without a white gauze mask covering nearly the whole face except the eyes, Debby, during the first 8 months of her life, had not seen the expression of a complete human face or the movements of a person's lips and mouth. The nurses, who had a strenuous schedule and a large number of children to care for, found time to speak to Debby only while they were dressing, undressing, washing, or feeding her. This meant that Debby was denied the many hours that a loving mother or private nurse will spend playing and talking with an infant.

As all the student nurses rotated regularly from department to department in accordance with their training program, the faces around Debby were continu-ously changing—as were the standards and patterns of training which the different young nurses applied to Debby's feeding and toilet training. The head nurse and the resident physician of each department, together with the chief of staff, were the only ones whose personalities and manner the child had experienced repeatedly and for any length of time. Besides the fact that Debby had no parental figures of her own, the circumstances of her upbringing gave her hardly a chance to develop permanent object relationships with parental substitutes.

Although the child's physical health was well taken care of, it easily can be imagined that her emotional and mental development would have to be abnormal. In fact, she had learned only the most elementary rules of everyday behavior. Her toilet habits, acquired—or not acquired—under the management of a variety of nurses, were far from reliable. Every quarrel among the children on her ward, every strong desire which she felt and expressed for anything—toys, dolls, or food—proved her to be a little savage, driven only by intense instinctual needs, without controls developed through education. Although she exhibited curiosity about the objects in her environment, her knowledge of the outer world, her motor skills, and her speech were severely retarded. However, in spite of all these serious limitations, Debby had a personal charm, an amusing and attractive way of doing things, which secured her the sympathy and affection of the children and adults around her.

Behind her occasional stubbornness, wildness, and aggressiveness one would expect to find a good deal of anxiety. One of the nurses reported an actual break-through of anxiety that had occurred two months before I came to the hospital. The ward in which Debby had her bed was to be painted. One day, coming back from the garden after playtime, Debby found the whole room emptied of furniture. Her bed had not been moved just to another corner of the room, as had happened before; it was gone. Debby was told that she had to go to another room and sleep in another bed. She reacted to this with a violent temper tantrum, screaming and crying. If we consider that she had nothing permanently belonging to her except this bed—even the toys she played with and the clothes she wore belonged to the hospital and were rotated among the children—we can well understand how desperate and overwhelmed by anxiety and confusion she must have felt when this central object of her orientation and of her attachments disappeared.[1]

I shall now quote briefly from my notes taken at the hospital.

February 3: Debby is able to pronounce all sounds of the German language correctly in isolation, but in spontaneous conversation she mispronounces almost every word, omitting or substituting a number of consonants. She expresses herself in 1- to 3-word sentences, using a primitive chain-like speech pattern. Her knowledge of the world outside the hospital appears extremely restricted. She seems to lack most concepts which would be familiar to the majority of her age mates. For example, she recognizes only white beds, white chairs, white tables and lamps. When I pointed out to her in a picture book brown chairs and tables, a colored easy chair, or a colorful lamp, she was unable to identify and name them. However, she loves looking at pictures with me. She reacts with obvious delight to any kind of stimulation: pictures, toys, bells, a music box, or words. I name the objects in the pictures, and she repeats every word most vividly, with accompanying movements of her whole body—jumping, laughing, gesticulating, saying every word over and over again. Because of her excitement her articulation deteriorates, becoming less correct with prolonged repetition. When we play word games together on the ward, the other children gather around our table and share Debby's pleasure, so that at times a whole chorus of children are repeating my words.

Debby calls every person in a white coat *Schwester* (sister) or *doctor*. At times when the other children have visitors Debby hears them call their mothers *mummy*, and she also calls out, "mummy." Every strange woman in civilian clothes is called mummy by her.

February 23: Debby was in bed with conjunctivitis. I sat at her bed and let her play with a music box. She was quite enchanted with it, calling out: "I want, I want!" When the music stopped she said: "Debby want more singing."

---

1. The late Susan Isaacs, with whom I discussed this case, suggested that Debby's bed may unconsciously have represented the "mother" to her, in the archaic sense of a primary love object offering familiarity and security.

Originally I had seen her twice a week, but from March on I could see her only once weekly. At my request the nurses tried to find a few minutes every day to speak with her and teach her the words in the picture books I had left for her. The older children on the ward, who understood very well that Debby was being taught to speak correctly, acted as my voluntary assistants and corrected Debby's speech in a most friendly and skillful manner.

April 24: Debby's articulation of German speech sounds is now completely correct in imitative as well as in spontaneous speech. She expresses herself in somewhat longer sentences of two to four words, and many of her short phrases and sentences are grammatically correct. Her vocabulary has increased markedly, and she knows and uses the names of many animals, flowers, and other objects in her picture books. One of the nurses took her for a walk in a nearby public garden, where they observed a squirrel, called *Eichkatzerl* in Viennese dialect. After this outing the children on the ward used to ask Debby: "What did you see in the park?" And Debby answered with much energy and expression: "*Eich-ka-tzerl!*" breaking up the long difficult word into three parts.

During April Debby was taken to an orthopedic hospital in the center of the city to obtain supports for her flat feet. A physician drove her and the head nurse downtown. Debby was extremely frightened when the car started; she cried and screamed. But a few minutes later she settled down in the car and played with her doll. In the unfamiliar orthopedic clinic she was quiet and shy; but on her way back to the children's hospital she was gay and lively, showing no sign of anxiety when the car started.

A week later the same nurse, Sister Gisela, took Debby downtown again to buy shoes for her. This time they went by streetcar. Debby was terribly excited during the whole excursion. She seemed very much afraid of the big red streetcars; she did not want to get on them and screamed in terror. After the nurse had persuaded her to get on and to sit down, she continued to sob in a desperate way. The same thing happened on their way home.

It was apparent that the unusual conditions of spending all her life in a hospital had seriously handicapped Debby's mental and emotional development. She lacked nearly all the experiences which are basic for most children in our civilization— experiences of mother and father; home and family life; ordinary furniture and common objects found in a kitchen and throughout a house; animals; street life, with vehicles, traffic, street noises, and crowds of people; shops and shop windows; working men; and so forth. The only vehicles which she knew well were German fighter planes, which were only too frequently seen during these early weeks of the German occupation. Whenever these big objects appeared, droning and shining in the blue sky, Debby with all the other children called out: "Plane, plane!"

Preparing for the Journey

Austria had been occupied in March 1938. The disorganization of life and the political confusion during the spring of that year, together with my own attempts to obtain a permit to leave Austria, were the main reasons for the irregularity of my visits at the children's hospital. By agreement with the hospital administration, I wrote to Debby's mother in April, pointing out to her the psychological dangers inherent in her child's growing up in a hospital and urging her to permit Debby's placement in a foster home. By that time the mother, alarmed by the political events in Central Europe, agreed that Debby should leave the hospital. She wanted the child to come to England to live in the home of a friend of hers, and she asked me whether I would be willing to escort Debby to England. This request from Debby's mother gave me a long sought chance of gaining a permit to leave Austria and to enter England as a visitor. I agreed to accompany the child to her country and hurried to prepare our voyage. Traveling had become extremely difficult by that time, and the business of procuring the necessary documents for Debby and myself left me very little time to visit the children's hospital during the last six weeks before our departure.

On May 1 I noted:

I have tried repeatedly to prepare Debby for the forthcoming trip, showing her pictures of children traveling in a train and looking through the window at trees, houses, and villages. Every time, Debby reacted in a negative, gloomy manner, shaking her head and saying decisively: "No, Debby won't, Debby won't, Debby won't travel."

As it was customary at the hospital, I had always entered Debby's ward wearing a white hospital gown over my clothes. In order to get Debby used to my ordinary clothes, I once entered her room wearing a regular hat and coat. Debby was already in bed for her afternoon nap. She pulled her blanket over her head, saying: "No, no, no!" Even when I sat down next to her bed, took my hat off and spoke to her, she did not want to look at me and kept hiding under her bed clothes. The nurses, who were fond of Debby and felt sorry to see her leave, told her frequently during that period that she would be going "on a trip to see Mummy."

A week later I took Debby with me for a walk outside the hospital. She took my hand and left the building with me without any sign of resistance. Debby walked very awkwardly; she had a peculiar way of putting her feet on the ground, and walking up and down an incline obviously was difficult for her. Throughout her life she had walked mainly on flat ground, from the toddlers' room to the balcony, or from the young children's department on the ground floor to the playground. She had rarely had the opportunity of climbing either stairs or hills.

We walked together toward the main street of the suburb, which was fairly busy with streetcars and other traffic. Debby was silent, and I commented on the things we saw around us. Sometimes she repeated words or phrases spontaneously after me: "Flower," "Pussycat," "Dog," "Debby is a good girl." Finally we sat down on a bench by the roadside, watching the traffic going by. Debby's face was very anxious. Her expression was so vivid that I myself could feel how threatening the streetcars were—bearing down upon us with all their rattling and ringing of bells, like big red monsters, unknown and frightening for the child. However, I remembered in time that it was my task to offer guidance and protection to the child, not to share her anxieties. I put my arm around her shoulders and explained in a calm voice and in short, simple sentences what was going on in the street. She sat very quietly on the bench and after some time she clasped my hand and said: "Debby go to bed." Then she added in a wishful tone: "Streetcar go to bed." I assured her that the streetcars would go to bed later on. We walked back to the hospital together, and she consoled herself with the words: "Debby go to bed, streetcar go to bed." Then she added: "Debby will eat meat," a statement the meaning of which I did not understand until a week later.

Debby repeated the remark when we were downtown again, buying clothes for her trip. Debby had always worn clothes belonging to the hospital, and her mother had now sent the money to purchase a small wardrobe for her. I met Debby and Sister Gisela downtown in a children's clothing store. Debby was very shy but she did not seem as frightened as she had been on other occasions. She had to try on several dresses, pajamas, coats, and hats. She looked very pretty in her new clothes, and the nurse and the saleswoman showed their pleasure. Placing Debby before a tall looking glass, they exclaimed: "Isn't that a lovely dress! Look, Debby, how pretty!" But Debby herself did not show the slightest sign of pleasure. Finally, when she was placed on a high seat to try on shoes and stockings, she burst into tears. Between sobs she repeated: "Debby will eat meat, Debby will eat meat."

Sister Gisela was able to explain to me the meaning of Debby's statement. Debby did not like to eat meat and had developed a habit of keeping it in her mouth for a long time without swallowing it. The nurses on duty often threatened her that they would call the head nurse, and occasionally Sister Gisela actually had been called and had scolded Debby. As Sister Gisela was one of the few permanent love objects in Debby's life, she must have played an important part in Debby's feelings and fantasies. The phrase "Debby will eat meat," apparently so unfitting to the actual situation in the store, could only be understood within the context of Debby's life situation.

We might interpret it in the following way: Debby does not like to eat her meat; Sister Gisela is called and scolds Debby, which arouses anxiety in the child; Debby promises to eat her meat, Sister Gisela is kind again and leaves the room; Debby feels relieved. Her promise—and sometimes the actual eating of meat—results in changing the angry, scolding nurses into kind ones and thus helps to restore the child's well-being. Debby then promises to eat meat whenever she is scolded and feels anxiety, later, whenever she feels anxiety in general. We remember that she made the same statement when she was frightened by the red streetcars and wanted to get rid of her anxiety. She expects now that these words will always have the result of relieving her of anxiety, of changing unpleasant situations into pleasant ones. Frightening situations seem to be created by and dependent upon the powerful adults, perhaps upon Sister Gisela in particular. In asserting her willingness to do what she does not like to do, Debby hopes to "placate the angry gods." In uttering this phrase, Debby uses language in a magic sense.[2]

The Journey

We started on our journey June 2. Sister Gisela and two other nurses brought Debby to the station, where I met her. Debby had been given one of the dolls she used to play with as a present; thus at least one familiar object was going with her. The large terminal was crowded with travelers and with German soldiers. Although I had booked reserved seats, we had to stand around for half an hour, hemmed in by a noisy crowd. Debby's face was strained with anxiety but she kept silent while Sister Gisela was carrying her in her arms. When the gates were opened eventually, the whole mass of people pressed ahead, shoving and pushing through the gates toward the train. In the midst of all these shouting and running men and women, Debby, feeling lost and desperate, began to cry. She did not sob loudly as she had done 2 months earlier when she found herself in a strange street-car. Her face expressed complete terror, and she whimpered softly with tears running down her cheeks. I had anticipated that she would be agitated and difficult to handle, but her actual behavior was much more saddening to watch. She behaved like someone who had succumbed to the frightful troubles of life without any hope of being able to defend herself against them.

Fortunately, our second-class compartment was at that time unoccupied and, as it turned out, we were to remain alone in it until we reached Cologne, at 4 o'clock the next morning. As soon as we entered the small compartment, Debby's tears stopped and her face brightened. She settled down in a corner and began playing with her doll, without any desire to look out the window. When the train began to move, she took no notice of the nurses waving goodbye outside, nor did she react to the movement of the train. We had two quiet, rather cheerful hours together playing with her doll and drawing pictures. At noon we had a picnic lunch in our compartment; then I laid her down on the seat. She fell asleep at once and slept for three hours.

On awakening, she did not seem astonished or confused to be in the place where she found herself. We had another snack in the compartment, played with her doll and with some roses that had been given to me at the station, looked at a picture book, and had a good time together. I began naming the objects in the pictures in English as well as in German: "*Eine Puppe*, a dolly, a dolly, *eine Puppe*." I didn't want her to be totally unprepared for hearing a strange language as soon as we landed on English soil. Debby repeated both the English and the German

---

2. We are reminded of ideas expressed by Sapir (1921) and by Vigotsky (1962), namely, that the meanings of words are not constant; they change as the child develops in accordance with different levels of consciousness and with the different ways in which thought functions. A true and full understanding of another person's, and particularly of a child's language and thought, becomes possible only when we understand the person's or the child's sphere of motivation, comprising his unconscious desires and needs as well as his conscious interests and emotions.

words after me quite happily, without much difficulty in articulating the new words. Once we went outside the compartment; we stood in the corridor looking out the window, naming things we could see outside, taking no notice of people who passed us in the corridor. Later, inside the compartment I put her on a chamber pot placed between the two benches so that she could hold on to them with both hands. Thus, after the anxiety at the station our first travelling day passed in a surprisingly agreeable fashion. About 7 o'clock in the evening I put her into her pajamas and wrapped her in my dressing gown. I gave her the doll and a rose to hold, and she fell asleep almost immediately. I turned the light out and went to sleep on the opposite bench.

Three times during the night Debby was awakened quite suddenly—once by the slamming of a door, then by a sharp whistling tone, and finally by the sound of hissing steam. Each time, she sat up and looked around with a bewildered expression, her eyes and mouth wide open. I said a few soothing words and put her back on her seat again, and she fell asleep.

The second day of our trip turned out quite differently from the first. At 4:00 A.M., in Cologne, many people poured into the train; from then on until we reached Calais, in France, the train was badly overcrowded, people standing in the aisles and luggage blocking the corridors. As Debby could no longer occupy a whole bench by herself, I had to wake her up and place her in the corner of her seat. There she continued to sleep, sitting up, until 6:00 A.M. When she opened her eyes, her expression became very gloomy. As our compartment was crowded at that time, I took her and her chamber pot into the toilet at the end of the corridor. She was very frightened, probably by the roaring noise coming through the waste pipe and also by the shaking of the train, which was more evident in the toilet than it had been inside our compartment. She cried aloud while using the pot and while being washed. Back in the compartment we had no chance to regain our cheerful atmosphere of the previous day. I took her to the dining room for breakfast, where we had a table by ourselves. As soon as we were somewhat isolated again from others, she became cheerful and smiling. She ate her breakfast very nicely and attracted the commendation of other travelers.

Afterward, as the morning advanced, the compartment to which we had returned became more and more hot, noisy, and crowded. Debby looked miserable, ill, and tired; eventually she began to cry. I tried my best to cheer her up, taking her on my lap and playing finger games with her, but with only passing success. Because of her fear of the toilet I apologized to our fellow travelers and let her use her chamber pot again inside the compartment. She was sitting on it when we reached Calais and the English Channel. Shouting porters walked through the train, and the passengers hurried toward the boat; in the midst of all the confusion Debby sat on her potty, crying. I had to pack up her toys and her belongings, get her off the potty, and dress her—all in the greatest hurry.

The way from the train along the pier and on board ship was an ordeal for Debby. She carried her doll and the withered rose in one hand, her other hand anxiously clutching mine. She tottered over the rough stones of the pier, crying bitterly: "Sister Gisela, Sister Gisela!" We had to climb up a steep gangway, the water lapping underneath us, and Debby had great difficulty in climbing. With the best of intentions a huge sailor took her in his arms to carry her on board. Debby was terrified, screamed, and kicked. I had to implore him to put her down on her feet again and let us walk slowly on board together. Climbing up the gangway, the child cried: "Where is Debby going, where is Debby going?"

Once on board ship I took her straight below deck into one of the cabins. I put her in a berth and lay down beside her, holding her in my arms. Debby relaxed, stopped crying, and soon was asleep. Half an hour later, when I was having a breath of fresh air on deck, a stewardess called me. I found a very miserable Debby inside the cabin; she had soiled herself. I had to wash her, change her clothes, and comfort her. I succeeded in lulling her back to sleep, but the same accident happened twice again before we reached Dover in England.

There I had to expose the terribly overstrained child to another ordeal, worse than that in Calais. Standing in the long queue before the immigration officer's room, and walking through the roaring luggage hall out to the train must have been an extended nightmare for Debby. Everybody tried to be kind and helpful, the passengers, the authorities, the porters, the customs officer. Friendly adults addressed Debby in English. But all their kindness was, of course, in vain. The child was so overwrought now that she simply howled.

It was a striking example of "catastrophic behavior" (Goldstein, 1940). Debby showed a subjective horror accruing from her past experiences, though in the objective reality no unfriendliness, threat, or danger—in the common sense of these words—existed. For a child of Debby's upbringing, with her lack of shared experiences and with no trusted parental figure to protect her, most of this journey must have been a succession of incomprehensible and horrifying events.

Eventually, we were inside a train again. We found seats in a corner opposite a young woman accompanied by a 6-year-old girl. Both spoke German as well as English. No sooner was Debby settled in her corner than the loud sobbing stopped. Her face became all smiles, and she started to play with the other little girl, who had a box of colored beads. A few minutes later when the train had started, I had a happy child at my side. The changes in her mood and behavior were most astounding: terror when she had to be in a crowd in an open space and immediate return to calmness and even cheerfulness as soon as she found herself in a small, relatively enclosed room.

During the journey from Dover to London Debby played with the little English girl. Together they looked out the window; and whenever Debby saw an animal—cow, sheep, or horse—grazing in the fields, she would clap her hands and exclaim in English: "Goats, goats!" I dressed her in a clean, pink dress and told her in German that we were now in England, that her mummy and her aunt lived in England, that she was going to live with her aunt who had a nice house, a garden, a baby, and a dog to play with. At this point Debby looked quite cheerful and well. Suddenly she began to sing a little tune of her own: "Debby goes to Mummy, Debby goes to Mummy."

We reached Victoria Station, London, where Debby had to live through the last stage of this traumatic journey. Needless to say, she started crying again as soon as we stood on the platform of the station. Her new foster mother was waiting for us, and together we went into an empty waiting room, where Debby stopped crying. The foster mother, Mrs. Grant, was waiting for her husband, who was going to drive her and the child to their home in the south of England.

Before leaving Vienna I had exchanged a few letters with Mrs. Grant, telling her about Debby's exceptional life history and the difficulties resulting from her upbringing. Now I talked with the foster mother for a few minutes, describing Debby's troubles during our journey. I gave her and Debby a few coloring books and crayons, and they began to play with each other. Then I left the station.

Debby's New Life

At this time I decided not to return to Vienna: instead, I applied for a visa to enter the United States. During the following year, while I waited in London for the visa to be granted, I saw Debby twice again. The first time was seven weeks after our journey, the second time eight months later.

Early in August I paid a brief visit to her foster home in the country and found a remarkably changed child. From a virtual infant she had turned into a serious little girl. In Austria she had worn a dirndl dress, and her hair was in pigtails; now she was wearing her hair loose, and she was dressed in a pale blue summer dress and sandals. I found her sitting on a rug spread on the lawn, having her tea outdoors.

Debby's foster parents, who had a charming English country house with a large garden, seemed to be kind and sympathetic young people. They hoped that Debby would forget all about her past. Debby had a room of her own, and a nursemaid looked after her and the family's 6-months-old baby. Mrs. Grant knew some German, but the nurse spoke only English. Mrs. Grant told me that Debby had no difficulty getting along with the nurse and was picking up English very well. I sat down beside Debby and spoke to her, first in German, then in English. She did not answer, but stared at my face with a serious expression, without any sign of recognition. I had only a short conversation with the foster mother, who seemed to be anxious lest my presence stir up memories of the recent past in Debby's mind. I left soon and called to Debby from the car. I gave her a box of chocolates, saying a few words in German to her. She answered: *"Danke"* ("Thank you") with a serious face, turned around at once, and walked back into the house.

I saw Debby the second time in February 1939. I had arrived by train and had to ask for directions to Debby's house. A nursemaid, pushing a baby carriage, with a little girl at her side, happened to walk by. She directed me to Mrs. Grant's house, telling me that they all belonged to the Grant household. Thus I discovered to my great surprise that the girl before me was Debby. She had become quite tall and looked almost like a child of 6. As we walked together to their house, I noticed that her gait was clumsy when she was walking uphill. Debby did not recognize me, and was rather shy and quiet. But once inside the house and in the presence of her foster mother, she became lively and cheerful, radiating her special charm. She bubbled over, talking English.

Mrs. Grant told me that, at first, while she was still talking in German to the child, Debby had made little progress with her English. When Mrs. Grant stopped talking German to her, Debby's English improved by leaps and bounds. At the time of my second visit she spoke English fluently; but she made some mistakes in articulation, which Mrs. Grant called her German accent. Debby pronounced *s* for *th* (in think) and *d* for voiced *th* (in there). While these mistakes are common among Germans and Austrians speaking English, it must be also remembered that confusion between *s* and *th* is fairly common among English and American children under the age of 6. Occasionally, Debby used German words in place of similar English ones, saying, for instance, "*Mein* darling" or "*mein* dress." Once Mrs. Grant overheard Debby saying to her playmate, the dog: "*Du bist Schwester Gisela*" ("You are Sister Gisela"). Mrs. Grant asked her: "Do you like Sister Gisela?" and Debby replied in English: "Oh yes, very much."

In her intellectual development she had just arrived at the state of "why" questions, so common among 4-year-old children. She was asking why questions from morning to night, but in addition she also asked many questions of the "What's that?" variety, which normally occur earlier in a child's life than "why" questions. Debby was indefatigable in asking: "What is that?" "What name has it?" "What do you call it?" repeating every new English word many times and enjoying it greatly, like a new toy. Mrs. Grant, fortunately, was as indefatigable in answering Debby's questions as Debby was in asking them. It was fascinating to watch how energetically Debby now was making up for the linguistic and intellectual paucity of her early life.

As was to be expected, her emotional development had not been free from complications. It had been rather difficult to feed her during the first few weeks at her new home. She had made a mess of her food and often had kept food in her mouth, as she had done in the past. By the time of my second visit, however, she not only had learned proper table manners, but she also seemed to enjoy eating and had become a very good eater. Her bed wetting had been much harder to cope with and had persisted over a longer period of time than her eating problems. Mrs. Grant, a patient and observant person, felt that most incidents of bed wetting had been connected with Debby's being emotionally excited the previous day. In the first few months after her arrival Debby had suffered from recurrent nightmares, during which she had often cried out: "*Kleidi anziehn!*" ("Put dressie on!") I was able to explain the probable meaning of this exclamation. I remember that I had repeatedly said ("*Debby wird jetzt ihr schoenes neues Kleidi anziehn*" ("Debby will now put her pretty little dressy on") when I had changed her dress on the Dover-London train, and I had used a similar phrase when I had to clean her and change her clothes after her accidents on the boat.

Debby had become familiar with the sight of cars, traffic, and people, but she had not been in a train since our trip to England. She liked shopping, although evidently she preferred small shops and became fidgety in large stores.

She seemed to be on excellent terms with her foster parents, whom she called Uncle and Aunt. Mrs. Grant told me that Debby responded well to suggestions and explanations, but she never obeyed simple orders. In the beginning she had appeared very negativistic, saying *"Ich will nicht!"* ("I don't want to!") in response to most demands or suggestions. This type of behavior had totally disappeared. She was fond of the baby and imitated taking care of it in playing with her doll. However, at the time of my second visit, she was not yet able to settle down to any activity which demanded sustained concentration, such as drawing.

Debby's mother had visited her at Christmas time. Debby had been prepared for her mother's visit, and had looked forward to it very much. When her mother arrived, mother and child had gotten along surprisingly well with each other. Afterward Debby continued to call Mrs. Grant *Aunt*, referring to her mother as *Mummy*.

During my second and last visit Debby gave no sign of remembering me. When I spoke to her in German, she stared at me with a very serious expression, then turned around quickly and left the room.

In a letter which I received from Mrs. Grant somewhat later, she wrote: "Debby is by no means what you would call an average child, and she needs very careful upbringing." From my brief visits I gained the impression that Debby's foster mother was sincerely interested in Debby and was willing to give her the continued affection and love she had been deprived of earlier in life. I doubted, however, that Debby would ever be able to "forget" her past, as her foster parents hoped.

Unfortunately, the vicissitudes of my own life, the outbreak of the second world war, and my emigration to the United States made me lose touch with Debby and her foster family. After the war I did not succeed in gaining further information about Debby's experiences during the war. I have often wondered what effects Debby's early, traumatic experiences may have had upon her later development and her personality.

COMMENTARY

Glancing over the observations made of Debby between January 1938 and February 1939, we might ask, first of all, what would be the proper *diagnosis* to encompass the specific features of Debby's unusual behavior and language development. In order to be more than a mere labeling device, a diagnostic statement must be based upon a set of interconnected observations, deductions, and hypotheses, related to a broader framework of theoretical assumptions; it should provide us with a better understanding of the general as well as of the specific features of each case and the dynamics of the significant variables; it should facilitate the formulation of a treatment plan and the choice of appropriate techniques for therapeutic or remedial action; finally, it should permit us to predict, within limits, the effects that a given form of therapy will have upon a given child under given conditions. If in a later stage of therapy the effects of the treatment do not agree with the predictions made, either the therapeutic techniques or the diagnostic formulations, or both, will have to be modified.[3]

In the course of our research studies we came to the conclusion that a three dimensional approach was most appropriate for the diagnostic evaluation of children with language disorders. The three dimensions to be considered are (a) the child's health and developmental history; (b) observations of the child's behavior and speech in both unstructured and structured situations, including the administration of speech and hearing tests, medical and psychological tests; and (c) observation and analysis of the environmental stimulation the child is receiving, with particular emphasis upon the patterns of adult–child interaction which the child is experiencing. A schema of this approach to diagnosis is presented in Figure 2.[4]

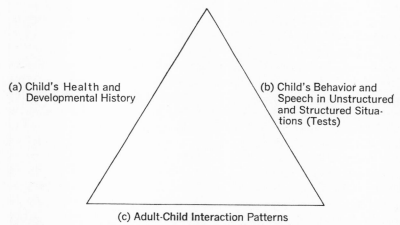

(a) Child's Health and Developmental History

(b) Child's Behavior and Speech in Unstructured and Structured Situations (Tests)

(c) Adult-Child Interaction Patterns

FIGURE 2.   DATA NEEDED FOR THE DIAGNOSTIC EVALUATION OF CHILDREN WITH LANGUAGE DISORDERS

If we attempt to apply this approach to our observations of Debby, we realize that the information we have is not sufficient to permit a comprehensive diagnosis of her condition. All we can engage in, therefore, is a bit of thoughtful speculation, as Nancy E. Wood has called it (1954, p. 5). The term *hospitalism* used by Spitz (1954) evidently is not satisfactory from a diagnostic point of view, as it refers to only one significant factor in the constellation of Debby's life: It

---

3. Darley (1964) and Wood (1964) recommended the formulation of a tentative diagnosis, to be followed by a period of "experimental treatment" devoted to further behavior sampling, manipulation of variables, and drawing of inferences and leading eventually to a more comprehensive diagnosis. The publications by these authors, together with Myklebust's *Manual* (1954), should be consulted for their detailed discussions of diagnostic problems and procedures.

4. See also Appendix XI.

suggests that Debby had spent most of her life within a hospital or an institution of some kind. Given this basic condition of institutionalized upbringing, we take it for granted that there are wide individual differences among institutionalized children—differences of constitutional endowment as well as differences in the specific object relations experienced with the available adults.

Unfortunately, because of my emigration I had no information concerning Debby's developmental history. Thus, we know nothing about her mother's pregnancy and delivery, though the transfer of mother and child to the particular hospital permits the inference that Debby was born prematurely. We also have no knowledge concerning Debby's health history, nor do we have information derived from tests of mental ability. We know that at the age of 3 years and 6 months she was severely limited in her cognitive development, retarded in the acquisition of language, clumsy and awkward in walking, and often hyperactive and disorganized in her behavior. In Chapters 12 and 13 we will describe children with multiple motor, perceptual, and language disorders whose symptoms resemble those observed in Debby, though all of these children grew up under normal conditions of maternal care. At this late date, however, and with the paucity of information we have, it is difficult to determine whether Debby's developmental lag was caused exclusively or primarily by her institutional upbringing or whether constitutional factors contributed to it. The facts, however, that she responded positively to verbal stimulation and that her speech improved rapidly once she received frequent and appropriate corrective feedback strongly suggest that environmental deprivation was the main reason for her delayed language development.

While we lack some vital information in the area of Debby's developmental history, we have numerous descriptions of Debby's behavior and speech observed in life situations; we also know a good deal about the kind of environmental stimulation and adult-child interaction she experienced. From these observations we can come to some understanding of Debby's object relationships, her language learning, and her modes of coping with new and strange situations and with severe crises in her life.

A number of observers, as mentioned by Bowlby (1951, Chapter 3), have reported that it was characteristic of children reared in institutions to be unable to enter into significant relationships with others, to accept love, and to enter into group play with other children. Fortunately, this was not true in Debby's case. We must remember, of course, that Debby was not one among many orphans in an orphanage or one of many foundlings in a foundling home. On the contrary, as the only healthy child among sick children, she had always been the object of special interest and the pet child of many staff members. Many adults had expressed their affection for Debby, and she had received care, help, and love from adults as well as children. What she had missed was a continuous relationship with one and the same significant adult. Except for her relationship with the head nurse, Sister Gisela, most of her relationships had been temporary and discontinuous; her perception of people was therefore diffuse and nonspecific, rather than individual and specific. To use an analogy, Debby's situation resembled that of a young child growing up in a very large family: the child's care is entrusted mainly to older sisters or maids, while the mother (Sister Gisela) is preoccupied with the chores of a large household and the care of many children and is accessible only sporadically.

However, while interaction with this maternal figure was infrequent, Sister Gisela was quite consistent in her style of interaction with Debby. A tall, handsome woman in her forties, she was a competent and kindly person with a firm, dependable set of values. It may have been this consistency in her behavior that helped Debby develop some form of primary object relationship; this in turn enabled her to relate easily to new people, provided she met them in a nonthreatening setting—within a hospital ward or a small, well-defined space. She related without difficulty to me when I began working with her—though she rejected me when I suddenly appeared in unfamiliar clothing—and later she related well to her new foster mother and the new nursemaid in England.

Following the principles stated in the introductory chapter, we expect a child's primary object relationships to play an important part in his learning of speech and language. We realize that it was not the absence of relationships but their discontinuity that interfered with Debby's speech and cognitive development. Another factor was the dissimilarity of style which the various caretakers demonstrated in their speech as well as in their handling of Debby.

In spite of this discontinuity and dissimilarity in verbal stimulation to which Debby had been exposed, she was able at the age of three and a half years to perceive all German speech sounds with sufficient acuity to repeat isolated sounds correctly after me. This fact suggests that no constitutional impediment interfered with Debby's auditory perception and discrimination. Beyond that, her memory for speech sounds and for their position in words increased rapidly once she experienced systematic verbal stimulation and corrective feedback.

The following factor should be noted. While Debby was still in the hospital, it was impossible to establish a situation in which one and the same adult could enter into extensive verbal interaction with her over a prolonged period of time. As I saw her only once or twice a week, Debby continued to interact verbally with many adults and children. However, through instructions to several nurses and some of the older children in Debby's ward, I had succeeded in establishing similarity in the style of interaction which Debby experienced. The nurses and children concerned with Debby's speech used the identical picture books and usually the same words they had observed me using in teaching Debby. Thus Debby received frequent and systematic language training and corrective feedback, though they were provided by more than one person.

From the rapid improvement in Debby's articulation once appropriate verbal stimulation was provided, we might hypothesize that immediacy and frequency of corrective feedback may be more decisive factors in a child's language training—at least in the learning of phonemic patterns—than interaction with a particular adult. The analysis of other cases to be presented later in this book will illuminate this hypothesis further.

Freud and Burlingham (1943, 1944) and Murphy (1962) have given many illustrations of the role of language in children's attempts at mastering the new and the strange, and in coping with crisis situations. As a child grows up, verbal communication becomes a most important tool in his exploration of the environment and his adapatation to reality. In periods of crisis, in particular, the child can ask questions and comprehend the explanations given to him. We have seen that Debby, with her limited verbal skills, reacted to stressful situations mostly with behavior disorganization, crying, or temper tantrums. Her primary defenses against threatening experiences were withholding or negation. A year after leaving the hospital, when she had made excellent progress in her mastery of English, these primitive defenses had largely disappeared.

Particularly striking was Debby's rigid and predictable reaction to the location in which she found herself: anxiety and even terror when she had to be in an open area with many objects, human and nonhuman, moving around in it; relief and calmness as soon as she was again in a small, well-defined space. We remember Debby's desperate outburst when her bed had disappeared from the ward. We know that all young children have a predilection for hiding in small enclosed spaces which they may find under a tree, under the dining room table, in the snow, or in a tunnel built of blocks. For Debby, who had no easy access to a maternal person for her protection, her small hospital bed with its rails around it had become the prototype of a protective area, providing her with security and inducing sleep. This meaning of her bed for her was reflected in her speech when she reacted to the anxiety-provoking streetcars, saying: "Debby go to bed—streetcar go to bed." If we accept Susan Isaac's interpretation[5] that Debby's hospital bed had acquired a protective, maternal quality for her, we will understand also the extreme mood swings which she demonstrated during the trip to England.

Of particular importance for Debby's adaptation to her environment was her change of languages. Verbal communication, which had been a minor tool of adaptation during her hospital life, became of major importance in her foster home. Several factors contributed to her rapid learning of English in the new environment. First, Debby was then almost a year older than at the time I had first met her. Second, she learned English as a second language after having grasped the meaning of language in her primary learning of German. Finally, she experienced for the first time in her life intensive language training, provided by her foster mother and the nurse. Both of them, aware that Debby was a beginner learning a new language, spoke to her in short simple phrases and provided her with constant corrective feedback. Furthermore, this teaching and learning of language did not take place in a crowded ward with ever changing people around her, but in a small well-contained household where a limited number of people interacted with Debby continuously. Thus the child simultaneously discovered people as differentiated, specific individuals with predictable behavior and learned to use speech as the primary means of interaction with these individuals.

---

5. See footnote 1, p. 25.

Obviously, Debby can not be called a bilingual child. The only time when she began to use two languages or labeling systems was during the few hours of the train ride from Dover to London, when we were in the company of the woman and child who spoke both English and German fluently. At that time Debby used the second language as another form of play (Stengel, 1939). We remember her foster mother's report that Debby's learning of English progressed by leaps and bounds once the foster mother gave up talking to her in German and used English exclusively.

This observation beautifully illustrates the role that identification with a love object plays in the acquisition of language. The learning of speech is not only a cognitive but also a deeply emotional experience for the young child; and, as is all emotional learning, it is accomplished through the process of unconscious identification (Stengel, 1939; Freud and Burlingham, 1943; Baker, 1948, 1955; Wyatt, 1949). The development of a strong, permanent relationship with a significant adult, her foster mother, was of primary importance for Debby's well-being at that point in her life; and the use of a language connected with the past interfered with her identification with the new love object.

We assume with Heinz Werner (1957) that for a young child languages are not abstract symbolic systems which can be interchanged at will; the meaning of language for the child is *holophrastic*, and the learning of language is embedded in a concrete and total relationship. Obversely, the same may be true for the teacher of the new language: Debby's foster mother, who desired so strongly that Debby should forget her past, presented the English language to Debby as a gift of love, fostering Debby's identification with her new family and her new country and at the same time promoting the child's repression of early memories and previous relationships.

From the foster mother's description we also derived glimpses of the ambivalent feelings Debby had developed for her first language. German had been the language of her first experiences of affection and love, and she transferred her affection to her new companion, the dog, when she addressed him in German: *"Du bist Schwester Gisela."* At the same time, memories of danger and anxiety appearing in her dreams and nightmares were expressed in German, as in the phrase *". . . Kleidi anziehn!"*

Looking back at Debby's unusual upbringing and experiences, we are reminded not only of the studies in hospitalism, mentioned earlier, but also of reports concerning the development of children growing up in communal nurseries. A. Rabin (1965) conducted a series of studies in which he compared the social and intellectual development of groups of children raised in a kibbutz, a communal settlement in Israel, with that of a matched group of Israeli children growing up in traditional family settings. Rabin pointed out that the kibbutz children experience "multiple motherhood." During his early years a kibbutz child is raised simultaneously by his own mother, who spends several hours daily with him; by the professional nurse who takes care of small groups of infants during the daytime; and by the night nurse, who is in charge of large numbers of infants. In comparing the two groups of children at the age of 2 years, Rabin found evidence that the kibbutz-reared children were significantly lower in social and language development than the home-reared children.

However, in contrast to most hospitalized children, in whom personality disorders are observed in later years, older children and young adults who had been reared in a kibbutz did not differ significantly from the control groups in intelligence, use of language, or social behavior. Rabin suggests that multiple motherhood may be most frustrating and inappropriate for infants during the early years of life. During the latency period and during adolescence the kibbutz children experience much adult affection and support, which, together with their strong intragroup loyalty, may contribute to their successful development in later years.

Debby also had spent her early years under conditions of multiple motherhood, and had been retarded in social and language development. We can only hope that in Debby's case also the affectionate support of her foster parents, which she experienced later, enabled her to overcome at least some of the effects of the deprivation which she had experienced in early childhood.

CHAPTER THREE

The Case of Nana: From Birth to
the Onset of Stuttering

In Chapter 2 we followed the development of a child through a crucial period in her life. We will now turn to the history of another child, Nana, whose learning of speech and language was disrupted temporarily by a period of stuttering.

The case of Nana—as I chose to call her—is based upon observation of my own child. I began my observations in 1942, a few days after Nana's birth, and continued them through the first 7 years of her life. I was familiar with biographical studies of children's language development published earlier (Preyer, 1893; C. and W. Stern, 1907), studies concerned chiefly with the growth of vocabulary in children, from the appearance of the first word to the age of 4 or 5 years. In contrast to that approach, it was my intention to observe Nana's language development, not as an isolated phenomenon, but in its dynamic interrelationship with other aspects of growth.

My observations, like those of other authors of biographical studies of child development, had to be made in the role of participant observer. Although my intimate relationship with the child precluded detachment, it gave me the rare opportunity of watching the child from day to day and gaining firsthand impressions during periods of developmental crises.

During the first three months of Nana's life I recorded my observations daily; later, I wrote weekly summaries of her development. During the period of her stuttering, from the age of 27 months to 34 months, I again took daily notes. In addition, I frequently recorded verbatim her monologues while playing, her conversations with others, and the stories and rhymes she made up. Descriptions of particularly striking or unusual behavior were written down as soon as possible after the occurrence. Reports from physicians and teachers and results of psychological tests, obtained at different age levels, complemented these records. While the original notes amounted to hundreds of pages, only a small portion of the recorded observations can be reported here.

Because of Nana's excellent language development, her stuttering came as a complete surprise. Her speech disturbance aroused in me strong feelings of anxiety and helplessness, feelings which I would encounter later again and again in the mothers of stuttering children with whom I came in professional contact. Beyond this, I was acutely aware of the doubtful validity of all existing theories on stuttering and the limited success of the various forms of therapy I had come across. Living with the child through this difficult phase in her development and observing, eventually, the gradual disappearance of her symptoms, I began to grasp for the first time the importance of the mother-child relationship in language development—as well as in its disruption. The insights gained through this personal experience were translated later into research hypotheses which, in turn, were tested in the studies reported in the second part of this book.

Looking through my records and diaries later, I found in them the "vivid, irreducible stuff" which makes case studies absorbing and enlightening, but also the methodological problems inherent in first-person documents, which have been stated by Gordon W. Allport in his well-known study, "The use of personal documents in psychological science" (1942). My records were rich in detail concerning Nana's social and intellectual growth, her personality, her play, and her language development, and they contained many examples of verbal interaction between child and parents. However, my descriptions were often "heavily saturated with mood," as Allport would express it; and they were incomplete in certain areas which one expects to find explored in depth in third-person case histories—for example, the personalities of father and mother, their feelings, and their relationship.

The question could be raised whether such personal and necessarily fragmentary observations merit publication. The answer can be found in a statement by Patrick Meredith of the University of Leeds, England. He describes the "two-way flow of information" that he considers desirable for an operational approach to research in child development. He points out that information derived from a family member will illuminate the specific and sometimes unique features of a case, while information gathered by a professional will aim at generalization:

Information from the family consists of "very particularized, unclassified, unformalized, anecdotal facts, a distillation from many hours of daily individual contact, necessarily biased, selective, erratic, perhaps spontaneous, perhaps contrived, perhaps inhibited. To expect something very different would be merely naive. . . . As in many other working situations the limitations of having to depend on information which is uncertain and incomplete must be accepted. Professional information . . . is necessarily more general, more scientifically authentic (though not always the last word), more formalized and systematic and often less readily comprehensible.[1]

Thus the information presented in Part I of this book, being personal and

---

1. Meredith (1964), p. 15.

anecdotal, had to be impressionistic in character and style, while the information in Part II, including the case histories presented there, will be more formalized, impersonal, and systematic. It is hoped that in the end these two forms of presentation will permit "a fusion of two complementary streams of information of basically different types."[2]

The case of Nana was included in this volume with the following purposes in mind: (a) to delineate the vicissitudes of Nana's language development within the context of the mother-child relationship; (b) to demonstrate in what manner her early psychosexual development, her use of language, and her modes of thinking were affected by the experience of stuttering; and (c) to direct the reader's attention to certain patterns of mother-child interaction that interfered with Nana's acquisition of language and to other patterns that had a therapeutic effect and served as models for therapeutic techniques, developed in later studies.

A linguistic analysis of Nana's learning of speech sounds, grammar, and syntax was not intended. Systematic studies of children's learning of phonemic patterns have been carried out by Grégoire (1937, 1947), Irwin (1941, 1946, 1947, 1949), Irwin and Chen (1943), R. Jakobson (1941), Lewis (1951), Mandell and Sonneck (1935), D. McCarthy (1930, 1960), Templin (1957), Wellman, Case, Mengert, and Bradbury (1931), and others. Studies of children's acquisition of grammar and systax have been undertaken by M. E. Smith (1926), Berko (1958), Brown and Berko (1960), Brown and Fraser (1964), Brown, Fraser, and Bellugi (1964), Miller and Ervin (1964), Slobin (1964a, and 1964b), and Brown and Cazden (1965).

In reporting here the case of Nana, an attempt has been made to separate observations from commentaries and discussions of therapy.

OBSERVATIONS

The First Three Weeks

Nana was the first and only child of healthy parents, both professional people in their thirties. Her arrival had been awaited eagerly. The mother's pregnancy was uneventful until the seventh month, when an attack of pyelitis led to a short period of hospitalization. There had been no evidence of left-handedness, hearing, speech, or reading difficulty in either the father's or the mother's family. In addition to English, both parents spoke several foreign languages.

The mother's delivery was prolonged but otherwise normal. She was under sedation during the last few hours, and the child was delivered by forceps. A pediatrician, examining the child at home on her twelfth day, declared that she was a perfectly healthy, normal infant. Nana was breast fed for 6 months and 19 days, and her vital needs for sucking, loving care, and mothering were amply

---

2. Meredith, *loc. cit.*

gratified. She began taking the mother's breast on the second day of her life, sucking vigorously. The mother enjoyed breast feeding and had an ample milk supply. A note in the mother's diary at the end of the first week reads:

> If Nana does not find the nipple at once she tries again and again, patiently, until she succeeds. She settles down to business, sucks vigorously, at times even hastily, and produces loud sucking noises and little lusty cries. . . . After feeding she usually falls asleep and looks extremely contented.[3]

Nana's first distinct smile appeared at 34 days, together with the beginning of a cooing form of vocalization. These utterances, which are difficult to transcribe, consisted of "comfort sounds" (Lewis, 1951), produced with relaxed vocal mechanism. The first consonants also appeared at this time, produced in the back of the mouth with the back of the tongue raised towards the soft palate: guttural *r*, *g* (as in *go*), *k*, a palatal *l*, and the nasalized sound combination *ng*; also the fricative *h*. Early comfort sounds occurred frequently after feeding, seemingly as a continuation of the sucking and swallowing movements in which the child had just engaged. Originally connected with satisfaction after feeding, these sounds soon became expressive of the baby's comfort in general.

Sucking the Pacifier

The child liked to be given a pacifier after feeding, to prolong the feeding movements until she fell asleep, and also while she was awake waiting to be fed. The satisfaction gained from sucking the pacifier apparently helped her overcome minor tension states. When she cried in apparent anger and was given the pacifier, she calmed down and made little chewing noises, the chewing of her pacifier accompanied by rhythmic sound production, such as *aa-aa-oo-oo-aa*. . . .[4]

At 3 months Nana sucked the pacifier mostly in the late afternoon while waiting for her feeding. She also sucked the rattle, the bead ring, and other toys; the mother's hand; or anything else that she could find near her mouth. Finally, at 4 months the pacifier lost all attraction for her. She had reached the stage where the new skill of grasping allowed her to put everything in reach into her mouth— be it a sheet, a spoon, a toy, or her blanket. At this stage the mother noticed two situations which tended to provoke anger in the infant: (1) frustration when a toy was too big for her mouth and she wanted passionately to put it into it, and (2) the unfulfilled desire for social contact and for things to look at.

---

3. Fries in her studies of the "congenital activity type" (1947), describes the differences in response to life experiences exhibited by the quiet, the moderately active, and the active infant. In view of Nana's behavior when feeding and of her general behavior at later stages of development, one would place her in the category of "congenitally active" children.

4. Froeschels (1925, 1948) emphasized the role of chewing in language development. His assumptions led to the development of "chewing exercises" as a therapeutic technique, used by him and his collaborators in the treatment of stutterers as well as of patients with vocal hyperfunctions.

Reactions to Auditory Stimulation—Changes in Feeding Behavior

Beginning on the nineteenth day, Nana liked listening to soft voices, quiet talk, little songs and lullabies. The sound of a guitar played by her father at Nana's bedside made her stop crying and kicking, and after some quiet listening she fell asleep. At 35 days she turned her head in the direction of a noise and with her eyes followed a person walking through the room.

At the age of 2 months Nana's feeding behavior began to change. Her mother recorded:

During the first 8 weeks Nana used to cuddle quietly in my arms while I fed her. Though she sucked vigorously, her body was passive. Now she moves her body, kicks her legs. She treats the nipple and the breast the way a little dog plays with a slipper, biting it, pulling it around, and barking at it. She makes little cries while drinking, even stops sucking to say her favorite syllable *ero*. If the nipple slips out of her mouth, she gets angry at it. Once she roared at it like a tiny lion, *whoon*.

Nana obviously was changing from primary oral pleasure to a more aggressive oral stage.

During the third month Nana began to produce playful cooing rhythms, *ero ero gero gattawoo, yawookawookawooka*. She smiled when her mother made funny noises at her, and mother and child began to have little cooing conversations. The mother talked to Nana, as most mothers do, in a gay and loving voice, sometimes imitating in her own voice the baby's cooing tones. The baby stared and listened, then answered with sounds, little cries, and high-pitched cooing, kicking her legs, waving her arms, wriggling her body, and smiling.

This form of overall response may be compared with Nana's more differentiated behavior in a similar situation at the age of 6 months. At that time mother and child liked to play hiding games. Nana pulled a blanket over her head; the mother called "goo-goo," in a tune descending from high to low pitch; Nana pushed the blanket off her face and produced a high shriek. The mother showed her pleasure every time the child's face reappeared; Nana, too, laughed aloud with pleasure, wriggled, and babbled excitedly. This game offered pleasant auditory stimulation as well as a delightful experience: losing mother and finding her again. Three weeks later—at 6 months 21 days—Nana responded with apparent recognition and shrieks of delight to the calling of her name, or to the original "goo-goo," both spoken by the mother in the same high-low tune.

COMMENTARY

Mowrer and Viek pointed to an observation made by John Whiting, who "noticed the almost universal tendency for human parents, especially mothers (both primitive and civilized), to babble, jabber, coo, and otherwise *imitate their infant's* own early vocalizations" (1945, p. 47, italics by the authors). Thus the mother's spontaneous imitations of the child's early sounds become conditioned stimuli for the child to utter similar sounds, and imitation of the child by the mother or father actually precedes the child's imitation of the parent. Piaget (1951), in his studies of the earliest forms of interaction between adult and child, observed such circular reactions between parent and infant occurring from the first month of life. He called these patterns of interaction "vocal contagion," defining them as merely a form of stimulation of the child's voice by another voice, without exact imitation by the child of the sounds which he hears. According to Piaget, vocal contagion precedes mutual imitation of sounds.

OBSERVATIONS

Fourth to Sixth Month

With the introduction of cereal and strained vegetables in her diet in the fourth month and the increased chewing and licking of rattles, rings, spoons, and toys, the muscles of Nana's lips and tip of the tongue became more active. Spinach or orange juice were blown into the mother's face with a delighted sound, *bbvv*, and the front consonants appeared gradually: the dentals *t, d, l*; the labials *b, p, v*; and the nasals *m, n*.

At 5 months 14 days Nana laughed aloud for the first time. Her voice at that time ranged from a very high, piercing and shrill voice (anger) to a full, low voice, which she used frequently for her playful vocalizing.

Around that time she also liked to utter a low-pitched grunt, produced with much abdominal and vocal pressure. This, however, was not a distress sound, but obviously was made for fun; she liked particularly to produce it while eating cereals or vegetables. Whenever the mother said "no, no," to this grunting, Nana grinned and grunted again and again. This was followed by a high little scream produced with soft vocal intonation. The mother then smiled her approval, "Yes, yes, this is nice." A game between mother and child developed out of this: grunting, disapproval; soft tone, approval. Nana seemed to like this game; it appeared to be a voluntary vocal response on her part. After the breast feeding, the mother usually propped Nana up on a pillow. Nana smiled and made a sound like *ha*, with the obvious intention to communicate and to provoke a cooing conversation with her mother.

Nana never suffered from constipation; apart from occasional attacks of intestinal infection and diarrhea, her digestion was always normal. The physician in charge of her agreed with the mother that "infants know what and how much they need to eat"; consequently, the baby was never urged or forced to eat. Nana, who was a strong, healthy, and handsome infant, was a good eater throughout early childhood.

From Cooing to Babbling

A number of important developmental events occurred during the sixth month of Nana's life: sitting up, turning over from stomach to back, weaning and adjustment to bottle feeding, drinking water and orange juice from a cup, and responding to her own name. Her speech activities developed from cooing to babbling.

Babbling began at 5 months 21 days. From single or separate sounds or short cooing phrases, such as *ho-go-li-va*, she proceeded to longer strings of sounds, which she produced with obvious pleasure: *babawawamamnabayayaya fch-fch-oijiji-edja hiii andjaja—aijajaja*. These strings of sounds were usually produced crescendo—from piano to fortissimo—and again decrescendo, often with a high-pitched climax toward the end. Nana played with sounds sometimes for as long as an hour at a time.

Vocal activities at this stage were most frequent when she woke up and when she was bathed and dressed. Eating also generally stimulated speech. Her eating pleasure was, however, not restricted to activity of the vocal muscles. She moved her legs, arms, hands, and fingers simultaneously, while producing rhythmic sucking noises. Eating, vocalizing, and whole-body movement all seemed to be one. There was also much vocal activity before, during, and after bowel movements. Thus vocalizing appeared to be connected primarily with "specific sensual experiences, tactual and muscular pleasures of singularly pleasurable character," or it served as "a channel for the release of surplus tension of various sources" (Erickson, 1940, p. 719).

The Weaning Period

At the age of 6 months Nana experienced the first major discontinuity or crisis in her life—the change from breast to bottle feeding. Weaning was carried through gradually over a period of 3 weeks.

During the first week only 1 breast feeding was substituted for by a bottle. When Nana's mother gave the infant her first bottle feeding, she held the child in the same position to which both had been accustomed during breast feeding. Drinking milk from the bottle, Nana produced the familiar rhythmic sucking noises which had accompanied her nursing. The sound of these sucking noises made the mother's milk flow, thus increasing the feeling of frustration which the mother experienced in offering the bottle.

On the fourth day the child reached out for the bottle and drank eagerly. Happy babbling followed each bottle feeding. On the sixth day Nana had two bottle feedings; she was restless, and bottle feeding became somewhat difficult.

On the seventh day of the weaning period the contact of the rubber nipple with Nana's mouth stimulated a good deal of babbling and the production of all kinds of vocal noises, but Nana swallowed very little milk. The mother tried to offer her milk from a cup. Nana reacted with much motor activity—blowing milk bubbles, babbling, and gurgling—but still drank very little. She woke up during the night, obviously hungry, and had to be breast fed. On the eighth day the child found a comfortable position for taking the bottle; she closed her eyes and drank with her familiar sucking noises.

From the eighth day on 2 of Nana's 3 feedings were given from the bottle.

On the fourteenth day the child was given a bottle for her first morning feeding. She took it, but did not look at the mother. Having finished the bottle, she turned her head away, which made the mother feel rejected. From the fifteenth to the nineteenth day Nana's first reaction to the bottle was to close her lips and turn away from her mother. However, when the mother in a friendly tone of voice coaxed her to drink, Nana turned her head back and drank her milk peacefully.

On the nineteenth day only one breast feeding was offered. The child showed little interest in drinking from the breast, interrupting her nursing repeatedly. The mother finally presented her with a bottle, from which Nana drank. Breast feeding was stopped on that day.

COMMENTARY

The early years of a child's life must be considered a period of the most complex and intricate learning experiences for both child and mother (Schur, 1960). Communication between mother and child begins at birth and develops into an ever widening network of messages. It develops through the stage of tactile communication and intimate body closeness to the more distant exchange of vocal messages, leading finally to the child's acceptance of words and sentences as symbolic equivalents of earlier tactile experiences (Shands, 1954; Frank, 1957; Schachtel, 1959). The importance of the mother's bodily closeness for the child's early ego development has been stressed by Frank (1957). Schachtel (1959) believes that the shift from the original predominance of the "proximity senses" (smell, taste, and touch) to that of the "distance senses" (sight and hearing) entails for the child a far-reaching change in his whole way of perceiving and experiencing people and the world around him.

During the weaning period both Nana and her mother experienced the loss of a unique form of bodily closeness, and both had to get used to a new and different relationship. The mother experienced feelings of rejection and loss. The child's turning away from the mother could be interpreted as withdrawl from a devaluated love object. However, when the mother spoke to Nana in a friendly voice, urging her to drink from the bottle, the mother's voice and speech were offered together with the bottle and were finally accepted as substitutes for the lost, or rather reduced, body closeness.

OBSERVATIONS

Repetitive Sound Patterns: The First Words

At 6 months 21 days Nana produced the sequence *ma-ma* very clearly while being fed her cereal. From 7 months 14 days on, the same sequence was heard frequently. When the mother heard this repetitive vocalization, she smiled and repeated it back to the child, who, in turn repeated it again.

The sequence *pa-pa*, spoken on the same pitch level as *ma-ma*, also appeared at that time. Brief repetitive sound patterns consisting of two or three syllables now became very frequent, such as *mama, papa, dada, nyan-nyan-nyan*, while the long strings of vocalization became less frequent.

Nana had reached the stage of "mutual imitation," as described by Piaget (1951). The mother often imitated the child right after Nana had uttered a particular sound pattern, thus closely matching her vocal utterance with that of the child. The child then redoubled her efforts and, stimulated by the other voice, imitated on her part the same sounds her mother was imitating.

Nana was now able to hold two objects at the same time, one in each hand, and she had reached the "throwing away" stage of motor performance. One day, at 7 months 26 days, Nana was playing outdoors in her carriage with three tin pie plates, enjoying the clashing noise, chewing the plates, watching them glitter in the sun, and, finally, throwing them down on the ground with a really big bang. After the third one had been dropped and had rolled out of Nana's sight, she waited, patting her hands and looking around for them; then she began making impatient noises which became rapidly more urgent. At last she broke into a loud *mama*. The mother picked the plates up and put them back into Nana's hands. Nana had done her first "voice magic," as Kipling might have called it; she was beginning to learn that her forming of a certain pattern of sounds would bring about need-satisfying action by one of the adults in her environment.

At the age of 9½ months Nana had reached another milestone of growth; she was able to stand up and to propel herself through the room in a half crawling, half rolling fashion. In addition, her first tooth had emerged, and 3 sound patterns—*mama, dada,* and *iti* (kitty)—had reached the distinctness of consistently used, meaningful symbols which we call *words*. Nana had crossed the threshold from pre-symbolic to symbolic language.

Early Symbolic Stage of Language Development: Naming

With the warm weather Nana's playpen was put outdoors in the yard near the sidewalk. Almost everybody who passed would stop and talk to her: the postman, the milkman, the garbageman, the women who went shopping, the old man with his dog, and all the children in the neighborhood, big and small. Nana enjoyed it immensely. She smiled and waved at everybody, walking around in her pen holding onto the rails, radiantly babbling back at her callers.

In addition to her parents, the persons who took care of Nana were Sophie, a young Austrian college student living with the family, and Mrs. Stone, an elderly American woman who came as a baby sitter. Approximately 80 per cent of the speech Nana heard was English; the rest was German. However, the adults usually addressed Nana in English.

Nana's acquisition of words progressed at the following rate:

9 Months 14 Days	3 Words
12 Months	6 Words
13 Months	10 Words
14 Months	22 Words
15 Months	31 Words

Speech Activities at 16 Months

JARGON TALKING

Nana produced a great deal of "jargon," which was nonsymbolic and not used for communication. It differed from the previous babbling in its very pronounced speech melody and modulation. In fact, it's prosodic qualities suggested adult speech.

USE OF WORDS

Six words which Nana used spontaneously had to do with eating:

Mi-a, when she saw, smelled, tasted, or wanted milk.
Butter butter, almost everything edible, except milk; also eating in general.
Appa appa, apple.
Oil, codliver oil.
Egg egg, egg.
Banana, nana, bavana, banana.

Seven words referred to "doing something"—activities or body movements:

Out out, going out, wanting to go out, or seeing somebody leaving.
Up up, getting up, wanting to get up, getting out of her carriage.
Down down, wanting to get down.
Hammer hammer, hammering on the pegboard.
Bad'n bad'n, in imitation of the German words "*Komm baden*," or *ba-ah* in imitation of "bath." Nana used either one when she was being undressed for her bath, was taken into the bathroom, or heard the water flowing into the tub.
Bye-bye, waving her hands, when she left the house or when somebody else left.
Home, coming home from a walk, seeing her house, walking through the door.

She used one word for a part of her own body: *Arm*.
There were 14 words for objects and pictures of objects, animals and pictures of animals:

Water, water in the tub, in the sink; hearing the water flow; later also referring to rain.
Bottle, her milk bottle, whether full or empty.
Paper, any scrap or piece of paper.
Tacktack, a watch.
Ball, her ball, a bib with a picture of a ball.
Button, button on her clothes, in a box; playing with buttons.
Pin, pin, safety pins.
Botth, box.

Bed, her mother's bed.

Dolly, a particular red doll.

Hot hot, in imitation of her mother's warning—used for fire, kitchen stove, a light, a burning match, hot food, eventually for an unlighted lamp.

Itty, kitty, real or in a picture.

Wowwow, dog, real or in a picture.

Du, duck, toy or picture.

Three words for people:

Mama, her mother, also need for help.

Dada, her father, the cleaning woman, other people who came and left again.

Baby, a baby in a picture book, every picture of a human face in a magazine, seeing herself in a mirror. When Nana wanted her mother to take the mirror out of her pocketbook and give it to her, she said *baby*.

Four words were used as exclamations:

No no, or German *nein nein*, accompanied by energetic shaking of her head when she refused to do something.

Ah-ah, produced with a glottal stop, for passing a bowel movement, urinating, or for her potty.

Bam bam, referred to a rhythmic game her mother had played with her; mother and child sitting on a bed had dangled their feet. *Bambam* gradually was used for other things which swung back and forth, but also for shoes. The word *choo* for shoe appeared at 17 months.

At the age of 15 months 21 days Nana spontaneously used for the first time two words in juxtaposition. One morning, in her crib, she said *down down butter butter*, meaning that she wanted to be carried downstairs to get something to eat. The afternoon of the same day, hearing water flowing into the bathtub, she said *bad'n bad'n water water*, using a German and an English word in combination.

UNDERSTANDING SPEECH

In addition to using words, Nana also seemed to understand the meaning of a few short phrases. She reacted to them in the fashion of a game. Asked "Where is your bear?" or "Where is your doll?" she would bring any object she had in her hand. Asked "Give it to mother," she would either give it to her mother or laugh and crawl away rapidly, holding onto her toy, saying "No no" or "Nein nein." Asked "Where is daddy?" when her father was in the room, she pointed to him.

COMMENTARY

If we try to list Nana's first words in meaningful groups, we are faced with considerable difficulty as to categories. Quantitative studies of children's vocabulary growth have been reported frequently in terms of word counts and numbers of words used in sentences at a given age (Preyer, 1893; Lindner, 1898; Ament, 1899; Shinn, 1900; C. and W. Stern, 1907; Bateman, 1914; Nice, 1917, 1925; M. E. Smith, 1926; K. Buehler, 1930; Fisher, 1934). In most of these studies children's speech activities were classified according to the categories used by older schools of logic and grammar.

Clara and William Stern were already quite aware of the artificiality and inappropriateness of these classifications. In *Die Kindersprache* (1907) the authors pointed out that grammatical, logical, and psychological categories which were, perhaps, compatible with the analysis of adult language could not be applied to the interpretation of language in children without clouding the true nature of the problem, particularly with regard to the very early stages of child language. The "primary symbols" (*Ursymbole*) of language, these authors suggest, do not yet possess a definitely specialized character. Out of a primary condition which is yet quite undifferentiated and primitive, the more consistent meanings of words gradually emerge in a definite sequence.

Dissatisfied with a merely grammatical analysis and interested in other, perhaps more significant, aspects of language in childhood, Piaget (1926) focused his observations on the role and function of the child's speech in relation to his environment.

All the earlier investigations have contributed indispensable material to our present knowledge of language development. Few of them, however, succeeded in avoiding the application of an adult mold and pattern in the evaluation of children's speech. If adult conversational usage is the criterion of correctness, language performance in childhood, particularly in the earliest stages, must by necessity seem incomplete, defective, incomprehensible and, at times, even bewildering. Such essential and specific elements of child language as rhythmic repetition, nonsense talk, or "commentary speaking"—to be discussed later—will either completely escape recording or will appear under the heading "irrelevant material." Our evaluation will probably become more compatible with the material observed if we watch out for *all* verbal manifestations at any given stage—particularly those that have more or less disappeared from conscious adult usage—and if we accept these manifestations as intrinsic items of children's communication.

In agreement with C. and W. Stern, Sapir (1921) and Werner (1957) point out that the first manifestations of speech in the young child are quite undifferentiated and primitive. They are indicative of images, rather than thought and ideas—images of a vague and unprecise character, the outline of which is still wavering and changing. They take in at one time a variety of meanings, then shrink and crystallize into words of a more definite and limited significance. For the first time in his life, the child begins to organize experience through speech signs.

At this stage the distinction between object, movement, image, and verbal symbol is not yet clearly established, and a high degree of concreteness still applies to all words. According to Werner (1957), early speech signs are still endowed with many concrete elements, and speech develops in the direction of the abstract only very slowly and gradually. Development toward the level of abstract language has to go through various stages, originating at the level where names are fused with the object they denote (Langer, 1942, 1962; Werner, 1957). As the process of naming advances, names gradually achieve the status of symbols representing the object. At the same time the expressive—or as Werner calls it, the physiognomic—quality of words may still remain alive in the background, a fact important to remember in therapeutic work with children.

All through the phase of naming the child is embarked on setting up a symbolic inventory of his experiences of things and relations, which is imperative before any ideas can be conveyed (Sapir, 1921). Groups of experiences which seem to have some common characteristic are tentatively lumped together into a particular speech sign. As an example, see Nana's use of *bambam* for swinging one's legs, for swinging movements in general, and for the object shoe. Under the influence of corrective feedback coming from significant adults, the child gradually becomes aware of significant differences in the realm of reality as well as in the realm of symbolic language. This cognitive process of increasing differentiation is reflected in the shifts in the child's usage of words.

A certain length of time and continued corrective feedback are necessary for this process of differentiation to occur. For example, when Nana was 18 months old, Sophie, the college student living with the family, came home one day with a new and very colorful umbrella. Nana called both the student and her umbrella *foffa*; the bright exciting object was experienced as part of Sophie. Transferring the color experience to other objects, Nana then called other colorful objects *foffa*—for instance, a Scotch plaid scarf. When she was taught the name *umbrella*, she began to call Sophie's umbrella *foffabyella*. At that point—18 months 14 days—Nana's word *foffa* referred to Sophie, to all umbrellas except Sophie's, and to certain very colorful objects. At 19 months Nana began to differentiate between colorful scarves and skirts, giving them separate names—*carf, kirt*—while she continued to use the word *foffa* for Sophie and for umbrellas. Finally, at 20 months, Sophie only was called *foffa*; all umbrellas were now called *byella* or *umbyella*, with the exception of Sophie's colorful umbrella, which continued to be *foffabyella*.

During the early naming stage, the child discovers the magic quality of speech signs, their power to revive images of the past (memory images) and of absent love objects, their faculty of expressing wishes in a more effective manner than mere crying and gesturing can do, and their propensity to induce adults to fulfill these wishes.

In summary, during the early symbolic stage the child begins to organize his experiences through the association of names with his sense impressions as well as with his memory images and wishes. The words used at this time are still largely undifferentiated, and their meaning is unprecise and shifting; object, movement, image, and verbal symbol are experienced as one entity. The child indulges in constant repetition of words, enjoying new words as if they were new toys. These endless repetitions are essential for the learning and "over learning" of verbal symbols. They are also pleasant and satisfactory, or "ego-tonic" (Erikson, 1950), for the child, providing him with an ever increasing sense of mastery.

OBSERVATIONS

Illnesses, Sleeping Disturbance, Motor Development

Between the ages of 13 months 12 days and 16 months 13 days Nana went through a difficult period in her development. Understanding these early irregularities in her behavior will help us evaluate the irregularities in her speech development later on; it will also bring some basic principles of child development to our attention.

Nana's difficulties began with a severe intestinal infection and diarrhea, which lasted for 4 days. Her pediatrician put her on a restricted diet, without milk. During 2 nights Nana woke up asking fervently for her *"mi-a,"* and a sleeping disturbance began which lasted for almost three months. Nana was awake for long periods every night, yelling, sitting up, or standing in her crib. When her mother came to pick her up and console her, Nana sometimes clung to her; at other times she pushed her mother's hand away and did not look into her face.

In the period following her recovery from the intestinal infection Nana suffered recurrent severe colds. Her motor development had reached a stage during which she crawled around a great deal and attempted to stand up alone and to take a few steps without holding on to somebody. Now she had to spend most of the day in her crib or carriage and was discouraged from crawling on the floor. During that period of illness she learned to pile 5 blocks upon each other; and holding a spoon in her right hand, she made attempts at feeding herself.

The sleeping disturbance continued, developing into a habitual pattern. The child was awake for hours every night. Standing up in her.crib, she cried and yelled, or recited the words *butter butter down down*.

Because of these nightly disturbances, Nana's mother felt increasingly exhausted. Unsuccessfully, she tried various approaches to get Nana to sleep, from rocking her to giving her sleeping pills prescribed by the pediatrician. The more her mother tried to calm Nana down, the more wakeful and noisy the child became. Nana's apparent "unwillingness" to sleep aroused anger in her mother. During her short and often interrupted hours of sleep the mother was hounded by a recurrent dream, which she recorded in her diary:

I dream that I have forgotten my child somewhere, or have lost her. I have left her in a friend's house, but I have forgotten the address of the house. I have to run through endless streets in a strange town trying to find the house in which I left my child, or through many rooms of a strange house in search of her, desperately asking people whether they have seen my child. In the end I find her again, experiencing a tremendous relief.

Aware of the aggressive feelings reflected in this dream, the mother felt guilty and dejected. She became increasingly tense and irresolute in handling the child, who in turn reacted with increasing restlessness.

Toward the end of the mother's pregnancy when her pyelitis had caused her to get up frequently during the night, father and mother had decided to use separate bedrooms. After Nana's birth this arrangement had been continued, and the baby shared her mother's room. Ten weeks after the onset of Nana's disturbance, the father suggested a rearrangement of the family's sleeping quarters. The parents again shared a bedroom and Nana's crib was put into a room across the hall. This arrangement had a very beneficial effect upon the mother, who enjoyed the renewed closeness with the father and also his help in looking after the child. No longer did she wake up at the slightest noise made by the child, and her nights became more restful.

During these difficult weeks Nana's imitative behavior at times had been quite striking. Nana liked to do the things she saw her mother doing, scribbling with a pencil when her mother was writing, or brushing her hair with her mother's brush. She also loved to imitate words, nonsense syllables, or funny sounds her parents made, and she played with words even if their meaning was unknown to her. The mere repeating of words apparently gave Nana great pleasure. While eating, she enjoyed saying the names of the things she ate.

Once when Nana tried to touch the hot stove, her mother had slapped Nana's hands very slightly, saying "no-no, bad." Nana, in imitation, slapped her own hand, saying *bad bad*. Two days later Nana was playing with a flower pot, and her mother said: "No, no, not for Nana." Nana continued to play with the pot until it fell down and broke. The mother scolded her and put her into her play-pen. The next day, standing again before the flowers in the living room, Nana said very loudly to herself *No no bad bad*, without touching the flowers. Her words and behavior indicated that she had introjected her mother's demands.[5]

Three days after the change of bedrooms Nana began to walk alone. She was then 16 months and 4 days old. Within a week she was able to run across the room unaided, and she began to climb the stairs alone holding onto the banisters. Ten days after the change of rooms and 7 days after she began to walk, Nana's sleeping disturbance had disappeared and she had regained the habit of all-night sleep.

COMMENTARY

Several factors have to be considered in analyzing this developmental crisis and its eventual positive outcome. The father's support and the change in sleeping arrangements apparently helped the mother cope with her own anxiety. In turn, her increased calmness in handling Nana helped in calming down the child. The timing of the disturbance with respect to developmental forces active within the child should also be considered.

These developmental factors have been investigated by Gesell (1929), McGraw

---

5. The importance of language for the development of the child's conscience or superego has been pointed out by Isacower (1939) in his paper "On the exceptional position of the auditive sphere."

(1935), Hendrick (1942), and Buxbaum (1947). They agree that motor abilities appear as a result of maturation of the neurophysiological apparatus necessary to perform them and that each ability appears at a very definite time in the infant's life. Their effective use, however, is not immediately established, but is practiced over a period of weeks. For example, during the weeks in which the child learns to achieve locomotion a considerable amount of his behavior will be concentrated in practicing the stages of learning necessary "to master space with his legs. But, when the child has learned to walk, the compulsion to repeat over and over a certain locomotor movement disappears, and the function is then at the disposal of the ego for use in a multitude of situations" (Hendrick, 1942, p. 42).

Three different stages in the development of motor abilities can be discerned: the *reflex phase*, characterized by its stereotypy and its close relationship to specific stimuli; *a period of practice and learning*, characterized by independence of stimulus, evidence of the need to practice repetitively, and increasing ability to modify the stereotyped pattern; and *maturity of function*, characterized by proficiency in using the apparatus at will without further practice. Hendrick pointed to the infant's tendency to be absorbed in a new activity for days or weeks and the often compulsive quality of the need to practice the unlearned function, a quality which will no longer be evident in the normal exercise of the proficient function later on. In his opinion *compulsive* repetition of an effort occurs (*a*) during a period of learning new patterns of a more complex nature, prior to the attainment of efficient performance or (*b*) when the exercise of a mature function is disturbed by anxiety or by external frustration or limitations imposed by other individuals.

Edith Buxbaum, in her studies of activity and aggression in children (1947), also discerned three stages in activity development. She stressed the innumerable repetitions in the second, the practicing stage. From her experience as a child analyst she concluded that during the process of learning, until the child has achieved control over his vital activities, his relationships to people are of the greatest importance. Buxbaum felt that various disturbances in children may be caused by interference in the practicing stage of activities. Such interference may be based upon or may lead to emotional disturbance between mother and child and may be responsible for a number of disturbances in vital activities such as eating, sleeping, speaking, or toilet training.

In Nana's case, her relationship to her mother had been unsettled and her locomotor learning interfered with during an important practicing phase. The sleeping disturbance, apparently caused by physical illness and hunger during the first nights, continued over a longer period of time because of the subsequent colds and the interference with her motor practice. Nana's compulsive standing up in the crib in the middle of the night, even when she was extremely sleepy, seems significant in this context. The disturbance disappeared when, with the father's help, a mutually supporting mother–child relationship was re-established and, simultaneously, the child mastered the important developmental task of walking alone.

OBSERVATIONS

Speech Sample, 18 Months: Rhythm and Repetition

When Nana was 18 months old, her mother recorded a sample of her spontaneous speech over a 15-minute period. Nana was looking at a picture book with simple pictures of objects, people, and animals. She took the book, climbed into a chair, looked at some pictures, then walked over to sit on the couch. The mother talked to her occasionally while taking notes.

Sits [climbs into the chair]. *Book book——buts buts buts tay tay gorsy horsy* [moves to the floor again]. *Sits sits* [back into the chair]. *Horsy book, horsy book——yam yam*[6] [laughs] *yam yam horsy! horsy!* [the horse in the picture is eating]. *What dat? what dat?——yam yam—— sibytaby house house house! no no no no—hum hum horsy horsy! yam yam.* [Turning the pages in the book, she continues in a singing tone] *horsy horsy horsy——horseee horseee* [wiggles in the chair] *yam yam* [stands up]. *Baby book! baby book,* [very loud and demanding] *baby book! baby book! baby book!* [Mother gives her the baby book. She takes it over to the couch, looks at some of the photographs] *panty baby.* [Mother says, "Put the book back, come here."] *Come come, baby book.* (She puts the baby book back on the shelf, takes the first picture book again, sits down on the chair with it, looks at the pictures, sees a baby clapping his hands *baka-cake, baka-cake* [looking at some other pictures] *mammy mammy lady lady——* [babbling] *awatawatawa. Aeropyane* [aeroplane] . . . *—apple—abowonono—fire fire!——Cup o'coffee, cup o'coffee! fire fire—mammy coffee.* [Seeing the picture of an umbrella] *foffa byella——book, bottle, shoe—foffa foffa foffa foffa—foffa foffa!——foffa foffa* [she continues in a singing tune] *foffa foffa?——foffa foffa——foffa foffa? foffafoffafoffafoffa—foffa gone——foffa—*(dreamily) *foffa . . . foffa . . . foffa? . . . foffafoffafoffa . . .* [she begins to tear a page. Her mother says, "No, no, don't tear it."] *No no no—foffa byella! foffa byella!—byella foffa, byella foffa—foffafoffafoffa.* [Mother takes the book away from her] *No no* [she jumps down from the chair, goes to the desk, gets a bunch of keys] *keys keys keys!* (Wants her mother's pocketbook which she calls bag] *bag bag.* [Hears the telephone ringing] *teyephone? te-ye-phone! te-ye-phone? teyephone!!* Out out [walks through the room carrying her mother's pocket book] *check book, check book, money money.*

The strong emphasis on *rhythm* and *repetition* in her speech was striking. It was not an imitation of adult speech; rather, it was an inherent, original rhythm, coming from the child.

The following examples will further illustrate this spontaneously rhythmical quality of Nana's speech. Her mother showed her a picture of a little boy taking a bath. Pointing to the faucets, the mother said in an explanatory tone, "Hot water, cold water." The child, repeating, immediately turned the words into a little sing-song: *hot water, cold water, hot water, cold water.*

Another day her mother, pointing to another picture, said "A ball and a bat." The child repeated in a singing rhythm *ball-a-bat, ball-a-bat.* After a while the beat changed into that of a ringing bell: *ball-bat, ball-bat,* with equal stress on both words.

---

6. At that time Nana's favorite expression for eating.

Transition from Words to Sentences

We remember that at the age of 16 months 14 days Nana had combined two words into the phrase *down down butter butter*. Phrases of this kind became more frequent during the next 6 months. The following are examples of such phrases.

Poseman poseman letter paper was Nana's announcement when she saw the postman coming.

When her mother was absent, Nana was frequently heard saying, *mummy gone back soon*.

Out the window meant that Nana wanted to look out of the window.

Sits! books! meant that she wanted to sit in somebody's lap and look at picture books.

Walking along the river, she exclaimed in a joyful tone, *water water boats ducks*.

Wanting to be taken to the river again the next day she said *tee-car* (streetcar), *boats, ducks*.

At night, getting ready for bed, she would say, *shoes off, kockings off, dressy off, dark night*.

Going to sleep, Nana often said in a singsong tone, *mummy seep* (sleeps) *daddy seep Bobby seep Helen seep Foffa seep shoe seep rubber seep teecar seep auto seep*, and so forth, until her mother would bring it to an end, saying ". . . and Nana sleeps."[7]

When Kathy and Lindy, two of Nana's playmates, left town, Nana said frequently *Katylindy choochootrain*. Four weeks later she seemed to have forgotten the 2 little girls, but she still liked to croon with increasingly blurred articulation *kadylindy-choochoo, ka-ylinnychoochoo*.

The first appearance of such phrases was quite striking. At 15 months Nana never put 2 words together. If her mother said in the morning "Daddy has gone away in his car," Nana would repeat either *daddy* or *car* or *gone*; but though she understood and used all 3 words, she never put them together in one statement. At age 16 months the faculty of putting 2 words together emerged.

At the age of 16 months 14 days a type of speech known as "analogical extension" also began to appear in Nana's communications. Before that, she had often spoken 2 words pronounced as 1, such as *bighorsy*. Now she began to take the word *big* out of the compound and combine it with other words: *big hat, big bag*, and so on. Similarly, she now used the word *coming* in relation to a variety of people: *daddy coming, poseman coming, Foffa coming*.

COMMENTARY

Juxtaposition, Word Order, and Stress

Nana's early infantile phrases represent a succession of images. Like a string

---

7. Nana's wishful reiteration brings to mind similar serial phrases used by Debby, our previous case, at the age of 3 years 5 months: "Debby go to bed, streetcar go to bed."

of beads or a row of building blocks the words follow each other in simple juxta-position. The phrase *out out hat hat mitten mitten out out*, for instance, presents an uncentralized structure, showing the "lack of hierarchization" that Werner (1957) considers characteristic for the mental life of young children. The child does not yet discriminate between the essential and nonessential parts of a situation; the parts appear homogeneous. They are named, and the names are coupled together in the form of a mere juxtaposition.

Sapir held that in all known languages juxtaposition is the simplest, most economical method of binding words together and of bringing them into some relation to each other without attempting any inherent modification of these words. "The very process of juxtaposing concept to concept, symbol to symbol, forces some kind of relational feeling, if nothing else upon us" (Sapir, 1921, p. 117).

On first sight, phrases such as *out the window* and *Mummy gone backsoon* seem to present the same presyntactic appearance of mere juxtaposition. However, a changing around of the words as if they were identical beads on a string would no longer be possible. The position of the words had become relevant, and thus the principle of word order has been established. The form of the verbal sequence has become as meaningful as the separate words of which the sequence consists.

We must also remember that the examples mentioned here are nothing but visual transcriptions of spoken speech. The structuring principles of stress and spacing, change of pitch and change of volume, in short, the expressive audible aspects of these phrases, are not represented in our transcriptions. If we analyze these early phrases as samples of actual spoken words, we realize that, with the appearance of *word order* and *stress*, they have become examples of a very definite configuration or pattern. Sapir considered word order the most fundamental and most powerful of all relating methods and stress the most natural means at our disposal to indicate the major elements in a sequence.

Brown and Fraser and Miller and Ervin systematically analyzed the appearance and grammatical structure of early "multiword sentences," which they considered examples of "telegraphic speech." Miller and Ervin found that the grammar of these early phrases was not identical with the adult model and that the children selected "the stressed utterance segments, which usually carry the most informa-tion" (1964, p. 13). Brown and Fraser found that "child speech is a systematic reduction of adult speech largely accomplished by omitting function words that carry little information. . . . The crude sense of the sentence is generally recover-able from the child's reduction for the reason that one profound dimension of English grammar is perfectly preserved in telegraphese, and that dimension is word order" (1964, p. 79).

Commentary Speaking

More than half of Nana's use of language at that time took the form of an unending verbal accompaniment to her own activities and to events as they occurred around her. Listening to Nana's speech, her mother was reminded of the manner of speaking a radio commentator uses, giving a running commentary, a description of events while they actually occur. M. E. Smith, observing the "conversations" of young children, used the same term in her report: ". . . very little of the young children's talk is conversation. It rather approaches monologue, being a running commentary on the child's own actions . . ." (1926, p. 21). Unlike the radio commentator, however, children apparently do not speak to inform other people of something or to describe something to them. We might ask whether children speak in order to inform themselves of something.

Daddy coming, water boats ducks, black doggy jump, Helen swing, Nana comb hair— these and similar phrases accompanied and described events while Nana was experiencing them; they were reactions to immediate sensory-motor stimulation. We might say that these commentaries served the child in coping with reality; they were a kind of defense against being overwhelmed by sensory-motor stimuli.

The young child finds himself part of an ever changing world, in the midst of a multitude of passing objects, people, colors, sounds, feelings. Gradually, through the process of symbolic transformation, experiences which were strange, vague, and sometimes frightening, become identified, differentiated, and meaningful. The procedures of naming and verbalizing experiences and feelings help the child to establish his first points of reference, which serve in developing a rudimentary orientation in the surrounding world. The continuous process of identifying and structuring reality through the usage of words emerges as one of the foremost features in ego development.[8]

This "repetitive commentary speaking," as I call it, appears to be by far the most frequent and psychologically the most significant usage of language in early childhood. It begins with the act of naming and continues all through the early symbolic and early relational stages of language development up to the complex level of advanced relational speech, which most children do not reach before the age of 5 to 7 years. All-important as this language function seems during the years of most intensive language learning, it is the one most remote from conscious adult usage.

Piaget (1926), in his early studies of language and thought of older children, observed that this type of speech was still very much in evidence at the age of 5 to 7 years. He called it "egocentric" as opposed to "socialized" speech and interpreted it as a sign of children's lack of "verbal continence," a "remnant of baby prattle." Discussing its function, Piaget came to the conclusion that "the whole of this monologue has no further aim than to accompany the action as it takes place" (p. 15).

However, this very fact that children need to accompany their actions and

---

8. Susanne K. Langer (1962) also stresses "the *formulation* of experience by the process of symbolization" (p. 62, italics by the author). She writes, "The great step from animal to man was taken when the vocal organs moved to register the occurrence of an image" (p. 51).

experiences with speech demands an explanation. Vigotsky, in his criticism of Piaget, presented an interpretation that seems more in accordance with a dynamic understanding of child development. Vigotsky found that Piaget's "egocentric speech" does "not merely accompany the child's activity but serves the purpose of mental orientation, of conscious understanding, of overcoming difficulties and obstacles; it is speech for oneself which serves in the most intimate way the child's thinking." He also observed that egocentric speech in children increases "when in the course of an activity difficulties arise that demand consciousness and reflection" (1939, p. 39).

Like Piaget, we want to know "What are the needs which a child tends to satisfy when he talks?" (Piaget, 1926, p. 11.) The need for symbolic transformation of reality is a uniquely human characteristic (Langer, 1942). It is this specifically human need that drives the child to accompany his experiences with a running commentary of verbal symbols. The infinity of experiences must undergo simplification (Sapir, 1921) and conventionalization (Schachtel, 1959), first through the process of naming, then through procedures that will set these names into mutual relations to each other. This continuous process of symbolic transformation, expressed in the child's commentary speaking, is one of the most important ways in which the child copes with reality.

The symbolic transformation of bits of reality into language serves the child in more than one area. Not only can immediate events be identified and thus become meaningful and coherent, the same procedure can be repeated even after the actual stimulation has passed. With the help of words, sensations and their feeling tone can be remembered and recalled. The day after her excursion to the river, Nana was able to revive her joyful experiences and express her wish to be taken to the river again, by using the phrase *teecar boats ducks*. The same desire to recall a fascinating experience and to repeat it found expression in *out the window* and *sits books*.

Her wish to be taken out of her crib and the memory of words used by her mother were combined in the phrase *come on, Nana*. Nana wanted her mother to say these words, taking her out of the crib. Using her potty, Nana also used her mother's words *good girly all done good girly*. In both instances language had become an instrument for identification with the mother.[9]

Finally, in Nana's repeated use of the phrase *Mummy gone back soon*, language became a vehicle for the working through of difficult, painful, or anxiety-producing experiences, a mechanism well known to therapists.

Thus language, even at this early stage, already has a variety of functions: to structure reality selectively and thus protect the child against overwhelming sensory-motor stimulation; to express wishes and desires; to make people do

9. These early examples of identification with the mother through the usage of words remind one of Ives Hendrick's hypothesis that identification begins wherever the child experiences some kind of envy of the power of the ambivalently loved person and that early identification is connected with the experience of being frustrated by that person in power (Hendrick, 1951).

things for the child; to communicate with others; and finally, to help the child cope with anxiety-provoking experiences.[10]

OBSERVATIONS

Development from 20 Months to 26 Months

When Nana was 19 months old her mother would put her on the potty or the toilet seat at regular 2-hour intervals and Nana often stayed dry during the day. At 20 months, however, she began to resist toilet training strenuously, screaming *no no no no!* whenever she was put on the toilet. At the same time she developed a passion for independence in general: she wanted to change her seat at the table during mealtime; she did not want to hold anybody's hand while walking on the street; and she refused to do many things that she was asked to do.

During the next 5 months Nana's mother made rather unsuccessful attempts at toilet training. At times the mother became impatient and angry, and she occasionally even spanked Nana. When Nana had wet herself or torn a book or done something else which she was not supposed to do, she either denied it, saying *I am a good girl*, or she anticipated the blame, saying *naughty, naughty, a naughty girl, don't do it!*

During the summer months Nana's play centered around water and sand. She loved washing doll dishes and doll clothes, helping mother water flowers, having a shower from the hose, or sitting in a bucket, splashing water. Hours at the beach, with its water and sand and freedom from do's and don'ts, were sources of never ending happiness.

At home she played with blocks, dolls, and pull toys, and she continued to find delight in looking at pictures in books and magazines. She spent approximately an hour each day with some adult describing pictures, telling stories, or reciting poems to her. She also liked to sit alone in a chair looking at picture books, chatting along in endless monologues.

One of her favourite picture books was the story of a flying pig,[11] a pig with wings, which her mother or other adults had read frequently to her. At 24 months looking at the pictures by herself, she carried on the following monologue:

Oh piggy piggy that piggy—that man that man that's a man——piggy in the wood—oink oink—dark night, wings wet—gets the wings wet—papapapa [babbling] *bumps in the water—here fish—fish crying—here fish crying—oo-oo-ooo* [playful imitation of crying] *here out—here is a girl, a man—swings—wings—here is a cow—sun—no sun—laughing sun—Clementina bumps down in the water—oh crying, oh Mummy—crying* [playful imitation] *there is a cow and a horsy, no*

---

10. M. E. Smith (1926) has pointed to individual differences in children's early use of language. Some of the children she observed found a distinct pleasure in the repetitive use of sounds and words, and they indulged in commentary speaking; others, placid, quiet or timid babies, indulged in no such voice play at all. The lack of enjoyment of speech and language in individual children, its possible origin and consequences, will occupy our attention in later chapters of this book.

11. O. Lebeck, *Clementina, the flying pig* (New York: Grosset & Dunlap, 1939).

swings—oink oink—that's a bird, sing, sing a sing—one a penny two a penny hot cross buns—that's a piggy in the woods, yes, a piggy with swings.

Around the age of 2 years she liked to make up songs of her own. These little songs often contained a mixture of nonsense words, memory images, snatches of nursery songs, and verbalizations referring to immediate sense impressions. The following is an example, overheard when she was 26 months old.

> *Brushes and ducks and brushes and ducks*
> *bricksies and brucks and bricksies and brucks*
> *and going to the country fair*
> *and going to the country fair—*
> *and talk to wix and wax and bins bins bins*
> *and Mary buys the sour cream*
> *and Mary buys the sour cream*
> *and bye baby bunting*
> *daddy goes a-hunting*
> *mummy buys a skin*
> *to wrap the baby in.*

While most of Nana's commentary speaking and chanting were done in the presyntactic mode, she also spoke occasionally in grammatically ordered sentences, particularly in conversation with others. At 22 months, when her mother asked her: "Where has Charley gone?" Nana answered: *Across the street.* Watching ducks in a pond, she asked them: *Could you come and play Nana?* Soon afterward she asked other children: *Could you come and play with Nana?* At 22 months she surprised her mother one morning by asking: *May I have the broom when I get up?* At 24 months she began to use grammatical forms such as *I wash myself, I wash my hands, Mummy washes herself, Mummy washes her hands.*

The length of her sentences increased from 4 words used in succession at 20 months to 6 to 9 words at 22 months, up to 10 words at 24 months and up to 13 words at 26 months. Her articulation of speech sounds was very clear and precise, though she could not yet pronounce all consonantal clusters correctly. In summary, one would say that Nana's speech development up to the age of 26 months had been very satisfactory, even advanced.

CHAPTER FOUR

The Case of Nana: The Period of Stuttering, and After

In this chapter as in Chapter 3, a period of two years of Nana's life will be presented; this will be followed by a very brief summary of her development in later years. The raw data concerning this period—recordings and diary entries—were extensive. Choices had to be made and made again, in order not to overtax the reader's interest and in order to keep the chapter a reasonable length.

The reality of life and development is highly complex and continuous and can never be reproduced completely. Whether a case history is written in the first or the third person, the writer—as Gordon W. Allport (1942) demonstrated—makes his choices both consciously and unconsciously, in recording as well as in editing. Such choices are dictated partly by the writer's theoretical frame of reference and partly by his own psychological dynamics. The validity of this as of any other case history will have to be judged by the internal consistency of the report and by its predictive power in reference to similar cases.

Because of the extensive period of time covered, gaps in reporting could not be avoided. Most of this chapter will be given primarily to observations; related commentary and the discussion of theoretical issues will follow in Chapter 5.

OBSERVATIONS

Onset of Stuttering, Early Symptoms, and Improvement (26½ Months to 28 Months)

During the month of December 1944 Nana and her parents were looking forward to Christmas. There was much talk about Santa Claus, and Nana helped her mother make paper chains for the tree. On the evening of December 22 Nana's mother cleaned out a dusty closet; during the night blisters appeared on the mother's hands. On the twenty-third the blisters spread to other parts of her body, and finally her feet began to swell so that she was unable to walk. Overnight the condition improved somewhat, but on the twenty-fourth the family physician found that Nana's mother had a bad case of hives.

Though the mother felt very uncomfortable, she was able to make preparations for the Christmas celebration, which they held December twenty-fourth. Around six P.M. the family and some friends gathered around the Christmas tree. While Nana and the visitors were standing around the tree, one of the adults asked Nana: "Which one of your presents do you like best?" Nana tried to answer, but seemed unable to speak fluently. She repeated the initial syllable several times before she was able to say a few connected words. Overhearing Nana's difficulties, her mother walked over to her and, taking her hand, led her to her seat at the table.

During the following night the mother's illness became much worse, and she had to stay in bed for five days. Her feet and hands were badly swollen, and for one day her throat was swollen also and she had trouble swallowing. The father, Sophie, and an elderly woman took care of Nana and her mother. Nana came into her mother's room several times a day, but was not permitted to stay long. Quite obviously, she was confused about the whole situation. Again she had difficulty initiating words. Compulsive repetitions of initial syllables appeared in her speech and became more frequent during the week. The cleaning woman, hearing these repetitions, said to Nana: "Don't do that, Nana, or you will have a stammer." Another time, trying to keep Nana out of her mother's bedroom, the cleaning woman threatened Nana: "Come on, leave your mummy alone. If you are not a good girl, your mummy will have another baby!" Thus separation from her mother was interpreted to the child as a punishment, or threat of punishment, for her own presumably bad behaviour.

Soon Nana transferred some of her allegiance from her mother to her father, calling for Daddy rather than Mummy when she woke up. On the sixth day the mother felt well enough to come down into the living room. Nana became very excited when her mother lay down for a rest on the couch, and she said repeatedly: "Mummy isn't sick, no, Mummy isn't sick again, you get up, you get up, you get up!" When Sophie offered to take Nana for a walk, she refused to go, saying: "No, no, I don't want to go out. I want to stay with my mummy!"

Nana's toilet habits were quite irregular during those days, and she often wet and soiled herself. Peculiarities of behavior also appeared: When she was tired or embarrassed, she turned her hair around her fingers; at other times her fingers were deep in her mouth.

On December 31 a houseguest arrived for the weekend. Nana's speech became worse; at times she was hardly able to speak at all coherently, repeating each word in a sentence three or four times.

After the visitor had left, Nana's parents discussed her difficulties and agreed that Nana had been overwhelmed by a succession of crisis situations. The excitement on Christmas eve, the mother's illness, Nana's separation from her mother, the number of people who had come to the house—all this, apparently, had seriously disrupted Nana's routine and her close relationship with her mother. The parents agreed on some therapeutic measures: Nana should have a very simple daily routine, and as much outdoor play as the weather permitted; there would be no insistence on toilet training for the time being; the mother would be with Nana as much as possible, and during her absence only Nana's old and trusted friends, Sophie and Mrs. Stone, would take care of her. Nobody should make any remarks about Nana's speech in her presence. The cleaning woman was asked not to come back, and friends of the parents were asked to visit after Nana had gone to bed.

During the first half of January Nana's stuttering continued. It was most noticeable when she strongly desired something but was not sure whether her wish would be fulfilled. She kept saying: "I I I wa-wa-want" or "let's let's let's let's . . .," and only after several repetitions was she able to express her wish in a connected statement. Nana appeared to be highly frustrated by her own halting speech. Under the impact of tension her symptoms changed from initial repetitions, often called "clonus" (Froeschels, 1925, 1948), to the drawing out of vowel sounds ("tonus," in Froeschels), or to a combination of both.

Nana's mother, observing Nana's conspicuous difficulties and also Nana's irritation about her own speech, said to her: "Nana, don't get so angry with yourself! When you get very angry and impatient you can't talk any more." Nana seemed to understand and accept these suggestions. The tonic and tonoclonic symptoms disappeared, but the initial repetitions continued to occur frequently.

Nana's mother had always been gratified by her child's excellent language development and her friends had often admired Nana's speech. Now the mother felt very upset and worried about Nana's stuttering and resented it when her friends and neighbors—and even the Fuller brush salesman—embarked upon giving her advice about her child's difficulties. However, during these trying weeks there were many hours each day when no stuttering was observed. Nana was happy and relaxed and spoke well when she played with her blocks, dolls, toys, and crayons. Playing outdoors in the snow had a particularly beneficial effect upon her. There had been heavy snowfalls, and Nana spent hours digging in the snow, rolling in it, climbing up snowy hills and sliding down again, having a completely happy time.

In January the mother experienced painful symptoms of pyelitis and was treated with sulpha drugs. However, she was able to take care of Nana during most of the day.

In spite of Nana's intermittent speech difficulties her language development, and in particular her learning of grammar and syntax, showed further aspects of growth. Often she introduced her sentences with "I say," "I think" or "I believe." She said, for instance: "I say, Daddy is one of the good mans I know." Talking about herself, she used either "she" or "I." Seeing herself in the mirror wearing an old snowsuit, she said: "She looks like a boy," using the construction *like a* for the first time. She became interested in the problem of sizes, remarking: "I have little hands, mummy has big hands." Seeing a newborn baby, she said: "That is a very little baby, Nana is a big girl." When she invited her mother to sit in her own little chair, her mother explained that the chair was too small. Nana replied: "No, it's not too small; it's big enough."[1]

One morning her mother said to her, "Oh Nana, I just had a lovely dream!" Nana asked: "Can you give me the dream, Mummy?" Her mother explained: "I cannot give it to you, the dream is inside my head." Nana looked at her mother and said pensively: "Mummy has a dream in her face."

From Nana's speech one gained the impression that she was beginning to differentiate between herself and the objects around her. As she became able to use words more extensively, her parents also got an occasional glimpse of her *early infantile fears and fantasies.*

At the age of 24 months, before the onset of her stuttering, Nana had already expressed fantasies related to eating things up and being eaten up, a type of fantasy which Susan Isaacs found commonly occurring in children during the second and third years and which she interpreted as arising from anxieties connected with "oral wishes of intense greedy love and hate" (1952, p. 93). Nana's fantasies were first observed at the home of a friend who had a little black dog called Mimmy. Nana was attracted by the dog but also afraid of it, saying: "The dog will bite me." The adults told her that Mimmy was a friendly dog, who did not want to bite her. Nana then said: "Doggy wants to bite you, no, no, doggy wants to bite you, doggy won't bite you, no, no. Nana bite the doggy, no, Nana won't bite the doggy, Nana won't bite Mummy, no."

In spite of her fear Nana was fascinated by "the Mimmy dog," and soon afterward, when she received a cat, she insisted on calling her Mimmy. At 25 months she heard two cats fighting in the yard and said: "Mimmy is going to eat Ginger up, Mimmy and Ginger fight, Mimmy is very angry." Her mother explained to her that cats do not eat each other up, even if they are angry. Repeatedly, Nana said in a half aggressive, half playful manner: "I am going to eat Mummy up, I eat Daddy up, I eat you all up." Her mother told her that people do not eat each other up, Mummy would not eat Nana up and Nana would not eat Mummy.

Soon after the onset of her stuttering Nana was heard to say: "I eat Mummy up—no, I eat Daddy up—no, I eat myself up." Another time she said: "I am going to pull my leg apart, can I pull my leg apart?" Often she exhibited a mixture of tender and aggressive attitudes toward grown-ups. She tried to scratch or beat her mother in a half playful manner, saying: "I am going to hit you with my paws"— like the fighting cats. Once she tried to hit her father, and when he prevented her from hitting him, she first hit into the air, then hit herself in the face.

At such times Nana appeared to be overwhelmed by aggressive and destructive impulses. Trying to cope with them, she directed them at one moment against

---

1. According to Sigel, "the concept of relative sizes is a difficult one to learn even though form discriminations are possible early. . . . The child must be able to abstract the size and see its relativity" (1964, p. 232). Words referring to size appeared in Nana's speech at a very early age.

her parents, at the next moment against herself. During such playfully aggressive scenes, stuttering of a tonic nature was often observed. One gained the impression that Nana's struggling to either express or repress her destructive impulses interfered with her production of speech.

At that time Nana was particularly attracted by a book with pictures of a bluebird flying around in search of somebody to play with. The bird meets, among other animals, a big black bear. Nana insisted on having the book read to her many times. At the age of 26½ months Nana "read" the book to her mother in the following manner:

> I read the bear to you. Peter and Polly stood in the window and the birdy flew and sang the wish to him and—[here Nana turned a page]. He said he pecked the pink bunny in his ear and said, would you like to come and play, and the bunny jumped and said oh no, oh no—[turning a page] he said to the ducklings would you like to come and play, no no no, we want to swim [turning a page] and the black bear—wee wee wee!—the birdy did not know it was the black bear—wee wee wee wee!—the birdy did not know it was the black bear—no, no, I am much too big. So [turning a page] Peter and Polly are sitting under the apple tree, will you come to play [turning a page] she brings him water to drink—I will read it again.
> [Here Nana started to read the book again from the beginning.] Peter and Polly stood in the window, Polly had ribbons and the birdy sang the wish to him [here she turned several pages until she came to the picture of the bear]. Wee wee wee! He did not know it was the black bear, see the great big teeth—wee wee wee wee!"
> [Nana insisted on reading the book a third time. This time her narrative form of speech began to deteriorate, she used more and more repetitive speech, exclamations prevailed, and she ended up saying] "No no no no, see the big bear, see the black bear, no no no. . . . [At that point her mother took the book away from her.]

If we follow carefully Nana's reading of the story, we realize that she was at one and the same time frightened and attracted by the big black bear and his great big teeth. She also tried to reassure herself: "No, no, I am much too big!"

Nana's fear of devouring and being devoured continued for many months to come. The specific meaning of this fantasy and its role in her emotional development could not be fully understood at this early stage.

By the middle of January Nana's communicative speech had become normally fluent again, and no symptoms of stuttering were observed during the following two weeks. By the end of the month Nana's parents felt much relieved and thought that Nana's stuttering had been a passing episode.

Renewed Difficulties (28 Months to 32 Months)

During the next 5 months, unfortunately, a number of events and circumstances again disrupted the relationship between mother and child, causing a prolonged crisis. This in turn was reflected in renewed deterioration of Nana's speech.

The following factors contributed to this crisis. Nana's mother continued to have painful attacks of pyelitis and had to be hospitalized twice for short periods of time. In spite of her health problems the mother accepted two part-time positions. As Sophie and Mrs. Stone were available only in the afternoon, a number of baby sitters and cleaning women had to take care of Nana during the mornings. Thus Nana was exposed to a variety of caretakers, who differed in their understanding of Nana's needs and in their methods of managing the child. To make matters worse, Nana's mother—contrary to her earlier intentions—felt that Nana should be toilet trained and weaned from the bottle at that time.

Because of the pressures of her work and responsibilities Nana's mother often felt tired, tense, and anxious, becoming at the same time more irritable and punitive in her reactions to Nana's toilet behavior. One morning, when Nana was 27 months old, the mother, in picking up the child, found that Nana had had a bowel movement in her crib and had smeared feces all over her blanket and the wall. The mother was disgusted and scolded Nana angrily. Nana reacted by saying: "Nana is a bad girl, she must tell Mummy when she has a stinky." After having been washed and dressed, Nana played on the floor, saying, "She is a good girl again."

Two days later a similar incident occurred. This time the mother was so frustrated and "mad" that she not only scolded but also spanked Nana. After this Nana stuttered through most of the day, speaking with tonoclonic symptoms.

Such discordant situations made the mother feel worried and unhappy; she blamed herself for mismanaging her child, thus causing her to stutter. However, the more guilty and depressed the mother felt the more inconsistently she handled the child, wavering between "sweet reasonableness" and sudden outbursts of anger.

On the Sunday following the two incidents just described, Nana's mother felt well and relaxed and the family spent a pleasant, quiet day together. Nana and her mother took a long walk and later played together in the house. Nana was given her potty and was told: "Now, Nana goes all alone on the potty." Nana herself took off her overalls and used the potty, then let her dolls and teddybear also sit on it. Nana's speech was excellent all through the day.

As mentioned earlier, Nana, from the age of 20 months on, had begun to exhibit a strong desire for independence. Now at the age of 27 months she insisted on doing all kinds of things unaided, even if the intended activity was beyond her skill, such as sewing on buttons. If, for instance, her mother took something from a shelf to give it to Nana, Nana refused it, yelling "I do it, don't help me, I do it alone!" until her mother put the object back on the shelf—whereupon Nana would climb on a chair and take it down all by herself. She wanted to dress, feed, and wash herself. In the kitchen she exclaimed: "I bake the cake! I wash the dishes!"

Parallel to this craving for autonomy she exhibited a strong desire to be continuously with her mother, saying: "Mummy can dress me—Mummy goes out with me—I sit with Mummy—Mummy reads a book to me!" If her mother was reading a book by herself, Nana would try desperately to get her mother's attention, even to the point of throwing something down or tearing something up.

During the month of February her speech vacillated between complete fluency, repetitive stuttering, and occasional severe blocking of speech. The home situation, the fluctuations of Nana's stuttering, and the conditions under which stuttering occurred may best be appreciated in looking at excerpts from her mother's diary.

February 6: I had to give a lecture in the evening. Mary, a high school girl, stayed overnight in our house.

February 7: I had to be away from home nearly all day. Jacky, a college girl, spent the day with Nana. I also had to go out in the evening. Nana stayed with her father.

Feburary 8: We had a tremendous snowstorm. I had to teach in one of the suburbs, had great difficulty with transportation and came home an hour later than expected. Mary, who had taken care of Nana, was upset because she did not know when I would be back. During the night Nana woke up and called for me. When I went to her room I found her with a preoccupied look on her face; she twiddled her hair around her fingers and spoke with marked stuttering.

February 9: It was Saturday and I was home all day. Nana spent most of the day playing outdoors in the snow; later she played with her toys in the house. She was cheerful and happy and no stuttering was observed. Actually, I have never observed Nana stuttering during playing and commentary speaking.

February 17: Putting Nana to sleep at nap time, I said to her in German: "*Du musst eine Decke haben.*" She replied: "Don't call it *Decke haben*, call it blanket." Later I said to her: "*Komm die Stiege herunter*," and she answered: "It is not *Stiege herunter*! No, no!" I explained to her that there were many languages that one could learn to speak and I mentioned that Mummy and Daddy sometimes spoke German with each other. [From then on she occasionally repeated a German phrase, but she never spoke German spontaneously.]

February 18: Until now Nana has been drinking milk from a cup when she sees other people also drinking from a cup at the table. However, she still goes to sleep sucking milk from her bottle. Today I persuaded her to go to sleep without her bottle. At midnight she woke up screaming for it.

February 19: In the morning Nana seemed rather disturbed; she spoke with some stuttering and refused to take an afternoon nap. I had to go out and Mrs. Stone took care of Nana. When I returned at 6:00 P.M., I found Nana extremely upset; she was crying and spoke with severe (tonic) stuttering. I had to sit with her alone in a room, hold her in my arms, let her have her bottle, talk to her, and tell her stories. It was 8:00 P.M. when she finally calmed down and fell alseep.

In reading these diary entries we get an impression of inconsistency and confusion. The mother wavered between strictness—in her insistence upon toilet training and weaning Nana from the bottle—and leniency—in giving in to the child's impulsive demands. Because of this inconsistency Nana was confused about her mother's wishes. Nana's clinging to her mother and simultaneous aggressiveness against her reflected the child's uncertainty about the mother's absences and returns. One may also wonder why the task of training her child in impulse control was so difficult for the mother.

In early March the mother frequently had to cancel her professional appointments because of ill health and had to spend many hours at home lying down. As the streets were covered with heavy ice, Nana only rarely played outdoors. Mild stuttering was observed intermittently in Nana's speech.

Because of the mother's poor health and the lack of adequate play facilities for Nana, the parents decided to send Nana to nursery school. She was then 28 months old. She attended nursery school from March 12 to March 15. Her mother stayed with her at school during the first day. Nana seemed to like the school and, in particular, enjoyed using the slides during outdoor play.

On the fifteenth Nana's mother had to go to the hospital for a 48-hour period. While packing her suitcase, the mother talked to Nana about the hospital and explained that she would have to sleep there 2 nights but would be back home on the third day. While the mother was away, Nana's father, Mary, Sophie, and Mrs. Stone took turns taking care of Nana.

On March 15 Nana developed a cold which gradually became worse and which kept her out of school for 2 weeks. On March 17 Nana accompanied her father to the hospital to bring her mother home. Meeting her mother, Nana was serious and unsmiling. At home the mother had to go right to bed and remain in bed during Sunday. Nana spent much time in her mother's room, and the mother told her "all about the hospital." During the next 3 days Nana asked a dozen times: "Mummy, tell me all about the hospital," and insisted on having the "hospital story" repeated with every detail.

Nana's speech had been neither better nor worse during her mother's absence, but her cold became increasingly bad after her mother's return. On March 22 Nana had a slight fever and had to stay in bed for 2 days while her mother took care of her. Nana's behavior was particularly sweet and friendly during this period, and her speech was completely fluent.[2]

At 28 months Nana began to ask frequent "why" questions.[3] She also began to use the conjunction *because*. A few days after her mother had returned from the hospital, Nana reminded her mother: "You cannot carry me upstairs, because I am too heavy."

In general, no severe stuttering (blocking of speech) was observed in Nana's speech between February 20 and April 18, although some hesitancy, with compulsive repetition of initial sounds and syllables, occurred almost daily. Severe stuttering occurred again on the latter date, when Nana once again suffered an attack of diarrhea.

Because of her intestinal infection Nana's pediatrician had recommended that she not eat fat or butter. At breakfast time her mother told Nana that she could not have any butter because she had diarrhea. Nana seemed quite upset about this restriction, and on her way to nursery school with her mother she spoke with marked stuttering. The mother asked the teacher to observe Nana's speech during the morning. When the mother came back at noon to get Nana,

---

2. I cannot resist mentioning here that this same phenomenon was observed again and again during our later work with stuttering children and their mothers: Whenever a stuttering child was ill at home and was nursed by his mother, all stuttering symptoms disappeared, as a rule. At the time of Nana's stuttering I did not yet fully understand the significance of this coincidence.

3. We remember that Debby (Chapter 2) began using why questions at the age of 4 years. The appearance of why questions in children's language has been reported by C. and W. Stern at the age of 2 years 10 months, and by Scupin at 2 years 9 months (see Piaget, 1926).

the teacher reported that Nana's speech at school had been quite normal. On the way home Nana insisted that she have butter for lunch. In the meantime the mother had realized that for Nana, the food restriction did not have the meaning of a medical, dietary prescription; Nana experienced it rather as a punishment for soiling herself. In order not to upset her further, her mother put a small amount of butter on Nana's bread.[4]

The mother had to go to work after lunch, and Nana stayed home with Mrs. Stone. When the mother returned a few hours later, she found Nana in a state of terrible excitement, crying and stuttering badly. Nana had had another sudden attack of diarrhea and appeared overwhelmed by the experience. Her mother finally succeeded in calming her down, and Nana went to sleep. Later the physician examined her and found no particular illness, except the diarrhea.

Apparently, when Nana had experienced another liquid bowel movement, she had expected to be punished again and not given any butter to eat. Her behavior recalled her reactions 7 months earlier, when she did not get milk to drink because of diarrhea. We must assume that for Nana, as for all young children, deprivation of food meant deprivation of maternal love.

Nana's cold continued during the remainder of April, and all together she attended nursery school only 8 times during the month. On April 22 Nana cried and complained: "My little ear hurts me." Nana had developed *otitis media* but was treated successfully with sulpha drugs. She stayed in bed 3 days, and her mother stayed home and took care of her. Again, during these days when she had her mother's undivided attention, he speech was excellent.

On May 5 Nana developed an "accompanying movement," a type of symptom frequently observed in the behavior of older stutterers. She began to hold her hand before her mouth while stuttering. Mrs. Stone had taught her to hold her hand before her mouth when coughing as it was "not nice" to cough at other people. Nana might have felt that her stuttering, like her coughing, was something "not nice" coming out of her mouth whether she wanted it to or not; hence, by analogy, she covered her mouth in order not to "hurt" other people.

Her mother was quite alarmed by this new symptom. She told Nana not to worry if sometimes she had to repeat a word, and she explained that all children repeated words more often when they were tired or angry; Nana did not need to hold her hand before her mouth when this happened. Nana spoke well for about a week, then held her hand before her mouth again during a stuttering incident. Her mother repeated her earlier explanations, and the mannerism, or accompanying movement, disappeared for good.

During the last 2 weeks of May Nana was eager to have her bowel move-

---

4. Piaget analyzed the meaning of *why* and *because* as used by children at different stages of development. For a child of 3 these are still poorly differentiated expressions, having in reality several heterogeneous meanings. The earliest whys are more affective than intellectual in character, and "instead of being the signal of verbal curiosity, they rather bear witness to a disappointment produced by the absence of a desired object or the non-arrival of an expected event" (1926, p. 164).

ments on the toilet; her speech was fairly normal during these 2 weeks. One evening, Nana went to bed with cocoa in her milk bottle, a drink which she liked very much. Waking up during the night, she found cocoa all over her bed. Apparently she thought she had had another attack of diarrhea. Calling for her mother to clean her up, she cried and again spoke with marked stuttering symptoms.

Toward the end of May Nana's mother had a conference about her with a child psychiatrist. The psychiatrist suggested that a child of Nana's age should not attend nursery school, as the group situation was much too strenuous for so young a child. The psychiatrist also pointed out that Nana's frequent colds migh well be her reaction to stress and might indicate her desire to stay home with her mother.

Undoubtedly, nursery school was very tiring for Nana. After school she usually was too tired to eat and fell asleep at once. Unfortunately, the mother suffered more pain herself at that time, and sending Nana to school gave her a chance to lie down during the morning hours. Nursery school was therefore continued.

The mother had become very distressed about Nana's stuttering. She felt unsuccessful in her maternal role and guilty because of her frequent irritability. Beyond that, she was increasingly exhausted and depressed.

Early in June, the mother's condition was so poor that she had to be hospitalized again for several days. This time it was diagnosed that she had a serious kidney ailment and needed a complete rest of several months' duration. The father rented a cottage at the seashore, and on June 20 he installed Nana and her mother at the cottage for an 11-week vacation.

COMMENTARY

Before turning to this new and important phase in the life of Nana and her mother, let us look back over Nana's history up to this point. Several major themes or "core problems" can be discerned.

Separation

Nana's stuttering had first appeared in a setting of social communication—the Christmas party—which was too difficult to handle for a child of her age. Whether her compulsive repetitions observed at that time should be called "initial stuttering" is a moot question; similar difficulties in communication probably are experienced by many children during the phase of early grammatical speech. Nana's difficulty became acute and longer lasting under the impact of the unexpected separation from her mother, that occurred soon afterwards.

Because of acute illness Nana's mother had become inaccessible to the child, and Nana experienced a break in a previously well-established speech chain. This disruption occurred during a critical period in Nana's language development, when she was learning to extend her communications from mere naming to grammatical speech patterns. A few weeks later, when Nana's mother again was able to spend more time with her, their patterns of verbal interaction were reestablished at the previous rate of frequency and intensity, and Nana's verbal skills gradually improved again. However, during the following months, when the mother's professional obligations caused her to be absent frequently from home, the originally intense verbal interaction between mother and child was further disrupted, and Nana's fear of losing access to her mother was reinforced. Nana reacted to the irregularities in her life with a mixture of anger and anxiety, clinging to her mother, as if insisting on being close to her.

Need for Mastery

Nana, from an early age on, had shown the characteristics of a "congenitally active," energetic child. Twice during her early years circumstances had interfered with her learning of a new and complex skill: The first time, her illness had interfered with her practice in walking; the second time, her mother's illness had disrupted her practicing of verbal skills and had deprived her of the familiar and dependable pattern of corrective feedback. Interference in the practicing stage of vital activities had caused disturbances in the child's behavior and had also led to emotional conflict between mother and child.[5] One might say also that her mother's inconsistent attempts at toilet training interfered with rather than facilitated the child's learning of sphincter control; Nana reacted with anger and stubbornness against these interferences.

Giving and Withholding

Nana had experienced oral deprivation several times; first during the period of weaning, then during the attacks of diarrhea when milk or butter had been withheld from her. Unavoidable as these deprivations had been, Nana had reacted to them with strong signs of frustration and anxiety. One could speculate that in the course of her early experiences giving and withholding—of food, of feces, of words—had become vitally important activities for her. They were imbued with love as well as with hate and fused with fears of devouring and being devoured, destroying and being destroyed.

Reactions by the Mother

Nana's behavior, occurring within an interpersonal network, can be appreciated only if we also consider the mother's feelings and her reactions to her experiences with Nana. Prior to the birth of her child the mother's self-acceptance had been based upon professional achievement. Difficulties in bringing up her child threatened the mother's self-confidence in her new, maternal role. Further-

---

5. See E. Buxbaum (1947).

more, proficiency in speech and language had been highly valued in the mother's own family; intensive verbal communication between herself and her widowed father had served as a strong, affectionate bond between them. Unconsciously, the mother experienced successful communication with others as a sign of love, and a breakdown in communication between herself and her child aroused considerable anxiety in her. Besides, her ill health had lowered her resistance to stress and further threatened her ego ideal and her self-confidence.

OBSERVATIONS

Let us now see how the change in their life situation affected these core problems in the relationship between mother and child.

Summer at the Beach: Gradual Disappearance of Nana's Stuttering Symptoms (32 Months to 35 Months)

SETTING AND ROUTINES

The time spent at the beach proved to be an important period for both mother and child. The mother's physician had made it clear that she was to consider herself a convalescent, that every physical effort on her part would be dangerous, and that an operation might become necessary if she did not comply with the physician's orders. The mother, who had a strong need for autonomy and independence and who always had thought of herself as a healthy and active person, finally began to accept the fact that she was ill and had to adapt to the restrictions imposed by her condition. Away from the city she gradually began to relax and soon came to enjoy her leisurely existence, free of professional obligations.

The mother's style of life had become considerably simplified; her pace had slowed down, and her activities were synchronized with those of the child. A cleaning woman did the limited amount of housework necessary. Nana woke up early and played around the cottage until her mother was ready to get up. Except for mealtimes, most of the day was spent at the beach. During cold, stormy weather, Nana and her mother stayed home together or visited neighbors in their cottages. Nana slept in the same room with her mother, and at night they went to bed at the same time.

As the mother was not allowed to swim or take long walks, she spent many hours resting at the beach, watching Nana play in the company of other young children. Nana greatly enjoyed playing in the sand and mud and wading in the warm shallow water of the bay. At low tide the children could wade far out, watching crabs and sea stars, collecting shells, carrying sand and water in their pails, or building castles on the wide sandbars. All the children owned little toy boats, which they let float in the water and dug into and out of the sand, and over which they fought violently, at times. Rolling down the high dunes was another exciting form of amusement. Jumping down from the rim of a boat into the sand was accompanied by a ritual: The children folded their arms and yelled, "Ready, on the mark, set fire, go," then they jumped. Altogether, the summer at the beach gave Nana an unprecedented opportunity for motor and muscular as well as social development.

During the first month of vacation Nana stayed very close to her mother. She enjoyed playing with other children while her mother was with her, but did not want to visit any of the neighboring cottages alone. By the middle of August, however, she had become thoroughly acquainted with her playmates; she enjoyed taking messages to other houses and loved visiting children in the neighborhood all by herself. Finally, she became so independent that she often disappeared completely from her mother's sight, trailing along with other children, seeking adventures in the dunes or in the shallow waters of the bay.

SPEECH

Nana's speech improved steadily. The disappearance of her stuttering symptoms occurred in the reverse order of their appearance (*Rueckbildung*). Severe stuttering, or blocking of speech, disappeared almost immediately after arrival on the island, while mild stuttering, or repetition of initial syllables, still occurred frequently during the month of July. It occurred mostly when Nana was excited and overstimulated, particularly when many children talked and yelled simultaneously and Nana had hardly a chance to make herself heard in the general upheaval. A relapse into severe stuttering, which will be described later, occurred during the month of August.

WEANING FROM THE BOTTLE

As Nana usually was awake quite early in the morning, she took a long nap every afternoon. She still drank milk from her bottle when she woke up in the morning, then again at nap time, and before going to sleep at night. Nana realized that the older children she played with did not drink from a bottle, while the younger ones did. However, when her mother asked whether she would like to drink from a cup the way Billy and Donald did, she would answer: "No, I want my bottle!"

One afternoon in August, the milk from the bottle flooded Nana's face. She brought the bottle to her mother, complaining: "Oh Mummy, I can't drink from the bottle, the milk makes me wet." Her mother pointed out to her that she was now a big girl with strong teeth, and that her teeth had made holes in the nipple. Nana seemed to understand this explanation completely. She put the bottle away and—much to her mother's surprise—never touched it again.

For several weeks after this event she refused to drink milk. Visiting at a friend's house she said in a sad voice: "I had a bottle but I am too big for it." But by the end of the summer she began drinking milk from a cup. After she had given up her milk bottle, she also gave up her regular afternoon nap, and from that time on she slept after lunch only occasionally.

TOILET TRAINING AND THE DISCOVERY OF SEX DIFFERENCES

Soon after arriving on the island, Nana stopped wetting her bed; she had become able to sleep for 8 to 10 hours without going to the bathroom. Early in August she also began to control her bowel movements, postponing them until she reached a proper place. At the end of the summer Nana was fully toilet trained.

The summer at the beach gave Nana her first experience of living almost continuously with a number of young children. As it happened, Nana played more with boys than with girls. Two boys living in the immediate neighborhood were her daily playmates: Billy, an aggressive, disturbed child of $3\frac{1}{2}$ years and Donald, a vivacious and outgoing three-year-old.

It was during July that Nana first seemed to become aware of sex differences, among the children. One day her mother found her standing before the toilet, trying to urinate like a boy. Her mother explained that only boys urinated standing up and that girls sat down. Nana replied: "But I *want* to do it that way!" The mother pointed out that boys had a penis and therefore urinated in a different way from girls. Nana insisted: "I want to do it this way, *I* have a peeny, I can do it like Billy!" She climbed up on the toilet seat and tried to urinate in a squatting position. Her mother told her that Nana's daddy and mummy liked having a girl and loved her just the way she was. Nana insisted however: "It's *fun* to be a boy!"

The next morning Nana ran around the room, obviously in need of going to the toilet. When her mother urged her to go, Nana exclaimed: "I don't know how to do it!" She insisted on climbing up on the toilet seat again and urinated in a squatting position; then she called: "Oh, it did not work. I made the floor all wet!" For a few days she seemed quite upset and baffled about the differences between boys and girls. It was a new discovery for her, and she had to experiment and find out what it meant.

At that time Nana reacted to all stories she heard about other people by asserting that she had done the same thing they had done. When she heard that a neighbor had lived in China, she said repeatedly: "When *I* was a little girl, *I* lived in China." When one of the boys mentioned that he had had a splinter in his foot, Nana said: "I had a splinter in *my* foot yesterday." Other children in her group seemed to do the same thing. It looked as if the children had to try out all kinds of possible identities and circumstances, to find out what they meant to them.

At bedtime Nana wanted to hear long stories about "When Nana was a baby," or about "When Mummy was a child." When her mother talked to Nana about her own childhood, Nana insisted on saying: "I was in Austria too . . . I went into the mountains too," and so forth. Occasionally, she asked questions about being born, or she asked: "Will I be dead like the dead fish?" Apparently, like Alice in Wonderland, Nana had embarked upon a search to discover the extent and the limitations of her own self.

TALKING WITH PEERS AND WITH STRANGERS

We have seen examples of Nana's speech in her monologues, or commentary speaking, and in talking to familiar adults, in particular to her mother. Other aspects of her use of language during the third year of life could be observed in her communication with other young children and also with strangers.

With her 3- to 5-year old playmates Nana shared the incorrect use of grammatical forms—incorrect by adult standards—such as "you was; I didn't do nothing; I selled, sleeped, swimmed, losed, leaved and so forth. The children also cherished "big" words such as "antiaircraftgun" or "payanyattention"—which they loved to yell and chant in chorus, and the "dirty" words—"stinky," "wee-wee," "doody"—which they used and repeated endlessly, much to the annoyance of the adults.

When Nana spoke to herself, her peers, or her mother, the listener who was more or less familiar with the context of her utterances could understand their meaning. The peculiarities and limitations of her use of language, at that time, became more evident when she talked to a stranger. One day when Nana and her mother were having a meal at a restaurant, a stranger sitting at the next table watched Nana playing with her little toy boats and asked her: "What do you call those boats?" Nana replied: "My mummy had a melon party, Donald and I had his hair washed, Mrs. Digiorno made horns from the soap, Donald and I were good children, we got the boats, we had our hair washed."

Nana was trying to translate her memory of an experience into words. The events she referred to were the following: The night before, Mrs. Digiorno, Donald's mother, had come to the cottage of Nana's mother to wash Donald's and Nana's hair. In doing this, she had shaped the children's soapy hair into little horns, much to their amusement. Both mothers had told the children that they were good children, because they had been cooperative in having their hair washed. Nana's mother had given a party for them, and they had all eaten watermelons. Finally, Donald's mother had given each child a toy boat as a reward.

A stranger, not familiar with the context of Nana's statement, would have found it difficult to connect her answer with his question. In particular, the time sequence of the events was not reflected in Nana's description; the listener would have gotten the impression that the melon party, the horns, the hairwashing, and the boats were all parts of one global, nonstructured experience.

IMAGINARY COMPANIONS

During the frequent periods of bad weather Nana played inside for long periods of time. She used blocks, dolls, shells, and household objects for all kinds of make-believe play. She pretended to go shopping, or cook; she painted shells and used them as dishes; she built a boat, a pier, or a house. During the last week of July Nana began to talk about an imaginary little sister, called Esther. Her mother had mentioned to Nana that she wished she could bring a little orphaned girl over from Europe to live with them. Nana kept talking about the sister; "Esther must live with us, she hasn't got a mummy and a daddy; we must buy her a little sunsuit, just like Nana's, and a bathing suit, just like Nana's, and a red hat and she must have a suitcase."

A week later Nana stopped talking about the sister and instead began talking excitedly about a cricket. By the end of July Nana's speech had become quite fluent; but now her mother observed with concern that repetition of initial syllables occurred in Nana's speech when she talked about the cricket. Nana's mother could not quite understand what the cricket story was all about. It seemed that the cricket lived with Nana and that Nana fed her and talked to her. The mother began sharing the story with Nana; together they talked about the adventures of the cricket—adventures that resembled Nana's daily experiences, such as rolling down the dunes, walking out to the sandbars, or riding on the big red bus. The mother told Nana that the cricket was their friend. Nana loved hearing and telling stories about the cricket. After a few days of sharing her fantasies with her mother, the stuttering symptoms disappeared again.

TEMPORARY CRISES AND RELAPSES INTO STUTTERING

Nana and her mother spent the first 4 weeks of their vacation alone together; then Nana's father came to visit them for a weekend. The parents, eager to talk to each other, fell into speaking German together, even in Nana's presence. Nana reacted to this with frequent and marked symptoms of stuttering. Soon the parents realized that Nana felt excluded—and rightly so—and that her stuttering was a signal indicating the distress and bewilderment she felt. Once the parents had become aware of this, they decided not to speak German when Nana was around and to have their private conversations at night, when Nana was asleep. In addition, the father spent more time alone with Nana, taking her on walks, playing and talking with her. After the father had left, Nana's routine, as well as her speech, returned to normal.

Two weeks later the father joined mother and child for a vacation. Remembering Nana's stuttering during her father's first visit, the parents decided that Nana's routine and her intimacy with her mother should be as little disturbed as possible. However, in view of the very limited space and the lack of privacy in the cottage, this was easier planned than done.

During the first week of her father's vacation, Nana again spoke with frequent repetition of initial sounds and syllables. There were also other signs of anxiety: She wet her bed 3 times during that week, and once she soiled herself. She was restless and excited in the evening, did not want to go to sleep, and would under no condition be left alone with a baby sitter. Several times she woke up and walked around in the middle of the night. One evening after Nana had gone to sleep, the parents were sitting outside on the porch talking to neighbors when Nana suddenly appeared on the porch. She wanted to sit on her mother's lap, and she said: "Mummy, I'm afraid!" When her mother asked, "What are you afraid of?" Nana answered: "I don't know. I want to know what the seagulls do at night and what all the stars are doing." Perhaps she also wanted to know what her parents were doing at night.

During that difficult period the mother overheard Nana carrying on an excited monologue: ". . . sleep cricket, have a bed in the corner, behind Daddy's bed, I go shopping, I bring you creampuffs as a present." As the monologues continued it appeared that Nana really did not like the cricket in the house and wanted her to sleep under the grass, outside. During this monologue rapid repetitions of initial syllables (accelerated clonus) occurred in her speech. The mother felt that Nana's fantasies about the cricket had to do with her anxieties and confusions concerning a possible sister and also concerning her father, who interfered with her easy access to her mother, which she had enjoyed all summer.

During the remaining days of the father's vacation Nana and her parents spent long, relaxed hours together at some of the more remote and lonely beaches on the island. This gave Nana a chance to become reacquainted with her father, to build sand castles with him, and gradually to include him again in her world and her network of communications.

By the end of the summer a friend gave Nana a little squeaking green gadget, which Nana called "my cricket." She carried it around with her for a while; at the same time she stopped talking about the cricket.

Nana's father returned to the city at the end of the month, and Nana and her mother followed two weeks later. During the long weeks spent at the beach Nana had made great strides in impulse control and ego development. She had given up the early infantile gratification of drinking from the bottle; she had become toilet trained; and her motor and social skills had developed concomitantly. Her command of language had progressed further, and her stuttering symptoms had disappeared.

The Year After (35 Months to 47 Months)

GENERAL DEVELOPMENT

The following year was a period of consolidation for Nana and her family. The father advanced in his profession; the mother's health had returned, and she was able to work part time.

Nana's health was excellent, and she did well both at nursery school and at home. The nursery school teacher commented that Nana was advanced in her command of language and in her reasoning power. She also showed much skill and imagination in drawing and painting. Nana was now taken care of at home by Joan, an American student who took Sophie's place after Sophie's graduation from college. Nana got along well with Joan; Joan's mother was a nurse, and she often talked to Nana about her mother's work.

Of the many observations recorded by the mother during Nana's fourth year only a few will be presented to illustrate her development and also the manner in which she coped with age-specific problems.

SPEECH SAMPLE

The following is a sample of Nana's use of language at the age of 3 years 5 months. The notes were taken while Nana played with her friend Will, who was 2 months older than she. The children were sitting on a rug, playing with dolls, trains, and blocks. One of the dolls was dressed as a nurse.

N. Let's smash it down, all of it! (*She pushes all the blocks down.*)

W. I build mine up again. (*He begins to build.*)

N. We have a nurse, a nurse.

W. Put it on my train.

N. No, I need it on *my* train, my train is sick. You don't need it on your train, people are not sick on your train, and I have a bed. I need a nurse.

W. You knocked all these down, you did!

N. (rather glibly). But I am a good girl. I did not mean to.

W. I am making a new train. I am making a new train.

N. And I am making a new train too, a new train. (*She sings while playing.*) Doodoo deedee ham ham hum hum. . . .

W. See my train!

N. See *my* train!

W. (*chanting*). See *my* train, see *my* train! I want to have a crib.

N. No, I need the bed. I have sickness all the time, you can have the desk. (*Nana gives Will the desk; she continues playing, singing.*) Glo-yy, glo-yy. . . .

W. I put the desk in for the clothes.

N. Our train has medicine.

W. All the trains have medicine, many people . . . and my toys, and many things.

N. (*sings*). Medicine and medicine.

W. I need the bookcase, you are not using it!

N. No, no, I need it. (*They begin to fight, both pulling at the toy bookcase.*)

W. I *need* the bookcase!

N. But *it isn't* a bookcase, it is a thing to put clothes in!

W. (*finds a little bead doll*). Oh, I have this, it is a little woman.

N. No, it is a little boy, Peter, Peter, Peter Pumpkin, my son John, went to bed with his clothes on.

W. I put him in pajamas. Do you wear pajamas?

N. Yes, my mummy and daddy have pajamas.

W. (*playing with a train*). I got a tankcar, I got a tankcar. (*He continues chanting.*) I got a tankcar. . . .

N. I have a tankcar too, I have a tankcar too . . .

The children's speech showed similar characteristics: They both used short, simple phrases and sentences; both enjoyed repeating their own words and phrases and repeating also what the other child had said. Their verbal interaction was at times a form of reciprocal imitation, and at other times it resembled a conversation.

PSYCHOSEXUAL DEVELOPMENT: FANTASIES AND FEARS, PROBLEMS OF IDENTITY AND SEX ROLE, COPING WITH AGGRESSIVE FEELINGS

While no trace of Nana's stuttering symptoms had remained, her behavior indicated that some of her earlier core problems still existed. She continued to be very much concerned about her mother's presence or absence. Though she was fond of Joan, frequently she asked her mother in the evening: "You will stay in the house, won't you?" Nana had a habit of getting up very early in the morning, and often she tried to get into her parents' bedroom to make sure both parents were available.

She continued to show signs of anxiety about eating up and being eaten up. When Nana was 3 years 5 months old, her mother noted in her diary:

It is surprising how many books for children deal with animals that eat others up or threaten to do so. Today Nana came home with a new picture book and asked me to read it to her. It had to do with a little duck that did not stop quacking. The duck was sent away by her family. In the woods she met an owl, a cat, and a fox. The little duck asked the fox: "Can you help me stop quacking?" The fox answered: "Yes, I shall eat you up, then you will stop quacking." The little duck was scared and ran away. Nana also seemed scared. She said: "Read it again, but leave the fox out. We don't want to hear about him!" Nana and I agreed that this was a very nasty fox, and that he should not eat anybody up because he talked too much. Soon afterward, Nana threw the book behind her bed and did not want to see it again.

One day in April, when Nana was 3 years 7 months old, the mother found her at the dinner table in an unusual mood, looking preoccupied, and with a stern defiant expression. Repeated questions brought only evasive answers such as: "I don't know . . . there was nothing." Finally, she tried to tell what had happened to her at school the same day. "They . . . they . . . that did not let me . . . they shoot . . . they shoot at me . . . they said I could not be a soldier because I had no star . . . they shot at me with sticks."

Her repetitions of whole words and the pauses she made between her words and phrases did not sound like stuttering symptoms, and Nana quite obviously was not aware of these repetitions. Rather, one gained the impression that she had great difficulty expressing in words—or encoding—her memories of a complex and upsetting experience. She seemed to grasp for words when she said: "I did not have a gun . . . there were no more big sticks . . . I walked all around the house . . . they said Nana cannot be a soldier. . . ."

Nana appeared overwhelmed by emotion and grief. After the meal was over, mother and child spent another half hour sitting at the table talking about Nana's worries, and their conversation continued while the mother brought Nana to bed. Nana used such unusual expressions as: "That's why I am so unhappy!" or "That's what makes me so sad."

Gradually, the mother began to understand that there had been a big fight among the children at the nursery school, and some of the boys had "shot" at Nana with big sticks. Nana's father had a friend, recently returned from the war, who had given Nana a star from his uniform as a present. For weeks Nana had proudly worn this star to school. Now she seemed particularly upset that in spite of wearing a star, she had been told that she could not be a soldier. She had felt rejected, an outsider; she also seemed frightened at being shot at and killed.

Her mother tried to reassure her, telling her that sticks were only play guns and could not really kill people. She was discussing with Nana whether or not she should shoot back at the other children, when Nana suddenly decided: "Tomorrow I won't wear my star to school. I want to be a Red Cross nurse." Just before Nana fell asleep, a visitor arrived who gave her a pretty pink apron as a present. At first Nana seemed little interested in the apron, then she suddenly declared: "Pink is almost white. Tomorrow I wear my apron to school and play Red Cross nurse!" She insisted that her mother draw her a picture of a nurse, with an ambulance and a hospital in the background. Finally, she put the picture on her pillow and fell asleep.

During the week after this incident Nana was difficult to live with. She seemed upset and disturbed and was at times very aggressive. She continued to play nurse almost without interruption. Joan had to make a nurse's cap for Nana, and all her dolls had become "patients." The dolls had either lost a leg or arm or they had broken their necks, and Nana had to bandage them again and again, innumerable times. She called her mother head nurse, and Joan "the other nurse," and she talked continuously of being on duty, or off duty. Her play had a compulsive quality, and eventually her behavior became rather annoying for the adults. At night she did not want to put her pajamas on, insisting: "No, Mummy, no Mummy, no, no! I must have my dress on and my apron." She finally agreed to "go on night duty" with her apron over her pajamas, and only then was she willing to go to sleep.

Her mother discussed the situation with the teacher and found that the teacher had been present when the "shooting" occurred. The teacher, who was somewhat overpermissive, had considered the whole incident a game and had expected that Nana would laugh about it. Actually, the atmosphere in the nursery school had become so aggressive that several parents complained about it. The teacher finally agreed that one of the children, a severely disturbed boy, should not come back to school for the remainder of the school year.

On the following Sunday a family friend who was a physician came to visit. Nana got very excited and told her a long story about her "patients" and their illnesses and how she had to take care of them. The physician went upstairs to visit Nana's patients and presented Nana with an old stethoscope. She examined all the patients, and taught Nana how to use the stethoscope. Finally, the physician assured Nana that all her patients were in very good shape and could get up the next day.

The same night Nana woke up at 2:00 A.M., crying and calling for her mother. At first she said that her throat ached and she wanted a drink of water. Then she said: "Mummy, I cannot sleep if these little things go in and out of my room!" "What little things?" asked her mother. "Dreams," answered Nana. Her mother replied: "What do you dream about?" Nana explained: "Naughty sticks, fighting!" Her mother had to stay with her for a while and tell her a story before she went to sleep.

In the morning Nana came to her father's bed and told him: "Daddy, I had a bad dream last night. I dreamed of little elves fighting with sticks, and there were children, big children and little children. They had a lunch and they did not let me come." Her father explained to her that in her dream she had remembered some of the stick fighting that had happened at the nursery school.

That evening Nana forgot all about her patients; she left them all in a heap on the floor and did not play nurse any longer. She was now less afraid of her own aggression and of being attacked by others, and she no longer needed to be a good nurse to reassure herself of her own goodness.

During this whole episode, which lasted about a month, no stuttering had been observed.

COMMENTARY

During this episode Nana, apparently, had struggled against intense feelings of aggressiveness and anxiety. According to Sigmund Freud (1926) the earliest anxiety in children is caused by the child's missing someone who is loved and longed for and feeling in danger lest his needs should not be satisfied because that person—his mother or her substitute—is absent. Melanie Klein added her observations of the anxiety aroused in young children by their own destructive impulses. From her experiences as a child therapist she concluded that the child's earliest ego defenses are "directed against the anxiety aroused by aggressive impulses and phantasies" (1952, p. 274).

The aggressive atmosphere in Nana's nursery school, tolerated by a teacher who neglected to set limits to the children's destructive impulses, had aroused in Nana fear of her own wishes to attack others and fear of being mutilated herself and destroyed. These anxieties were reflected in her dreams and in her compulsive play with her dolls, who—in her fantasy—had become mutilated patients. Giving up her role as a soldier and embracing the role of a nurse was a form of atonement; it protected her against her destructive impulses and also against being shot and killed.

At that stage of her development Nana had found two ways of expressing her intense feelings without relapsing into stuttering: one, acting out her fantasies through play; the other, verbalizing her fears in her talks with her parents. At the age of 3½ she no longer experienced her parents as extensions of herself; they had become whole persons, and her relations to them had been stabilized. This *trust* in her parents enabled Nana to externalize her anxieties, expressing them in words and sharing them with her parents. As Melanie Klein stated: "Externalization of internal danger-situations is one of the ego's earliest methods of defense against anxiety and remains fundamental in development" (1952, p. 279).

FOLLOW-UP (4 YEARS TO 21 YEARS)

At no time during the following 17 years did Nana have any relapse into stuttering. She continued to be a "congenitally active type." She became very skillful and creative in drawing, painting, and designing, and she was an excellent student. As a child she was often stubborn and easily angry. In the first grade she was slow in beginning to read, but she became a good reader from the second grade on and eventually an ardent reader. She was not good in spelling, mostly because she did not like to pay attention to spelling rules.

In later years she proved to be very determined in doing what she had set out to do, working hard toward a goal once she had chosen it. In spite of a severe illness and hospitalization during her fourteenth year, she graduated from high school with high honors and later graduated from one of the leading Eastern colleges. Having become increasingly interested in writing and the use of language, she decided to make a career in journalism.

CHAPTER FIVE

The Case of Nana: Theoretical Issues

THE ROLE OF REPETITION IN LANGUAGE DEVELOPMENT

In order to discuss Nana's history we must, first of all, define our criteria of stuttering. We will ask the questions what kind of repetitive speech should be taken as symptomatic of stuttering and what kind occurs normally in a child's early language repertory.

Developmental Repetition

As we consider Nana's language development through the first 4 years, we become aware that repetitive speech occurred on all levels of language development. It differed in form and frequency with the age of the child and with the purpose of her verbal activities.

At each developmental stage the child tended to repeat a unit of speech characteristic of that particular level. At the presymbolic, or babbling, level she repeated sounds or strings of sounds: *nyam nyam hagliwo mana mana mana yooyoo*. . . . At the early symbolic level she engaged in almost unending repetition of words. As noted earlier, at the age of 18 months 14 days Nana said, while looking at a picture book: *Book book buts buts horsy horsy sits sits baby book horsy book what dat? What dat?* Beginning with the early relational level the child repeated phrases mostly. At the age of 26 months 14 days, Nana said, looking at a picture book: *All streetcars, all streetcars, all the horses, all the horses, lady sleeping, lady sleeping in the bed, I see the houses, see the houses.* . . .

Repetitions of characteristic developmental units should be considered as developmental repetitions. There are, of course, no sharp lines of demarcation between different linguistic phases, nor do the repetitions characteristic of earlier speech levels disappear completely with the appearance of more advanced forms of speech. As Heinz Werner said: "Development does not proceed from one definite and permanent level to the next; it rather oscillates around relatively stable levels of integration reached by an individual at a certain point in time."[1] Temporary regressions to earlier levels—as observed in play situations—must not necessarily be interpreted as signals of learning difficulty, provided the child is able to advance again without seeming effort to the more complex level. It is important to notice that all these varying forms of repetition are produced with ease, without any sign of stress, and with apparent pleasure and playfulness.

Compulsive Repetition

The onset of stuttering is characterized by the appearance of compulsive repetition of initial sounds and syllables, occurring at a stage of development when the child tries to express himself in connected speech (the early relational level). These compulsive repetitions must be differentiated clearly from the developmental repetitions. The linguistic units repeated under the influence of frustration or anxiety are no longer representative of the child's normal stage of language development; they are different in kind from developmental repetitions. Compulsive repetitions do not serve as building stones in the construction of larger syntactic units. The child is no longer able to shift freely back and forth between simpler and more advanced language patterns. An example of compulsive repetition is *I I I wa wa want to to to th th throw the c c c clay away*. The child appears to be aware of and irritated by these involuntary repetitions. He experiences them as ego alien.

If the disruption of speech continues, the symptoms become more complex and eventually the syndrome of stuttering as a full-fledged speech disorder emerges. As the child tries harder to express himself, he produces his compulsive repetitions with increasing muscular tension; this in turn leads to rapid repetitions in some instances, while in other instances the speech tempo will be slowed down. Finally, blocking or withholding of speech may occur as symptoms of a more advanced difficulty. Speech production may then sound like the following example: *IIIIIIIII . . . I I th th think it was my my my mmmmmmmmmmmmmmmmmm-other*.

Self Repeating and Other Repeating

In order to appreciate fully the role of repetition in language learning, we must take into account not only the different forms of repetition occurring at different developmental stages, but also the different modes of speech in which repetition occurs.

Nana at times repeated her own words and phrases and at other times repeated the words of others. The latter form of repetition is usually referred to as *imitation*.

---

1. Address before the Massachusetts Psychological Association, 1955.

In our records of Nana's language we found many instances of self-repetition. It occurred most frequently during monologues or commentary speaking, when the child was alone or thought she was alone. It also occurred at times in the presence of other children or even in the presence of adults. Such repetitions are characteristic of the mode of speech which Vigotsky (1939) called "speech for oneself." The child translated into words, or encoded, her immediate experiences, sense perceptions, feelings, or memories. In doing so she provided her own verbal input—she experienced internal feedback—and this in turn stimulated her to repeat further her own verbal utterances.

Repetition of others, or imitation, occurred whenever the child turned from talking for herself to talking with a speech partner, using *social* speech instead of *egocentric* speech.

Slobin (1964a) investigated the role imitation of the mother's speech plays in the child's acquisition of syntax. He found that the child imitates the mother's speech differently at different age levels. It should be added that the mother, taking her clues from the child, also imitates the child's speech differently at different times, thus providing various and changing types of corrective feedback for the child.

Slobin pointed out that mothers frequently expand the child's utterances, adding those grammatical elements left out in the young child's "telegraphic" mode of speech. For example, if the young child says "wheel come off," the mother may reply, "Yes, the wheel has come off again." Analyzing the data derived from the observation of two children, aged 18 months and 27 months, Slobin found that the mothers repeated the children's words 30 per cent of the time, and the children repeated the mothers' words only 10 per cent of the time. As the children became older, this mutual imitation decreased in frequency. From the age of 3 years on the children seemed less and less prone to imitate, and the verbal interaction between mother and child became more an actual conversation than a form of mutual imitation.

Slobin raised the question whether there might be a *critical age* at which children are especially prone to imitate the speech of significant adults. One might ask the complementary question, whether corrective feedback from significant adults might be of particular importance during certain critical stages of children's language development and whether the absence or the withdrawal of corrective feedback may have a differential effect upon children's language learning, depending upon the stage of development during which they occur?

Compulsive repetition of initial sounds and syllables occurred in Nana's social speech, yet hardly ever during commentary speaking; we must assume that the feedback expectancies differed in these two situations. When the child spoke for herself, she experienced internal feedback and did not expect feedback from her mother. Speaking for herself, she used short, simple utterances, often consisting of single words or of phrases; and often she repeated these utterances before proceeding to the next statement. The span of her verbal utterances was brief and in accordance with her verbal ability at any particular time. In contrast to this type of verbal behavior, speaking to an adult meant that she attempted to stretch the span of her utterances and to change from the simple telegraphic mode of speech to the more complex syntactic mode.

It appears that talking for oneself is a simple, repetitive, nonstrenuous activity, whereas talking to others demands a greater effort. Making this effort, the child expects to receive *external* or corrective feedback, to be provided by his adult speech partner. If the child's expectations are disappointed and the external feedback is not forthcoming, he may experience difficulties in formulating his statements. He then may repeat certain words or initial syllables while he continues to search for the appropriate word to follow in the sequence.

In summary, the child simultaneously develops two modes of speech: social speech, or speech-for-others, and egocentric speech, or speech-for-oneself. These two modes of speech differ considerably in their psychological significance as well as in their linguistic structure.

Vigotsky, as early as 1939, stated that egocentric speech—which I have called commentary speaking—is speech-for-oneself and serves the purpose of mental orientation. He suggested that the child's early egocentric speech gradually disappears from overt usage, changing to "inner" speech. According to Vigotsky, the structures of social and of egocentric speech differ more and more from each other as the child grows older. While social speech becomes increasingly complex, speech-for-oneself remains grammatically incomplete; it even has a regressive tendency. As Vigotsky put it: "Self-understanding is possible with a minimum of words" (1934, p. 42).

Repetition of words or of whole speech units (phrases) occurs frequently in children's egocentric speech (commentary speaking). It can be observed also in the speech of adults talking to themselves aloud and even in the social speech of people of low intelligence or a low level of education. It disappears more or less from the overt social speech of most adults, particularly those of some education.

Emotional Aspects of Compulsive Repetitions

Let us now look once more to Hendrick's assumptions (1942) concerning the occurrence of compulsive repetitions. Hendrick stated that compulsive repetitions occur either (1) during a period of learning new patterns of a more complex nature, prior to the attainment of efficient performance, or (2) when the exercise of a function is disturbed by external interferences, anxiety, or guilt.

It is well known that many young children go through a phase of frequent repetition of sounds and syllables at approximately the time when they are beginning to learn grammatical speech. This phenomenon has prompted Wendell Johnson (1955) and others to speak of a period of "physiological stuttering." It has led them to advise parents to "leave the child alone" as he would eventually "outgrow his non-fluencies."

Our interpretation differs from Johnson's. Hendrick's first assumption would explain the occurrence of such phases of increased repetition; we would expect the disappearance of these involuntary repetitions as the child masters the new and complex skills of grammatical speech. Normal as such temporary difficulties in language development may be, their outcome will be, however, quite different if the child experiences feelings of anxiety, anger, or guilt in connection with his involuntary repetitions.[2]

Incidental stuttering occurs frequently in many speakers, adults as well as children. Feelings of anxiety, anger, or guilt usually are not experienced during such incidents.

For example, in a recent lecture which I gave in German before a German audience, I attempted to describe mothers who push, oppress, or dominate their children. In German, I tried to formulate this in the following manner: "*Es gibt Muetter die das Kind bedr . . . bedr . . . bedr. . . .*" The three words possible in this context were: *bedraengen, bedruecken,* or *bedrohen.* Not having spoken German for some time, I was unable to decide quickly which of these three words would be most appropriate within the context of my lecture. All three words began with *bedr.* It is of interest that the compulsive repetitions occurred exactly at the point where a choice between these words had to be made.

Similarly, I recently overheard a radio speaker say: ". . . this would only cau-cau-confuse people, cause confusion among people." The similarity between the initial syllables of *cause* and *confuse* interfered with the speaker's encoding process, making a choice of words more difficult and causing involuntary repetitions.

The following example will serve to illustrate the possible emotional aspects of compulsive repetitions. A principal had a conference with the parents of a boy with school problems. For several months the teacher, the principal, and a counselor had given the child a great deal of assistance and his learning and behavior had improved considerably. The principal anticipated that the parents would express their appreciation for the help the child had received. Instead of this, the mother opened the interview with an attack against the teacher and against the school in general. When the principal reported the incident he stated: "My disappointment and my anger were so intense that I was unable to answer her immediately in a calm manner. Trying to control my feelings and uphold my professional role, I stuttered: 'Bu-bu-bu but I I don't understand what you mean!' "

In this particular instance the compulsive repetitions were caused by the fact that a very rapid change in the speaker's verbal planning was called for. The principal, who had been "set" for a friendly interview, experienced sudden and severe anger. His anger and irritation interfered with his ability to shift rapidly from one verbal schema to another.

---

2. Baker (1948, 1951, 1955) has demonstrated that a factor of repetition compulsion operates in all written and spoken language. Through the statistical analysis of large numbers of connected words, spoken by various speakers, he came to the conclusion that similarities in the initial sounds of words—vowels or consonants—induce the speaker to repeat a word immediately after its first use, or—if no direct repetition occurs—to choose a word very similar to one just used in the same utterance.

It appears that a variety of intrapersonal and interpersonal conditions may interfere with a speaker's encoding facility. The speaker who is set to speak does not always pause while he searches for words; his motor speech mechanism, once innervated, may continue to function in an involuntary manner while he struggles to find the appropriate words to be used in continuing his utterance (groping for speech). Conditions causing such interferences may range from fatigue, illness, or lack of familiarity with the topic, the language, or the audience to feelings of anger, rage, anxiety, or guilt.

Maclay and Osgood (1959) described four types of hesitation phenomena commonly occurring in spontaneous English speech. They differentiated between "unfilled," or silent, pauses in speech, and "filled" pauses and repetitions. Hesitation intervals in speech were most prolonged and the tendency for a filled pause or a repetition was most evident at points of high uncertainty, when the choices to be made were most complicated.

Goldman-Eisler (1958, 1961) further analyzed the psychological difference between filled and unfilled pauses and came to the conclusion that the 2 phenomena reflected differential internal processes. *Cognitive activity* was accompanied by an arrest of external action for periods proportionate to the difficulty of the cognitive task—the unfilled pause—whereas *emotional attitudes* were reflected in vocal activities of an instantaneous or explosive nature, producing filled pauses. Goldman-Eisler agreed with Maclay and Osgood that *ah* or *m* sounds, or repetition of initial syllables, were speakers' reactions to their own prolonged silences at points of difficult decision. She observed that the speech of her experimental subjects was most hesitant when a speaker's choice of words was highly individual and unexpected. These findings confirmed her earlier assumptions that "outgoing emotions such as jealousy, sex, aggression, and wishes formed an excitation inhibition syndrome measurable through the process of speech" (1958, p. 66). She further observed "considerable differences among individuals in the silence they can tolerate without breaking it with vocal activities" (1961, p. 24).

While Macley's and Osgood's findings, as well as those of Goldman-Eisler, were derived from the study of adult speech, their observations—with due regard for differences in level of maturation and learning—contribute to our understanding of speech difficulties in children. In the speech of an adult, whose encoding system is well established, such hesitation phenomena will not be the forerunners of prolonged or permanent speech difficulties. In contrast to this, a young child possesses only unstable and primitive verbal schemata and depends largely upon external feedback for proper verbal functioning in social situations. Conditions interfering with the child's customary feedback patterns are apt to cause overt, though temporary, disturbances in the child's verbal expression. If such disturbances become fused with feelings of anxiety, anger, or rage directed toward a significant adult (parent), the compulsive repetitions may become increasingly frequent and severe and may be the forerunners of more complex symptoms of disordered speech.

THE PSYCHODYNAMICS OF STUTTERING
IN EARLY CHILDHOOD

We are now in a position to formulate several hypotheses concerning stuttering in young children.

Stuttering is not a deficiency or disorder in the child's total language behavior. Rather, it is a difficulty in the child's attempt at communicating with a significant adult.

Corrective feedback from a significant adult is of particular importance during a learning period when the child changes from a simpler form of encoding, such as "naming," to a more complex form, such as the learning of grammatical patterns. This change will occur in individual children earlier or later and more or less rapidly, in accordance with the child's innate ability and with the parents' particular involvement in the child's language development.

During the learning of social speech patterns, the child develops specific expectancies concerning external feedback. If external feedback is disrupted frequently, or suddenly withdrawn, the child—unable to depend solely on his internal feedback—may react with frustration and confusion and may show signs of obvious difficulty in social speech. The more stable and intense the child's habitual feedback experiences with a significant adult (mother) have been, the more likely it is that withdrawal or loss of customary feedback—without provision of an acceptable substitute—will interfere with the child's speech performance.

If and when the child experiences the loss of expected feedback as a loss of parental love, he may react with a mixture of anger and anxiety to the disruption of parent-child communication. Such intense and contradictory feelings in a child will interfere further with his ability to communicate, leading to the excitation-inhibition syndrome, described by Goldman-Eisler. The overt manifestations of this disturbance will be hesitancy, difficulty in word finding and in the planning of verbal schemata, inability to function on a relatively advanced level of social communication, regression to earlier forms of infantile repetition, and pauses filled with compulsive repetition of initial sounds and syllables—in short, the syndrome commonly called "stuttering."

THE DYNAMICS OF NANA'S STUTTERING
AND ITS DISAPPEARANCE

Our analysis of the role of repetition, imitation, and feedback in language development has led to the formulation of some general hypotheses concerning the nature and dynamics of stuttering in early childhood. We will now attempt to identify the specific factors responsible for Nana's stuttering.

Going over Nana's early developmental history, we came across three periods of *crisis*: first, the weaning period, age 6 months to 6 months 21 days; second, the sleeping disturbance, which lasted from 13 months 12 days to 16 months 13 days; and third, the period of initial stuttering, lasting from $26\frac{1}{2}$ months to 28 months.

Lindemann (1944, 1956) and Caplan (1955, 1959, 1961) proposed the so-called crisis model of mental health and mental disorder, which will be helpful in the analysis of Nana's developmental disturbances. The crisis approach emphasizes the importance of periods of discontinuity and disequilibrium in human living. Crises are inevitable in human life; they may range from brief periods of upset to more extensive periods of seriously disturbed equilibrium. During crises occurring in early childhood, mother and child have to develop methods of coping with new and often difficult circumstances. Crucial changes in behavior and in relationships may take place during such periods, and novel methods of dealing with stress may be called for.

Crises may have a positive or negative outcome. Mother and child may emerge from a crisis with a new repertory of successful coping techniques; benefiting from this learning experience they will gain in ego strength during the process. In less fortunate instances the period of crisis may lead to a decrease in the mother's caretaking ability simultaneously with increasing disorganization in the child's functioning. As Caplan stated: "Crisis represents both a danger and an opportunity" (1961, p. 13).

All 3 crises in Nana's early history were characterized by temporary disarrangements in the communication network between mother and child, first on the preverbal, later on the verbal level. Each time "patterns of mutual regulation" (Erikson, 1950) had to be changed. The mother had to realize that her prevailing manner of feeding, handling, or training the child, had become inadequate and that a shift in their interaction pattern was called for. During each of these crises the mother experienced painful and incapacitating feelings of helplessness and guilt. However, as her anxieties were balanced by her inherent love for the child and by the child's inherent health, endowment, and growth tendencies, each of these crises had a positive outcome.

The onset of Nana's stuttering occurred at a time when her mother, because of acute illness, had become inaccessible to the child; Nana consequently experienced a break in a previously well-established speech chain. This disruption of communication coincided with a critical period in Nana's language development, the change from mere naming to the learning of grammatical speech patterns. Nana's anxiety concerning separation from her mother was expressed clearly in the statements she made when her mother was well again: "Mummy is not sick, you get up, you get up!" and: "I don't want to go out, I want to stay with mummy!" (p. 65).

When Nana's mother was again able to spend time with her child, their patterns of verbal communication were re-established at the previous rate of frequency and intensity. Nana received the accustomed feedback from her mother, and the disorganization in her verbal behavior gradually disappeared.[3]

---

3. In our clinial work several parents mentioned that one of their children had gone through a period of initial stuttering, occurring under circumstances not unlike those observed in Nana's case. According to the parents' reports, the symptoms had disappeared again without professional intervention as soon as the mother *spontaneously* intensified her verbal interaction with the child, taking care that communication was carried out on the child's developmental level.

The first limited crisis in Nana's language development was followed, unfortunately, by a more extensive disruption in mother-child interaction. This was accompanied by a more serious disorganization of Nana's speech, lasting for almost 8 months. Decisive factors in Nana's prolonged stuttering had been the mother's repeated inaccessability because of illness, fatigue, and overwork, and also her futile attempts at toilet training, which led to intense conflicts between mother and child. Beyond that, the child's expressions of anger and aggressiveness, together with her overt symptoms of stuttering, had activated latent anxiety in the mother, leading to increasing rigidity in her defenses.

In analyzing the child's difficulties, we must remember also that language learning and language disorders do not occur as isolated phenomena, but at all times are interrelated with and affected by other aspects of the child's development. Nana experienced her stuttering during the third year of life, when her thinking was still preconceptual and prelogical (Piaget 1951, 1954). For children at this stage of development "all kinds of events may be related one to the other . . . not on an . . . accurate cause-effect basis, but rather because of juxtapositions in time and space" (Sigel, 1964, p. 218). Nana's use of language was still halfway between communication with others and the egocentric monologue (Piaget, 1951). Words still represented primarily subjective internal images colored by individual symbolisms, rather than concepts which are general and communicable; objects still were connected with other objects in a prelogical, magical manner, through a kind of direct participation in fantasy; and her prelogical reasoning, influenced by desire, frequently lead to distortion of reality. Nana's early infantile thought processes were reflected in her infantile anxieties: fear of loss of the mother, fear of being left alone and empty, fear of being attacked and overwhelmed, fear of losing autonomy, fear of devouring and being devoured, fear of one's own anger, rage and destructive impulses.[4]

As Nana's mother became inaccessible to her, the threatened loss of her mother as a dependable speech partner increased Nana's infantile anxiety of losing her mother's love and care. In this context it seems of particular significance that Nana's speech was always perfectly fluent when she was ill and her mother took complete care of her—a phenomenon that we encountered later again and again in our clinical work with young stuttering children and their mothers.

Having examined the factors which interfered with Nana's speech performance, we will now turn to those which facilitated it and which had a therapeutic effect. The mere presence of the mother apparently did not always suffice to diminish Nana's anger, anxiety, and stuttering. If the mother was preoccupied or tense, her negative feelings acted as barriers between her and the child. The mother's presence was helpful to Nana only when the mother was in tune with the child, comfortable in her manner of communication with her and empathically sharing Nana's feelings and interests. The summer at the beach provided the ideal setting for renewed closeness, "mutuality of relaxation" (Erikson, 1950), and

---

4. See Erikson's discussion of "The Fear of Anxiety" (1950, Chapter 11).

harmonious intercourse between mother and child. As the mother was able to give the child her undivided attention, disciplinary conflicts were at a minimum, and Nana's speech improved steadily.

Nana's own aggressiveness as well as the manner in which Nana's mother reacted to it had a particular bearing upon Nana's stuttering.[5] Nana had severe difficulty speaking when she was angry at her mother and at the same time afraid of losing her mother's love. She stuttered when she expected her mother or other adults to be angry with her because of her "badness." She also stuttered when the mother, on her part, showed uncontrolled anger. Such situations, imbued with anger and aggressiveness, were the core situations triggering off Nana's stuttering. At a later stage of development her anxieties concerning her own speech had become generalized, and stuttering occurred also at other times when the core situation was no longer in evidence. Whenever Nana's mother succeeded in handling Nana's aggression calmly and without counteraggression, Nana's tensions were relieved and Nana's speech became normally fluent.

Of particular therapeutic importance was the sharing of stories between mother and child—for instance, the cricket story. These stories were not traditional children's tales told by the mother, however; the stories were initiated by Nana, they were Nana's fantasies spoken aloud. The mother listened to the fantasies without interfering. She not only took her cues from the child and matched her words with the child's themes, but also protected the child against the anxiety aroused by the fantasies. *To be helpful, it was not necessary for the mother always to understand the symbolic meaning of Nana's fantasies; sharing her stories with her mother meant to the child that the mother accepted her feelings.* In this manner the mother intuitively practiced a form of child therapy without interpretation of unconscious symbolism. This type of therapy will be elucidated further in Chapters 7 and 8. It has been used with great ingenuity by the Swiss educator and child therapist Hans Zulliger (1953, 1957, 1959).[6]

---

5. Isaacs (1937) described the intensity and fierceness of the young child's anger and rage, together with his intense anxieties of destroying others with his aggressions and of being destroyed by them.

6. A therapeutic technique which has some similarity to Zulliger's has been developed by Richard A. Gardner, who introduced *mutual story telling* in child psychotherapy (Gardner, 1968a and 1968b). The therapist induces the child to tell a story of his own invention. He then tells the child another story, using the same characters in a similar setting, but suggesting "healthier resolutions" of the conflicts that the child presented symbolically in his own story. Like Zulliger, Gardner does not interpret the child's unconscious fantasies directly. In responding to the child's story with one of his own, he accepts the child's feelings and points out possible alternative approaches to the child's problems. The technique can be used with a tape recorder, or it can be adapted for use with dolls or toys. If used wisely, this ingenius procedure should be helpful in therapeutic work with children approximately 6 to 12 years of age.

PART II

Developmental Speech and Language Disorders in Children

CHAPTER SIX

Group A: Stuttering Children

A Developmental Crisis Theory of Stuttering; Report on an Experimental Study[1]

In the case of Nana stuttering was interpreted as a developmental disorder, or a deviation in language development. It is important to differentiate between children who, like Nana, present the *primary* symptom of developmental stuttering, and those whose stuttering appears in combination with other disorders of speech and language (*secondary* stuttering). I suggest that the term *developmental stuttering* should be used if in the child's history we find normal, even advanced language development prior to the onset of stuttering. Stuttering can appear also as a secondary symptom in children with severely defective articulation or as a part-aspect within the complex syndrome of a multiple motor, perceptual, and language disorder.

In the research studies which will be described here and in Chapter 11 an attempt is made to clarify the essential difference between developmental, or primary, and secondary stuttering. Unfortunately, this differentiation has rarely been made in the voluminous literature on stuttering.

THEORETICAL ISSUES

Many theories concerning the nature and origin of stuttering have been proposed over the centuries, beginning with Hippocrates' idea that incongruence between thinking and speaking causes stuttering—a belief which is still surprisingly popular—and Aristotle's opinion that the cause of stuttering was a defective

---

1. Sections of this chapter are based on a doctoral dissertation submitted to the graduate faculty of Boston University, April 1958 (Wyatt, 1958a) and summarized in *Language and Speech* (Wyatt 1958b). I wish to express my appreciation to Professors Chester C. Bennett, Austin W. Berkeley, A. William Hire, and Albert T. Murphy for their assistance in the original investigation.

tongue. Cures prescribed for the disorder have varied likewise—from de l'Isère's Muthonome, an instrument for the regulation of the rhythm of the stutterer's speech, to surgery of the muscles of the tongue, propagated by Dieffenbach in Berlin in 1841, to the "psychic" treatment advertised by Madame Leigh in New York around the same time. A summary of earlier theories and forms of treatment can be found in Froeschels' *Lehrbuch der Sprachheilkunde* (1925).

Froeschels' description of the symptomatology of stuttering (1934) deserves attention. According to him, the initial form of stuttering is always repetitive. While repetitions seem to be rather effortless at the beginning, they are produced with increasing effort and tension until finally, at an advanced stage, intensive tension may lead to a complete disruption or blocking of speech production. Froeschels hypothesized that the child's awareness of his difficulty and his conscious attempts to overcome it were the cause of the developing vocal and articulatory hyperfunctions. He called the repetitive form clonus, the blocking, tonus, and the frequent mixture between the 2 forms, tonoclonus.

Froeschels further described how the tonic symptoms gradually become prevalent; grimaces and contractions of other muscles of the body appear, called accompanying movements (*Mitbewegungen*). In cases of several years' duration the late form of slow tonus may appear, together with embolophrasic sounds or syllables: utterances produced at the beginning or within a sentence which are not essentially connected with the words to be spoken. Some patients learn to substitute less conspicuous for more conspicuous symptoms. The avoidance of dangerous words may lead to a twisted or stilted sentence structure. Tic-like motions—such as tapping the floor with one's foot—may partly replace the more striking symptoms of articulation, thus leaving speech proper comparatively undisturbed, though often slow and halting. Froeschels called this advanced stage of stuttering "disguised stuttering" (*kaschiertes Stottern*).

Froeschels' terminology was derived from the medical vocabulary, in which the term clonus is used for a spasm with violent successive muscular contractions and relaxations and tonus indicates a continuous muscular contraction. The choice of these terms would seem to reveal an implicit assumption of a physiological disturbance as the basis of stuttering.

Currently prevailing theories can be classified into several groups.

Genogenic Theories

In genogenic theories the stutterer is considered to be biologically different from the nonstutterer. The most widely known among these has been the theory of "mixed cerebral dominance" proposed by Travis (1931) and Orton (1937), according to which stuttering is caused by a conflict between the two hemispheres of the brain. In later years Travis shifted from a neurological to a psychodynamic approach to stuttering, however (Travis, 1940). Cobb (1944) believed in a combination of lack of cerebral dominance and anxiety neurosis as the cause of most cases of stuttering (genogenic and psychogenic origin). Van Riper (1942) shared the belief in an underlying weakness of the central coordinating system, a condition which he calls dysphemia. Asperger (1956) discussed stuttering in children only in connection with organic brain damage.

Psychogenic Theories

Psychiatrists and psychoanalysts, focusing on the stutterer's personality rather than on his speech patterns, have classified the disturbance among the psychoneuroses (Schneider, 1922; Coriat, 1928; Blanton and Blanton, 1936; Fenichel, 1945); or among the borderline disorders (Glauber, 1953). The stutterer has been described as afraid of his own aggressive impulses; the prevalence of strong unconscious anal-sadistic and oral-aggressive attitudes has been stressed.

Fenichel (1945) included stuttering among the pregenital conversions. He mentioned the unconscious anal-sadistic significance which speech has acquired for the stutterer. Speaking, in many cases, means an aggressive act directed against the listener. In some cases of stuttering the function of speech itself represents an objectionable instinctual impulse. Fenichel pointed to the outstanding therapeutic difficulty inherent in the fact that speech, the very instrument of psychoanalytic therapy, is disturbed. He presumed that somatic compliance in the affected organs may be combined with psychogenic factors so as to bring about this pregenital conversion.

Glauber (1953) came to the conclusion that the pathology of stuttering was embedded in the parent-child relationship. He observed in his cases the presence of strong ambivalence, especially in the form of sadomasochism. Appelt (1929) applied the principles of Adlerian psychology to an interpretation of stuttering as a form of psychic infantilism, the complex expression of a compensatory system and of attempts towards security. Stein (1953) and Barbara (1954) discussed stuttering as a psychosomatic disturbance; Barbara tried to adapt Horney's principles of psychotherapy to its treatment.

Combining the neurological with the psychological approach, Despert (1946) used the cross-sectional method for a study of the psychodynamics of stuttering. Her research included neurological examinations and motor, psychometric, and Rorschach tests, as well as the study of play, drawing, dreams, and fantasies of 50 stuttering children. No specific hypotheses were formulated and no specific personality traits could be described as characteristic of the stutterer. Obsessive-compulsive trends were found in some cases. The most common finding was anxiety, which was found to be preceding and pervasive, not secondary to the speech difficulty.

Developmental Theories

In developmental theories the stutterer is considered not inherently different from the normal speaker. The change from normal to abnormal speech is seen as a gradual one, related to home situations in which early environmental pressures intensify a child's feelings of insecurity and anxiety.

Froeschels (1943) stressed the normalcy of the repetition of syllables in the speech of the young child; Johnson also emphasized the fact that the beginning speech in children is "normally nonfluent." The child repeats sounds, or parts of words, or whole words or phrases and "besides engages in various other types of hesitancy" (Johnson, 1948, p. 197). In his "semantogenic" theory Johnson insisted that the reason for the onset of stuttering was not within the child but "inside the parents' heads," in the parents' attitudes and reactions to the child's speech and in their labeling of his normal nonfluency as stuttering. While for Froeschels the source of the pathogenic development appears to be centered within the individual himself, Johnson's position, similar to that of Glauber's, may be called a parent-centered or environmental theory.

Busemann (1927, 1953), E. Wiesenhuetter (1955, 1958), and Flosdorf (1960) combined a devlopmental with a social-psychiatric approach in their interpretation of stuttering in children. Busemann believes that stuttering indicates an affective crisis (*Affektkrise*) and is rooted in the "period of stubbornness" (*Trotzperiode*) occurring in early childhood. He stresses that stuttering, an expression of a disorder in the speech function, is at the same time a sign of a disturbance in the child's relationship with his environment. Wiesenhuetter treats stuttering as a childhood neurosis having it's onset during a crisis of maturation (*Reifungskrise*), usually in the fourth year of life. The personality of the stuttering child becomes "arrested on the path to maturation." Flosdorf shares Wiesenhuetter's and Busemann's basic assumptions concerning the origin of stuttering. His extensive clinical work with older stuttering children will be discussed in the following chapter.

Other Recent Approaches

Wischner (1950) considered stuttering as a "learned anxiety reaction system" and interpreted the stuttering symptoms as originally accidental or consciously executed movements which through continual reinforcement ultimately become integrated into the total stuttering pattern.

An attempt to integrate the behavioristic and the psychodynamic frames of reference can be seen in Sheehan's "approach-avoidance conflict" theory of stuttering (Sheehan, 1953, 1954). In Sheehan's view stuttering is the result of opposed urges to speak and to hold back from speaking. The holding back may be due either to learned avoidances or to unconscious motives. Two principal hypotheses are presented: the conflict hypothesis and the fear-reduction hypothesis. According to the former, the stutterer blocks or stops whenever conflicting approach and avoidance tendencies reach an equilibrium. Conflict may occur at several levels: word, situation, emotional content, relationship, and ego-protective levels. The fear-reduction hypothesis maintains that the actual occurrence of stuttering reduces the fear that elicited it sufficiently to permit release of the blocked word, resolving the conflict momentarily and enabling the stutterer to continue. Treatment proceeds through an integration of psychotherapy and speech therapy.

Other approaches have been concerned with feedback. Lee (1951) suggested that stuttering might be related to a defect in the perceptual monitoring of speech processes. If the monitoring of ongoing speech involved a closed feedback loop, then any failure in the feedback would lead to a repetition of the signal—a particular word—until the appropriate information reached the monitoring system and the speaker could proceed. Cherry and Sayers (1956) and Yates (1963a and 1963b) applied the principles of delayed auditory feedback (DAF) to the analysis of stuttering in adults. Neely (1961), comparing the disturbances characteristic of stuttering with those produced by DAF, found great differences between them, however. He concluded that an adequate account of stuttering behavior could not be found in the auditory feedback mechanism.

Finally, Goldiamond (1964) treated stuttering and fluency as manipulable operant response classes and attempted to modify the symptoms of stuttering in adults through the use of operant techniques.

DISCUSSION OF THEORETICAL ISSUES

This review of currently prevailing theories discloses a wide variety of opinions concerning the nature and treatment of stuttering. In a number of theories it is assumed a priori that disturbances in the behavior of an individual must have their cause within the individual himself (intrapersonal theories); others stress environmental conditions impinging upon the individual (environmental or interpersonal theories). There is, however, very little detailed or precise knowledge as to the nature of those conditions which would be significantly related to the speech disorder under discussion. Such highly nonspecific factors as excitement, fear, hostility, tension, emotional stress, parental attitudes, and educational practices have been held responsible for the child's speech difficulty. Busemann (1927, 1953), E. Wiesenhuetter (1955, 1958), and Flosdorf (1960) are the only authors who consider the notion of critical periods in development and the crucial role timing plays in developmental disturbances.

The major weakness of most studies seems to lie in their lack of conceptual schemes for systematizing the data and bringing them to bear on crucial psychological problems. Without the prior assumption of a particular set of constructs that dictates the selective organization of experience, the number of possible variables to be studied is practically unlimited and research tends to become nonspecific and unwieldy.

Theorists who interpret stuttering as a deviation in child development neglect, as a rule, to apply principles of general validity in genetic psychology to its study. For example, in most of the theories the nature of continuous change, which is inherent in child development, has not been sufficiently acknowledged. Speech or stuttering in young children, in older children, and in adults has been treated essentially as the same kind of phenomenon. Similarly, attitudes or feelings of parents toward their stuttering children have often been interpreted as if they were permanent fixtures of the parents' personalities, not changing over time.

Genetic psychologists have pointed out that psychological categories change their nature and meaning in the course of development, thus becoming qualitatively different from one age to the next (Stone and Church, 1957). Werner (1957) demonstrated that each new and higher stage of development is fundamentally an innovation, not merely an addition of certain characteristics to those of the previous level. Piaget (1954) has shown that the child's perception of reality, including the perception of his parents, undergoes a radical change during the early years of life. Similarly, changes in parental attitudes toward one and the same child and, consequently, changes in the parents' perception of the child have been demonstrated in studies conducted at the Child Study Center, Yale University (Coleman, Kris, and Provence, 1953).

Piaget (1951) also analyzed the successive stages of sensory-motor learning dependent upon imitation of a model. Mutual imitation between mother and child can be observed during the early stages of language learning. In the advanced stages of imitative learning sensory-motor patterns become internalized, and the child no longer depends upon the presence of the original model; he has become capable of imitating internally a series of models in the form of images (see also Berlyne, 1957).

Piaget's observations agree with the studies by McGraw (1935), Hendrick (1942) and Buxbaum (1947) mentioned in Chapter 3 of this book. These authors observed three phases in the development of motor abilities: the reflex phase; the period of practice, during which the child gives evidence of a need to practice repetitively; and, finally, maturity of function. Interference with the learning of an activity during the practicing stage may lead to the appearance of compulsive repetitions (Hendrick); it also may be expressed in inhibition or in fixation in the practicing phase of functioning (Buxbaum).

Shands (1954), following the stages in the child's early use of symbols, hypothesized that more indirect contact with the love object becomes possible by means of signs and symbols. These permit the relationship to remain real to the child at a greater and greater distance from the love object.

Baker (1951, 1955), finally, considers "reciprocal identification" between speech partners as the core mechanism operating in all speech relationships. One-sided withdrawal of reciprocal identification when the partner is unprepared for it may have a traumatic effect upon the partner and leave him in a state of acute and intense frustration.

In summary, we conclude that previous research into the nature and origin of stuttering has been hampered by the application of scientific models of explanation which (a) do not fit the interpersonal nature of language processes and (b) do not account for the continuous change inherent in child development. Utilizing certain concepts and assumptions derived from genetic psychology, from the psychology of language, and from psychoanalytic ego-psychology, we have formulated a *developmental crisis* theory of stuttering.

THE DEVELOPMENTAL CRISIS THEORY OF STUTTERING

In this theory developmental stuttering is interpreted as a disturbance in the learning of speech and language. The "learning of stuttering" is embedded in the normal learning of speech patterns, from which it begins to deviate at a certain point. The theory is expressed in the form of six basic assumptions.

1. The acquisition of language by the child, though dependent upon maturation of the organism, is essentially a learning process. In this process the mother (or her substitute) serves as the primary model and provider of feedback for the child attempting to learn the language patterns which are specific for a given culture. Thus primary language learning occurs within an interpersonal matrix of mutual imitation, reciprocal feedback, and reciprocal identification between mother and child.

2. A continuous, uninterrupted, and affectionate relationship between mother and child, combined with frequent and appropriate verbal interaction between them, provides the optimum condition for successful language learning in early childhood.

3. Language learning goes through a series of interrelated stages. Each new and higher stage of development represents fundamentally an innovation, not merely an addition of certain characteristics to those of the previous level. In individual children and under specific circumstances, shifting from a less differentiated to a more differentiated level may produce a crisis in language learning.

4. Increasing mastery of the patterns of symbolic language permits the child to sustain the relationship with the mother at a greater and greater distance in place and time. Once the child has reached the stage of internalizing the basic linguistic patterns of the model, he can reproduce them also if the model has been absent for some time. Eventually, autonomy of the function will be reached when the child can dispense with the original model. He will then be increasingly able to modify the linguistic patterns at will, and he will turn to a variety of different models (people) for additional learning. The child's interpersonal network of communication changes gradually from a dualistic to a pluralistic one.

5. The child's relationship to the original model (mother or her substitute) is of particular importance during the practicing stage of a new function or activity or during a period when the child is learning new patterns of a more complex nature, prior to the attainment of efficient performance. A disturbance in the mother-child relationship occurring at such a critical period may lead to compulsive repetition of effort, to fixation in the stage of development at which the disturbance occurs, and to activation of the kind of hostility which the child's particular phase of development puts at his disposal.

6. A disturbance in the customary patterns of verbal interaction between mother and child occurring at the time when the child is in the practicing stage of early grammatical speech may make it difficult for the child to continue language learning successfully. It may lead to a regression to earlier forms of language behavior, expressed through the initial symptoms of stuttering. Unable to sustain

his identification with the mother at a distance, the child feels increasingly anxious and angry at his mother. These feelings of anxiety and anger may lead to a gradual change in his perception of the mother and to a further and more complex disturbance in his relationship to her. The eventual result may be depressive anxiety and subsequent defensive mechanisms, together with the symptoms of advanced stuttering.

THE EXPERIMENTAL STUDY

Method and Procedures

From the theory presented the following general hypothesis was deduced. Once stuttering in a child is established we expect to find demonstrable signs of a disturbed mother-child relationship. Further we expect that in a comparison between stuttering and nonstuttering children of the same sex, age, and intelligence we will find that the stuttering children differ from the nonstuttering children in the disabling experience of this disturbed relationship.

In order to test the validity of this hypothesis, a method was designed which would permit investigation of the feelings of stuttering children and at the same time permit a demonstration of the difference in the feelings of stuttering and of nonstuttering children.

The experimental group (E) consisted of 20 stuttering children between the ages of 5.6 and 9.6 years, with an I.Q. of 90 or above as determined by the Goodenough Draw-a-Man Test (1954). In each case the diagnosis of stuttering was made first by the individual referring the child to the experimenter, then by the experimenter. The control group (C) consisted of 20 nonstuttering children matched as to age, sex, and intelligence. In order to establish a homogeneous sample of stuttering children, care was taken not to include any child with additional known pathology, either of medical, psychological, or social origin, in the E group.

Children in the E group were referred from three Eastern public school systems, and from two speech clinics. The children in the C group came from Eastern public and private schools.

The E group consisted of 70 per cent boys and 30 per cent girls, and the C group of 75 per cent boys and 25 per cent girls. The hypothesis of homogeneity of groups with regard to age and I.Q. distribution was tested by Fisher's t test and found tenable.

Three dimensions of the feelings of stuttering children were investigated:

1. Distance anxiety. Intense need for physical and emotional closeness to the mother.

2. Devaluation of the mother. Intense feelings of anger directed against the mother and subsequent devaluation of her as a helpful and trustworthy person.

3. Fear of disaster. Intense feelings of helplessness and fear of impending disaster.

Three special hypotheses were formulated:

Hypothesis I. Stuttering children experience intense distance anxiety more frequently than nonstuttering children.

Hypothesis II. Stuttering children experience intense feelings of devaluation of the mother more frequently than nonstuttering children.

Hypothesis III. Children in the advanced stages of stuttering experience intense fears of disaster more frequently than nonstuttering children.

The interpretation of the third dimension called for a subsidiary hypothesis, IIIa: The experience of intense fear of disaster tends to be confined to children in the advanced rather than the initial stage of stuttering.

It was assumed that children would be only partly conscious of their feelings of anxiety and anger concerning their mothers and that these feelings could not be discussed with them directly. It was, however, assumed that through the use of projective tests the children's feelings could be elicited in the form of fantasies, the content of which would be apparent in the form of verbal responses to the test stimuli.

The Dependent Variables

The dependent variables chosen, distance anxiety (DA), devaluation of the mother (MD), and fear of disaster (FD), were defined as follows:

Distance anxiety (DA). The child shows the need for closeness to the mother, he is afraid of losing closeness with her or access to her, he is anxious because he feels he is not close enough to her.

Mother devaluated (MD). The mother is devaluated as a love object. The child is disappointed with his mother; he perceives her as frustrating, angry, aggressive, ugly. She departs from his ideal; she cannot be trusted. The child expresses angry feelings and hostile wishes toward her.

Fear of disaster (FD). The child has uncanny feelings about the world around him; he feels that he himself, or his home, is threatened by accidents or destruction; he fears the whole world will fall apart.

The Instrument

Preceding the experiment, a preparatory study was carried through. This was for the purpose of developing a suitable instrument to elicit specific fantasies that would permit valid inferences concerning the child's feelings for his mother. We decided against the complete administration of an already existing projective test, as this might have provided us with only a small segment of the kind of content in which we were interested. In order to obtain a sufficient sample of specific fantasies related to our predetermined set of variables, we had to find a set of stimuli that would be highly sensitive toward the differential variables in which we were interested and, thus, would channelize the child's fantasies in a specific direction.

A combination of projective tests was developed, called the Mother-Child Relationship Test (MCR Test). This consisted of 8 pictures taken from well-established projective tests—the Thematic Apperception Test (Murray, 1953) and the Children's Apperception Test (Bellak and Bellak, 1949)—and of a story completion test called Episodes. The latter consisted of 4 story stems (Numbers 2, 3, 4, and 5) taken from the Duess Fables (Duess, 1946) and 5 original story stems that were developed for the purpose of this study. A transcript of the MCR Test can be found in Appendix I.

In administering the MCR Test, it was found that the combination of a picture and a story completion test had specific advantages. Most children produced satisfactory responses to both types of test. Some children, however, in both the experimental and the control groups, had difficulty producing spontaneous verbal responses to pictures, but responded easily to the more structured interpersonal situation of the story completion test. Once the experimenter had initiated the story, these children were quite willing and able to carry on from there. On the other hand, a few of the stuttering children spoke fluently when they did not have to look at the experimenter and could associate directly to the pictures, but they had great difficulty coping with the interpersonal situation during the story completion test. In general, a combined type of test rather than either a picture or a story test alone seemed to be the best means of eliciting usable responses from stuttering children.

All children were tested at the respective school or clinic from which they had been referred; thus they were familiar with the surroundings in which the testing occurred. The administration of the MCR Test was preceded by that of the Goodenough Draw-a-Man Test (Goodenough, 1954). This permitted a quick appraisal of the subject's intelligence and was also found helpful in establishing rapport between child and experimenter. Children whose stuttering symptoms were so severe that they were unable to produce coherent responses had to be excluded from the experiment.

The children's responses to the MCR Test were written down verbatim. Later, the handwritten test records were typed, eliminating from the transcript all formal indications of stuttering, such as repetition of sounds or syllables or notation of extensive pauses. Each record was identified with the initials of the child tested. The records of the E and the C groups were combined and arranged in alphabetical order.

Scoring Procedure

A set of scoring rules was worked out for the scoring of the three dependent variables DA, MD, and FD.[2] Each response was scored on three degrees of intensity:

---

2. The scoring rules for the MCR Test can be found in Wyatt, 1958a.

Score O. No evidence of the variable was found in the response.

Score L (low). The variable was evident in a mild form, sometimes in the form of a playful or joking expression, with mild affective loading.

Score H (high). The variable was evident in an intensive or excessive form with high affective loading.

Six themes or scoring categories were identified for the variable DA; 14 for the variable MD; and 4 for the variable FD, a total of 24 scoring categories.

The test responses were scored first by the experimenter, then by two independent judges.[3] The raters were presented with the transcripts mentioned above, which did not permit the identification of stutterers on the basis of recorded speech symptoms. The number of 250 words for a single record was arbitrarily set as the minimum quantity necessary to permit a meaningful interpretation of test responses. Three stuttering and two nonstuttering children produced records with less than 250 words, which were not used in the final experiment.

The number of records was 40 and the number of scores was 1800. The raters reached complete agreement on 1634 scores, partial agreement on 154 scores, and no agreement on 12 scores. Allowing half credit for partial agreements, the raters reached a 95 per cent agreement.

Statistical Tests and Results

It was assumed that stuttering and nonstuttering children would not differ in experiencing mild feelings of distance anxiety and devaluation of the mother and mild fears of disaster. These would be expressed in test responses to the MCR Test calling for a score of L (low). It was expected, however, that stuttering and nonstuttering children would differ in experiencing such feelings in intense form, which would be expressed in test responses calling for a score of H (high). For the purpose of statistical testing of the hypotheses, the percentage of H scores within all scorable responses was computed for each variable and the raw scores derived from each variable transformed into proportional scores, representing the proportion $H/(H + L)$. These proportional scores were computed for each record as the basis for comparing the E and C groups.

This study was so designed that hypotheses I, II, and III called for a comparison between the E and C groups; the subsidiary hypothesis, IIIa, called for an intragroup comparison between the 2 subgroups of the E group.

Hypotheses I, III, and IIIa were tested by a 2 × 2 test of independence, yielding a χ^2 with 1 df (1 tail test). The Yates correction for continuity was applied for the calculation of χ^2 (Edwards, 1951). Hypothesis II was tested by the Kolmo-

---

3. Doris Gilbert, then at Harvard University, and Donald Klein, then at the Wellesley Human Relations Service, Incorporated, served as judges.

gorov-Smirnov Test for two samples (Goodman, 1949). The result of the statistical test of Hypothesis I was found to be significant at the .005 level of confidence; the result of Hypothesis II was significant at the .1 level only; the result of Hypothesis III did not quite meet the requirements for significance at the .05 level, while the result of Hypothesis IIIa was significant at the .05 level.

DISCUSSION

The value of this study cannot be determined by considering quantitative results alone. A qualitative analysis of the responses of both groups to the MCR Test is equally important, as it can help us to deepen and refine our clinical understanding of the stuttering child.

Hypothesis I

We hypothesized that stuttering children experience intense distance anxiety concerning their mothers more frequently than do nonstuttering children. The correctness of this hypothesis was borne out by the highly significant result of the statistical test of Hypothesis I. The crucial psychological difference between stuttering and nonstuttering children of the same age, sex, and intelligence lies in the experience of intense distance anxiety in stuttering children and in their intensified need for closeness with the mother.

Examples of the original responses to the MCR Test given by stuttering children will convey the specific quality and intensity of this kind of anxiety.[4] Among the responses which were scored high *DA*, the most striking ones were those which we summarized under the headings "Theme of the Endless Search for the Mother" and "Theme of the Lost Child." The Theme of the Endless Search has the quality of a nightmare; it conveys feelings of desperate anxiety and helplessness. Responses in which the child mentions that the mother is finally found contain expressions of intense relief. The Theme of the Lost Child likewise indicates the child's intense anxiety and his awareness of the great distance between himself and his mother and the obstacles in the way of getting close to her.

A girl of 5 years and 8 months said in response to Episode 6: "The mother died. Susy cried and cried and cried so hard." This was followed by her response to Episode 7: "Susy found that that was her real real mother and that other mother was not her mother. She was so glad!"

A boy of 5 years and 6 months answered to Episode 6: "Some bad man took the mother away and dumped her off a submarine. Tommy got his father and his brother and he went searching the whole ocean, but the mother had been caughted in a big whale."

The following story, told by a boy of 5 years and 10 months in response to

---

4. In conjunction with reading the responses, the reader should consult Appendix I.

Episode 6, conveys with particular clarity the nightmare-like quality of the Theme of the Endless Search.

The mother had gone some place and Tommy tried to go and find her in all the neighbors' houses and he could not find her and he keeped going in the neighbors' houses and then Tommy had to go down to the pond and every place; he has to make sure his mother had not gone there and fallen in—Well, so he had to dive in his bathing suit and put on a tube so he would not fall in and then so he dived in with the tube and so he had to go over the pond and then so he could not find her in the pond and he had trouble getting out of the water. And then so he could not take the tube off his waist so he would not fall in, so then he could swim and he took the tube off and he swam and then the pond was not very deep and he put his feet on the bottom; it was steep and he could not get up—He finally got up and then he went back to see if his mother was there and she was there and so he said "I thought you were not in the house"—And the mother said, "I was hiding in the closet."

Symbolic images used frequently by stuttering children were of the kind the door was locked, the house was locked, all houses are locked everywhere. In other instances the child sees his mother behind a closed window but cannot get at her, or the mother is moving away in a moving van and the child tries in vain to follow her. All these images convey strikingly the stuttering child's feeling that the mother is inaccessible and that he is helpless in the face of insurmountable obstacles.

Hypothesis II

We hypothesized that stuttering children experience intense feelings of devaluation of the mother more frequently than do nonstuttering children. This hypothesis was found tenable at the .1 level only. A qualitative analysis of the test responses will help us in our interpretation of these results.

Feelings of devaluation of the mother existed in both groups and were expressed in a variety of ways: She disappoints the child, departs from his ideal; she cannot be trusted or relied upon; she does not feed the child; she is aggressive, destructive, mean, or nasty; she does not cherish the child's gift; she damages or destroys the child's property. Hostile feelings against the mother also were expressed in both groups in the form of stories describing serious conflicts between mother and child.

The mother's hiding, the willful disappearance of the mother, was a frequent response given by subjects in the E group. The stuttering child seems to experience separation or distance from the mother—which may be caused by life circumstances beyond the mother's control—as an unfriendly, teasing, or hostile act on her part, to which he reacts with intense anger. The following excerpt from the record of an $8\frac{1}{2}$-year-old stuttering boy presents a good example of the way in which the stuttering child's anger at his mother is directly related to his distance anxiety.

Probably his mother went shopping with his sister or some people . . . so Tommy got very worried, it was getting very late and the door was locked to the house and finally, finally his mother came home. And I have something else, write it: And Tommy was very mad at his mother and scolded his mother, and that's all.

In comparing the test responses of the E and the C groups, we were impressed to see how gleefully nonstuttering children expressed all kinds of aggressive fantasies concerning their mothers, from scrambling eggs upon the mother's head to throwing stones through her windows. Projection of angry or hostile feelings upon the mother and seeing her as mean, coercive, or unfair person was also quite common among the responses of the nonstuttering children. However, these normal children in the C group did not at the same time express the intensive fear of losing access to the mother that was so strikingly evident in the E group. The stuttering child, then, seems to be locked in a perpetual difficulty: The original distance anxiety leads to increasing anger and hostility against the mother; and the aggressive feelings, while common to the whole age group, lead in the stutterer to fear of abandonment as retaliation by the mother, thus reinforcing and increasing the basic distance anxiety. It is *the combination of distance anxiety and anger* that makes the stuttering child different from the nonstutterer, rather than either his anxiety or his aggressive feelings seen in isolation. Because of the constant mutual reinforcement between his feelings of anxiety and anger, the stuttering child often also has particular difficulty in the management and control of his aggressive feelings.

Subsidiary Hypothesis IIIa

We hypothesized that the experience of intense fears of disaster would tend to be confined to children in the advanced rather than the initial stage of stuttering. This hypothesis was confirmed at the .05 level of significance. This result, together with the results of hypotheses I and II, contributes further to our understanding of the psychological status of children in the initial stage of stuttering. The combination of intense distance anxiety and anger directed against the mother appears characteristic for young children at the early stage of stuttering, whereas fear of disaster will rarely be encountered in these children.

Hypothesis III

Hypothesis III as well as the subsidiary hypothesis IIIa dealt with the emergence of fears of disaster in stuttering children. We hypothesized that children in the advanced stages of stuttering should experience intense fears of disaster more frequently than nonstuttering children. This hypothesis was found to be tenable at less than the .05 level of significance.

Inspection of the data revealed that our third variable, FD, differed qualitatively from our first and second ones, DA and MD. Fears of disaster were either experienced at a high degree of intensity or not at all. Thus we seem justified in concluding that with the appearance of intense feelings of disaster a crucial—and under certain circumstances perhaps morbid—change has occurred in the child's inner world. In view of the intensity and the apparently crucial role of these fears, a further psychological analysis of their nature seems indicated.

Responses scored high FD were mainly of 2 kinds. Responses in the first category expressed the child's feeling that the whole world seemed to change, to become threatening or to fall apart. These fantasies seemed permeated by a great deal of free-floating anxiety; the child felt threatened by a general but vague fear that could only be alluded to through symbolic expressions. Responses in this category read: Rocks fall on the house, the roof caves in, the floor of the house is rotten; the cave is locked up, nobody can get out; the water froze to ice, the boy was frozen to ice, the world is covered with water, with ice; a witch made everything disappear, made the world disappear.

In the responses belonging to the second category the child himself felt threatened with complete destruction. Responses read: The child dies from poison (in some cases the poison is given by the mother or by a witch-mother); he dies from an accident; he is taken to the hospital and dies; he falls down a cliff; he falls down into the toilet, is flushed away, goes down the drain. The child is being eaten; the whole family, including the child, are all eaten up or destroyed. In some instances the child has a nightmare-like experience—gets killed, or cannot move (feet stuck in the mud)—explicitly because he disobeyed his mother.

While the responses in the first category express a general devaluation of the world, the second category represents fears of retaliation or punishment meted out by the mother leading to destruction of the child's self. These feelings are not unlike those described by Melanie Klein in her theories concerning "the depressive position" (Klein, 1950; Zetzel, 1953).

According to Klein, the feelings of the infant from the very beginning of life are bound up with people or parts of people in his immediate environment. Of these people the most important is the mother, and close to her in importance, the father. As the child experiences them, his perceptions and memories are organized into concepts of enduring objects within him. These whole objects (mother) or part-objects (for example, the mother's breast) will appear good or bad to the infant depending on how far they satisfy his immediate needs or frustrate them. He wishes to incorporate the good object and attack the bad one. His wish to attack the "bad mother" is projected onto the object, leading to a fear that the object will attack him. In fits of rage the differentiation between good and bad may be abolished; the child's own inner world then becomes a very dangerous place in which the objects he loves and wishes to preserve can be destroyed. The interchange between reality and fantasy, between inside and outside, leads to the building up of a system of objects and to deep unconscious fantasies of love, hate, and persecution; it also causes depression.

Klein considers the existence of depressive tendencies as a normal phenomenon of infantile life. Disappointment in the parent at a later stage of childhood leads to a revival and reactivation of these early depressive tendencies. Klein also relates the pathogenic effect of such disappointment to the mental stage of the child at the time of the disappointment. The significance of the disappointment in the mother and the extent and depth of the later depression will depend on the child's own fantasies in which he will elaborate and distort the actual reality situation.

Disappointment in a significant love object as the cause for depression has also been stressed by Erikson and by E. Jacobson. Erikson (1950) sees a "failure in the child-mother relationship of mutuality" as a reason for depression in children. E. Jacobson (1946) defines disappointment in a love object as a state in which expectations of gratification from an object are not fulfilled. Such disappointment leads to disillusion, to devaluation of the parental object, and to withdrawal of libido. Jacobson also points out that experiences of disappointment in the mother are unavoidable in child development; the mother has to inflict early disappointments in the course of weaning and toilet training. Disillusion regarding the parents plays a significant and necessary though painful part in the child's adjustment to the realities of the external world. Whether this process of disillusionment has a constructive or destructive effect upon the child's ego depends on the severity of the disappointment and on the stage of development at which the disappointment occurs. Extreme deflation of the parental image occurring early in the child's life deeply affects the child's ego. As at an early age the imaginary magic power of the parent is the main source of support for the child's developing selfhood, devaluation of the object leads to fears of self-destruction. "Once the object is devaluated the child will react from then on to any disappointment with a narcissistic hurt. He will become sensitized . . . to failure in his ego functions and react to them as to disappointments coming from a love object, with a devaluation of the world" (Jacobson, 1946, p. 132).

Combining these interpretations of the nature of depressive feelings in children with the insights gained from our experimental study, we can now refine our original theory.

The stuttering child has experienced a disruption of the patterns of complementary verbal behavior, which are so vitally important for the learning of language. Not yet able to master social language without corrective feedback and unable to sustain his relationship to the mother over distance, he reacts to these experiences with anxiety, anger, and, eventually, with devaluation of the love object. In his overt behavior he alternates between excessive clinging to the mother, expressing his distance anxiety, and acts of aggression against her, expressing his frustration and anger. He has experienced ego failure, and he re-experiences it every time he tries to express himself in words. He experiences this ego failure as an ever renewed disappointment in his expectations of help and gratification from the mother, causing him intense feelings of helplessness.

Whether or not these combined experiences will lead eventually to a reactivation of the early infantile depressive position, to a devaluation of the world, and to fears of impending disaster, may depend on 2 interrelated factors. The first is *the child's degree of anxiety tolerance*—an aspect of his ego strength—which in turn depends on the severity of earlier disappointments in the mother, disappointments experienced during the prelinguistic stage of development. The second determining factor must be seen in *the mother's symptom tolerance*, in her reactions to the child's stuttering and to his alternately demanding or aggressive behavior. The interrelationship between these 2 factors, the child's anxiety tolerance and the mother's symptom tolerance, will determine the appearance or nonappearance of depressive anxiety and the choice of defensive mechanisms. The outcome will be different in each individual case.

In view of our findings we would expect a high degree of similarity in the psychological status of all children in the initial stage of stuttering, with distance anxiety as the outstanding and significant psychological mechanism. We would expect an increasing diversity in the psychological status of children in the advanced stages of stuttering, with feelings of depressive anxiety as a possible but not necessary aspect of the stuttering syndrome, and with subsequent diversity in the development of defensive mechanisms.

ILLUSTRATION OF THE PSYCHOLOGICAL ASPECTS OF STUTTERING

In concluding this discussion we present one more excerpt from the test responses of an older stuttering boy, age 8 years and 5 months. It contains illustrations of the psychological concomitants of all phases of stuttering considered in the theory.

TAT 5: Mother was looking for her little boy, but she couldn't find him. He was playing hide and seek—so she almost tore down the house looking for him. Soon she found him underneath a chair. It was her best chair too . . . he had made holes in it . . . mother got *very* mad . . .

Episode 1:
. . . [Tommy] had not picked up his room . . . she [his mother] got very very very very angry . . .

Episode 5:
I once had a dream about a witch coming on a broomstick and catching my best friend . . . and there was a whale . . . and I fell in the water—and it was full of dead fish.

Episode 6:
She [the mother] had gone shopping. He waited for her but she did not come home, so Tommy decided to go look for her and she—he went down and there was a big sale going on and she—and there was cars all over the road and Tommy walked through and then he saw his mother but she was in a store and the store was closed and she could not get out. So Tommy took a big rock and he threw it in the window and then he started kicking the window and then he decided that it was not a good idea, the owner of the store would be mad at him and so he stopped and tried to get in the door and he pulled and pulled and all of a sudden the handle came off and then he could not go in even if he wanted to—And he saw a window at the top of the store and he said, "I'm going to go in this window." And he kept climbing and climbing and soon he got through the top and he found out the window was locked and he could not get down and so he tried to break in the window and just when he broke it in he fell down, down, down and he just caught onto something just when he hit the cement—And he dropped off and landed on his feet and so he tried to climb it again and he got to the top and he walked in the window, but he found out that the door that led to the stairs was locked and he could not get down there— This was a storeroom and he saw a sledge hammer and banged it right in the

door and the door fell all the way downstairs and then he walked down the stairs; he took the sledge hammer and he saw another door and that one was locked too and he hit with a hammer but it would not break down—So he hit again and again and oh—it broke down but he saw an angry man looking at him when that door broke and the man said, "Why are you breaking down my store?" He said, "I was trying to get my mother!"—"Your mother is not in here!"—"She isn't?"—Then he walked down and looked where his mother was—but it was only a dummy that he had seen. And when Tommy got out he walked home and he saw his mother and she was very angry because she had heard that Tommy had broken down the man's store and he had a spanking that day and he could not go out and play.

Episode 7:
[She was] cleaning up her house.
[She said] "I don't have any food."
So Tommy said, "You must be a very poor lady."
The lady said, "I am"—So Tommy said, "I go home and get some food for you."
So he ran home, he got the food and he gave it to the lady and the lady was very happy that he did.

Again we find the theme of the endless search, with obstacles in the way of the child trying to find the mother. We observe his intense disappointment when he eventually finds her: "It was only a dummy!" We can also see how his anger against his mother is projected upon her: She herself is being perceived as being "very very angry." At the same time the child seems to sense that the mother on her part searches desperately for him, trying to re-establish the lost relationship with the child. The beginnings of depressive feelings can be found in the story of the "dead fish." Finally, we see already the emergence of defensive mechanisms: The child's anger is partly displaced from the mother upon the father, who is seen as an angry man who keeps the child away from his mother. In the last response the child makes restitution to his mother in the hope that this will undo the consequences of his anger and re-establish his original positive relationship with her.

SUMMARY

A theory has been presented concerning the origin and nature of stuttering in children. Stuttering has been considered to be a disturbance in the child's relationship with a significant adult, interfering with his primary language learning. The disorder has been analyzed within the interpersonal matrix of the mother-child relationship. Three operational hypotheses were derived from the theory, and the tenability of those hypotheses was investigated by means of an experimental study. The importance of distance anxiety combined with anger against the mother, as paramount psychological problems of the stuttering child, has been demonstrated. The emergence of depressive anxieties and fears of disaster in the advanced stages of stuttering has been considered.

This theory should have implications for further research as well as for therapy with stuttering children. Further research will be necessary to elucidate the problem of individual differences in the reactions of children at different age levels to temporary separation from the mother or to losing access to her. Research is also needed to determine the safety limit, or the period of time during which children at different stages of development can be exposed to loss of customary feedback without experiencing disruption of language development. The ways in which children and mothers cope successfully with temporary separation and distance from each other should also be studied.

The extent and frequency of depressive anxiety in older children in the advanced stages of stuttering should be investigated, together with their choice of defensive mechanisms. For therapeutic purposes it would be important to know, in particular, whether or not the mother's defense mechanisms concerning her involvement in the child's stuttering—such as denial of his disturbance or the wish to make him repress his hostility—influence the child's choice of defensive mechanisms and thus the development of the stuttering syndrome.

Three propositions of importance for therapy can be deduced from this study:

1. The mother of the stuttering child must be included in the therapeutic process.

2. Therapy with a stuttering child should be initiated as soon as possible after the appearance of compulsory repetitions.

3. Therapeutic techniques have to be specific and must be different for children of different ages and in different stages of stuttering.

Therapeutic methods based upon these principles were developed and tested between 1958 and 1964. These methods and their results will be described in the following chapters.

CHAPTER SEVEN

Therapy with Stuttering Children and Their Parents

THERAPY STUDIES

The Pilot Study

A one-year pilot study, *Patterns of therapy with stuttering children and their mothers*, was carried out at the Wellesley Public Schools from 1958 to 1959.[1] Under this project 20 stuttering children, 16 boys and 4 girls, and their mothers received therapy. All children were of normal to superior intelligence. Their ages ranged from 2 years 9 months to 15 years 6 months.

It was the purpose of this study to experiment with several patterns of therapy considered appropriate for the treatment of stuttering children and their mothers and to evaluate the treatment results. An attempt was made to develop successful patterns of treatment which would also prove to be economical in terms of therapeutic investment.

The assumption underlying this study was that developmental stuttering in young children represents a disorder in language learning, coincident with a disruption of the relationship between mother and child. In older children, with a long history of stuttering, however, rigid defenses have been established, and stuttering has turned into a personality disorder, on the one hand, and into a disturbance in interpersonal relations, on the other. In view of this dual conception of stuttering, it seemed mandatory to develop different forms of treatment for children at different age levels.

Three specific treatment patterns were developed for children of different ages. Therapy with *preschool children* was focused upon the mother. In the

---

1. The study was partly supported by the U.S. Department of Health, Education, and Welfare, National Institute of Mental Health, Small Grant M-2667-A. For reports about this study see Wyatt, 1959, and Wyatt and Herzan, 1962.

presence of mother and child the therapist demonstrated games of "word matching" and "mutual imitation," derived from observing effective interaction between mothers and young children and between preschool teachers and children. The mother was encouraged to spend more time each day alone with the stuttering child in an affectionate setting of bodily closeness. Mother and child were to talk with each other in simple short sentences, in an atmosphere where each one had the other's full and undivided attention. In sessions with the mothers alone their feelings of helplessness and frustration regarding their children's stutterings were explored and they were helped to understand and to manage the children's fearful, clinging, or aggressive behavior.

In the case of a *school-age child* the therapist saw mother and child separately in weekly sessions. The work with the mothers was similar to that described above, with less emphasis upon word-matching techniques. In sessions with the child the therapist encouraged the child to verbalize his feelings of anger and anxiety, and through the medium of a meaningful relationship with the therapist, helped him to cope with these feelings.

Therapy with *older children and adolescents* resembled more traditional psycho-therapy. "Divided management" was used. Children were seen once a week by the therapist. Mothers were seen once or twice a month by a parent counselor, who coordinated her work with that of the child's therapist.

In this pilot study, I was in charge of all diagnostic and therapeutic procedures. I also counseled all mothers with the exception of the mothers of the 2 oldest children, who were seen by the assistant school psychologist and by a social worker. Helen M. Herzan was the psychiatric consultant.

At the beginning of the pilot project we had hypothesized that younger children (under 7 years of age) should show marked improvement or return to normal speech after a smaller number of therapeutic sessions than older children. This hypothesis was confirmed. Ten out of 12 children under 7 years of age, but only 5 out of 8 children over 7 years, showed marked improvement or return to normal speech within treatment periods ranging from 4 to 12 months. The number of therapeutic encounters for the improved cases ranged from 4 to 14 in the younger group and from 10 to 33 in the older group, a difference which was significant at the .01 level.

The results of this study supported our hypothesis that developmental stuttering is a preventable disorder of psychosocial origin. The years between $2\frac{1}{2}$ and $4\frac{1}{2}$ in a child's life emerged as the critical period for the onset of the disorder. These findings seemed to agree with Penfield and Roberts' (1959) concept of the "biological time-table for language learning"; the authors assume that the most intensive language learning occurs between 2 and 4 years of age.

The Research Study

Following the pilot study, a more extensive research study, entitled Treatment of Children with Nonorganic Language Disorders, was carried out at the

Wellesley Public Schools.[2] In this project, which lasted from 1961 to 1964, the research in therapy with stuttering children and their parents was continued with a larger number of cases, more therapists, and improved techniques for diagnostic assessment and treatment. Information gained from the pilot and research studies was pooled and will be presented in the following pages.

In addition to stuttering children, 2 other groups of children with developmental language disorders were also studied in this project: children with severely defective articulation in the absence of hearing loss and children with motor-perceptual and language disorders. Our experiences with these two groups will be reported in Chapters 11, 12, and 13.

The Setting

The setting was the town of Wellesley. In 1960 the town had 26,000 inhabitants, and in November 1963, 3,430 children were enrolled in the elementary schools. While the median income of the residents was higher than that of other towns in Massachusetts, the socioeconomic range was sufficiently wide to permit the study of children from the lower and upper as well as from the middle classes. Parental education ranged from less than a high school diploma to more than a college degree. A large number of general practitioners and medical specialists practice in the town, and many of them referred cases to our project. Six social and health agencies are represented in the town, among them the Wellesley Human Relations Service, Incorporated, which originally was established as a pioneering project in community mental health. Several staff members of that agency, who served as mental health consultants in the Wellesley Public Schools, cooperated with our project.

The Wellesley public schools system has been rated among the better school systems in Massachusetts. Administrative policies are enlightened and progressive, teachers are well trained, and classrooms are not overcrowded. Our research aims and techniques were discussed repeatedly with administrators and school personnel, and we obtained full administrative sanction.

We were also permitted to use the school facilities. Although preschool children and their mothers were seen first at home, most of the testing and therapeutic activities involving children and mothers were carried out in the elementary school buildings. Children from kindergarten to grade 6 were seen during school hours in their own school buildings. Preschool and junior high school children were seen after school hours.

Staff and Staff Training

Four therapists and 2 parent counselors participated in the project at various times. (The names of the participants are given in the Preface.) Two of them had

2. The study was partly supported by the U.S. Department of Health, Education, and Welfare, National Institute of Mental Health, Research Grant MH-4643. For reports about this study see Wyatt and collaborators, 1962, and Wyatt, 1963, 1964, and 1965.

advanced degrees in counseling psychology, 2 in speech and hearing therapy; 1 was a former teacher and 1 an experienced social worker. Therapists with different backgrounds were used, because we were searching for new approaches to the treatment of children with developmental language disorders and we did not think that any single profession had a monopoly on the best possible methods for work in this field. Rather, it appeared that all our therapists and counselors, regardless of background, needed training in the type of therapy proposed.

Staff training was carried out in various ways. All therapists and counselors attended weekly supervisory group sessions, conducted by Helen M. Herzan, the consultant in psychiatry. The chief investigator also had regular conferences with Dr. Herzan. All therapists and counselors met weekly with the chief investigator for administrative conferences. In addition, all staff members met frequently with consultants and guest speakers to discuss research techniques and problems of methodology.[3] Frequent conferences were held also with teachers and school administrators. Therapists and counselors working with stuttering children and their parents reported about each session with a child or parent in a written summary. Staff training in process recording was carried out for several months to provide uniformity in the data for later analysis and evaluation.

Sample and Diagnostic Procedures

Between January 1961 and January 1964, 262 elementary school children (kindergarten to grade 6) were referred by their teachers to the regular school speech therapy service and were given routine speech examinations. Group hearing tests were given routinely by the school nurse to all children in the second, fourth, and sixth grades. If a child's behavior and verbal responses indicated the need for an individual hearing test, the child's family was informed and the test was given by an audiologist or otologist, at the parents' expense.

From this pool of school referrals children who presented symptoms of stuttering or severely defective articulation were selected for research purposes. Preschool and preadolescent children were referred by local physicians and public health nurses.

Sixty-two children, 53 boys and 9 girls, were selected for extensive diagnostic study, and 53 of these received therapy under the research program. The children's ages ranged from 2 years 6 months to 14 years. All children except one lived at home with both parents.

All children receiving therapy had normal hearing and were of normal to superior intelligence, as measured by group tests of mental ability given routinely

3. Our staff benefitted from discussions with Roger Brown, Professor, Harvard University; Katrina de Hirsch, Director, Pediatric Language Clinic, Columbia-Presbyterian Medical Center, New York, N.Y.; William J. Freeman, Coordinator of Community Services, Wellesley Human Relations Service, Incorporated; and Donald C. Klein, Director, Boston University Human Relations Center. We are grateful to our guest speakers, who were most generous with their time and advice.

at the Wellesley Schools.[4] Where such test results were not available, individual intelligence tests were administered.[5]

If a child showed other symptoms than stuttering or had other difficulties in addition to stuttering, a number of additional tests were administered. For example, we used The No-Howe Speech Test for English Consonant Sounds (Smith, 1957), the Peabody Picture Vocabulary Test (Dunn, 1959), the Developmental Articulation Test (Hejna, 1955), and The Bender Gestalt Test for Young Children (Koppitz, 1957). In certain cases we also used perceptual-motor tests, such as those devised by de Hirsch (1957), Frostig and Horne (1964), Kephart (1960), and Wepman (1958), and an informal rhythm test similar to the one mentioned by de Hirsch, Jansky, and Langford (1965 and 1966). Projective tests, such as the Mother-Child Relationship Test, described in Chapter 6, and the Draw-a-Person Test (Machover, 1957), were administered also in many cases.[6]

For diagnostic purposes and for the evaluation of treatment results a Definition of Terms was worked out, a copy of which can be found in Appendix II.

The Intake Interview[7]

A detailed developmental history was obtained in each case. Before treatment with the child was initiated, the child's mother or both parents had a conference with the research psychologist, who conducted an intake interview. The interview was clinical, or semistructured, in nature.[8] The topics to be covered had been chosen in view of our research interests in cooperation between our therapists and medical consultants. The information gained during this interview was transcribed later onto a standardized Intake Form, a copy of which can be found in Appendix III.

The intake interview with parents emerged as an important methodological practice that should be useful not only for research purposes but also for practical therapeutic ends. It served to pinpoint the factors in the child's family background or in his own developmental history that were related to the onset of his speech difficulty and that might be important to the course of therapy. It also helped us to differentiate between those children whose symptoms appeared to result primarily from an interruption in the development of communication between mother and child and those whose symptoms resulted primarily from neurological damage or cerebral dysfunction of some variety.

---

4. California Short Form Test of Mental Maturity, S-Form (Sullivan, Clark and Tiegs, 1957).

5. The Stanford-Binet Intelligence Scale (3rd Revision), Form L-M (Terman and Merrill, 1960); the Wechsler Intelligence Scale for Children (Wechsler, 1940); and the Measurement of Intelligence by Drawings (Goodenough, 1954).

6. For further discussion of these diagnostic procedures see Chapter 13.

7. The following section is based upon a paper, "The Intake Interview," presented by Harriet M. Stanton at the 38th Annual Convention of the American Speech and Hearing Association, New York, N.Y., November 1962 (see Wyatt and collaborators, 1962).

8. See Dohrenwend and Richardson, 1963.

In the following example the difficulty had a nonphysiological cause. Jim, age 6, was a handsome, healthy boy whose mother recalled no difficulty either during her pregnancy or at the time of his birth. He had never had a serious illness, and his development of walking, talking, and caring for himself had been entirely normal. He was, indeed, learning to speak well at $2\frac{1}{2}$ years of age, when his baby sister was born. During his mother's stay in the hospital he was left with a woman who was a relative stranger, who took good physical care of him but had little understanding of children. Shortly after his mother's return home, the maternal grandmother became seriously ill. For a period of several months the mother, although she remained in the home and cared for her children, had little emotional energy available to satisfy their needs. While the mother was dimly aware that Jim was showing signs of stuttering, she was too distracted to pay much attention to it.

An example in contrast to Jim was John. He was 6 also, but he was a clumsy boy with an odd gait. Although he was in first grade, he had not yet learned to hold his pencil properly. John's mother stated that she had had difficulties throughout her pregnancy and was afraid several times that she might miscarry. John was born a month prematurely and spent the first 2 weeks of his life in an incubator. Although his general development had been satisfactory, at the age of 2 he had had a serious illness with high fever, which was accompanied by a convulsion. He began to talk at about 18 months, but his articulation had always been poor. In the last 2 years he had developed a strong tendency to repeat himself, which was labeled stuttering by parents, teachers, and physicians. In John's case careful consideration had to be given to the possibility that his so-called stuttering might actually be related more to probable neurological damage than to emotional factors.

A diagnostic differentiation of this kind has implications for the choice of treatment. For Jim the therapeutic procedures used with young stuttering children were recommended. For John, however, certain educational measures aimed at helping him use more effectively what abilities he had seemed more appropriate. His speech was treated only as one of a number of difficulties, all stemming from the same source.[9]

The intake interview also proved valuable in determining factors which might be of importance in the course of therapy. Let us return to Jim and compare his family situation with that of another child, Roger. Information about the parents' background suggested that Jim's parents, Mr. and Mrs. Smith, were mature, sensible, intelligent people. They reported that their own childhood had been happy, and they still maintained fairly close relations with both sets of grandparents. Mr. Smith was a professional person who rarely changed jobs, the family had moved only once during Jim's life. The family enjoyed vacation trips together, usually to visit grandparents, uncles, or aunts. So far as the mother knew, no member of either family had ever had a speech or hearing difficulty. Mrs. Smith

---

9. See Chapter 12.

had been advised to overlook her son's stuttering; but she had come to feel that this was not a useful attitude, and she was very eager to receive help for him.

In contrast to this was the case of Roger and his family. Roger's mother, Mrs. White, reported that her husband's father died when her husband was a young child and for several years he was brought up by his grandmother. He rejoined his mother when she remarried but he never felt close to his stepfather. In adult life he had almost no contact with any of his relatives. Mrs. White herself had an older and a younger brother. Her older brother was a severe stutterer, with whom various methods of treatment had been tried. Mrs. White remembered vividly the concern of her family about this problem. She had also been indoctrinated by her brother concerning possible attitudes on her part which might have caused her son to stutter. Mrs. White, an intelligent, well-educated, conscientious mother, had spent a great deal of time ruminating about her brother's suggestions; at the same time she had tended to follow the advice of friends and physicians with whom she discussed the situation and to ignore or deny that her child had any difficulty.

Plans for therapy with these children and their parents were influenced by our evaluation of the probable ease or difficulty in handling the families involved. Information about the background, attitudes, and experiences of the 2 sets of parents was useful to the therapists in deciding what areas were most likely to require attention and what probable attitudes and difficulties in treatment they were likely to meet.

The intake interviewer used a special intake form. The form contained specific categories, such as information about the mother's and father's families, the patient's siblings, and his developmental history, school history, and speech development.[10] The taking of the case history required skill in dealing with people. To know how to direct a conversation to get at the areas of special interest presupposed both training and experience in this type of interviewing.

At the beginning the purpose of the interview was explained to the mother, and she was assured that any information she might give would be treated as strictly confidential and would not be shared with the child's teacher or any other school personnel not directly associated with the therapeutic program. The mother was encouraged to talk about herself, her family, and her child as she had seen him developing. At times direct questions were interspersed to bring an interview back onto the track of our particular interests.

Some parents found it so difficult to talk about themselves that most information had to be obtained in response to direct questioning. Most parents, however, began to talk spontaneously about some aspect of their child's behavior or about his speech problem; the rest of the interview developed out of this initial response, rather than out of a technique of question and answer.

In an interview of this sort there were, of course, areas in which it was easier to obtain information than in others. For example, many mothers knew little about the conditions surrounding their child's birth. They did not know the nature of

---

10. A copy of the Intake Form can be found in Appendix III.

anesthesias that were used, and frequently they knew little about their child's condition at birth. Other relevant information might not occur spontaneously to a mother, even when she was directly questioned about it. For example, questions were always included in the interview concerning possible separations of mother and child during the years when the child's speech was developing. A mother would sometimes declare with conviction and sincerity that she had never been away from the child; however, by the time of her first session with the therapist, she would spontaneously recall a separation from the child, when hospitalization or a death in the family had necessitated her being away from home. In other instances, discussion of the intake interview with other members of the family resulted in the mother's being reminded of situations in which she had been separated from the child, if not physically, at least emotionally. If, however, no efforts were ever made to obtain this sort of information in a structured purposeful way, it might never come to light, simply because the parent would have no way of knowing it might be relevant.

Thus the intake interview served several purposes: (1) to obtain information about the child's medical and developmental history and the onset of his speech disorder, (2) to gain relevant information about the family situation and its probable contributions to the child's speech problem, and (3) to induce the parents to accept the kind of professional help we offered.

We were aware that parents' retrospective reports concerning children's births and early development were not completely accurate (see Pyles and Mac-Farlane, 1934; Pyles, Stoltz, and MacFarlane, 1935; Mednick and Shaffer, 1962; Wenar, 1963). We attempted, therefore, to check the information received in 2 ways. First, the reports of all initial interviews were inspected by our pediatric consultant, who, on the basis of available data identified each case tentatively as (1) presenting evidence of neurological dysfunction, (2) being suspect of neurological dysfunction, or (3) presenting no evidence of neurological dysfunction. In cases considered suspect of neurological dysfunction, the consultant attempted to gain further information from the child's physician or from the hospital where the child had been delivered. In some instances he assisted the parents in obtaining a neurological examination of the child.

The second check on the information was made by the therapists working regularly with the parents. The therapist was in a position to evaluate the accuracy of the mother's statements. If a mother did not recall significant facts during the

TABLE 2—DIAGNOSTIC CATEGORIES

A	Stuttering Children	24
B	Children with Severely Defective Articulation	18
B¹	Children with Severely Defective Articulation and Stuttering	11
C	Children with Multiple Motor Perceptual and Language Disorders	9
		62

TABLE 3—AGE DISTRIBUTION AMONG GROUPS

	A	B	B[1]	C	Total
Under Seven	10	18	11	6	45
Over Seven	14	0	0	3	17
	24	18	11	9	62

TABLE 4—SEX DISTRIBUTION AMONG GROUPS

	A	B	B[1]	C	Total
Male	22	12	11	8	53
Female	2	6	0	1	9
	24	18	11	9	62

initial intake interview but recalled them later during therapeutic encounters, the information was then added to the material recorded on the Intake Form.

On the basis of our diagnostic criteria, we found that our sample of 62 children who had been seen for diagnostic evaluation could be subdivided into categories, as shown in Table 2.

The distribution of age and sex in these four groups is given in Tables 3 and 4.

THE NATURE OF COMMUNICATION THERAPY

In developing our methods of therapy, we drew upon our knowledge of dynamic psychology, of child development, and of language behavior in childhood. Our work with mothers and children was influenced by the writings of L. Jacobson (1949), Burlingham (1951), Furmann (1957), Sander (1962), Mac-Namara (1963), and others. Certain aspects of our therapeutic procedures were derived from the studies in "crisis-intervention" by Goodrich (1961), Klein and Lindemann (1961), and Waldfogel and Gardner (1961). Our interest in the role of fathers in children's language development and in communication therapy was enhanced by Ostrovsky's (1959) study of the father's influence upon the development and the education of the preschool child.

In developing therapeutic procedures, we were interested not only in the stuttering child's overt language disorder, but, equally, in his covert psychological difficulties, derived from the disruption of the mother-child relationship. It would be erroneous to assume, though, that communication therapy with stuttering children and their parents is nothing but a variation of psychotherapy, however skillfully executed. We must remember that if a disruption occurs in the area of complementary verbal behavior between a young child and a significant adult, it affects an individual not yet capable of independent verbalization of experiences.

Once the relationship between child and love object has been disrupted, a contact disorder ensues that will most likely be transferred to other newly forming relationships and will predetermine their meaning.

An adult—therapist, parent, or teacher—who is capable of attuning himself to the child's level of communication may, however, succeed in establishing a therapeutic relationship; this will in turn serve the child as a starting point for the development of further complementary relationships. In order to succeed in making his communication a therapeutic one, the more mature teaching adult must adjust his level of communication to that of the less mature learning child. The adult must respond to the clues given by the learner, be alert to the learner's verbal and nonverbal messages, and provide the learner with corrective feedback. *The helping adult has the double role of assisting the child in coping with his feelings of anxiety and aggression and, at the same time, of communicating on any level which may be appropriate and comfortable for the child in verbal distress.*

The following example of spontaneous therapeutic communication between a kindergarten teacher and a stuttering child illustrates these principles.

Miss B., a very gentle and skillful young kindergarten teacher, referred Betsy to the therapist because of Betsy's marked difficulties in communicating. The therapist first observed Betsy in the classroom during "show and tell period." Betsy talked with marked hesitancy, frequent repetition of initial sounds and syllables, occasional prolongation of vowel sounds, and in an unusually slow tempo, thus presenting symptoms of moderate stuttering.

The teacher had reported that when Betsy and her mother came for their first child-mother-teacher conference, prior to the beginning of school, Betsy was the only one among 26 children in the same situation who did not say a single word during the whole visit. Once in school, it had taken her several weeks before she began speaking to her teacher.

Following the classroom observation, the teacher, Betsy, and the therapist went together into an empty room next door. The therapist, who was a stranger to the child, sat quietly in a corner while Betsy's teacher spontaneously established a situation of closeness between herself and the child. Miss B. sat down, holding Betsy close to her so that she and the child each had an arm around the other. The teacher held a picture book in her lap—the story of a kitten—and she began looking at the book with Betsy, talking about the pictures. Both of them at first excluded the observer from their interaction.

The teacher began to describe the things that happened to the cat in the pictures. The objects and events in the book were on the child's level of interest and experience, and the teacher used early relational language to describe the pictures—simple sentence structure with chainlike linking together of one short phrase to another. "And what does the kitty do here? He is getting out of his box, see—out of his box—and here, here he climbs over the box, over the box—here—and here, he jumps down, down into the grass." From time to time Betsy spontaneously fell in with the teacher ". . . . out of his box . . . over the box . . ." and, laughing out loud, ". . . . jumps out of the box!"

Turning to another page, the teacher translated an aspect of the picture, roundness, into words: "And here the kitty goes round and round, round and round . . ." Immediately, Betsy moved her hand round and round, following the cat in the picture around the tree. At the same time she intoned in a chanting manner: "Round and round and round and around the tree. . . ."

Teacher and child thus demonstrated the ideal communication situation: Both adult and child were attuned to each other, and reciprocal identification between the speech partners was established through acts of mutual imitation.[11] From time to time the teacher participated in the child's motions and gestures as well as in her speech; in addition, she communicated with the child on the prelinguistic level through body closeness and touch. Thus a pattern of multilevel communication between adult and child was established. The teaching and learning of linguistic structures were embedded in the genetically earlier complementary behavior of bodily closeness, touch, and gesture—a matrix out of which the conscious command of symbolic language emerges only gradually.[12]

Finally, the moment had arrived at which Betsy felt ready to invite the strange, new person to participate in this game of word matching. She began to look sideways at the therapist, then back at her teacher. The therapist, responding to the clue, "tuned in," asking the child a question formulated on her level of language development: "And what is the kitty doing here? Is the kitty outside in the snow?" Betsy, not yet looking at the strange person but looking at her teacher, answered: "Yes, the kitty is in the snow. He must be cold—in the snow." After several minutes of such indirect communication, Betsy spontaneously walked over to the therapist, ready to talk to her directly. Thus the child was given time to assimilate the stranger gradually and used her teacher, a familiar love object, as an intermediary in relating to a new person.

In later conferences with Betsy's mother, the therapist helped the mother communicate with Betsy in ways similar to those used by the kindergarten teacher, which made communication comfortable for the child.

The aim of this form of therapy is the re-establishment of a positive mother-child relationship and the consequent acquisition of normal speech by the child. Therefore, the therapist's procedures should be so designed and organized that the mother is not replaced by the therapist in her role as the primary speech model; the therapist only complements and guides the interactions between mother and child. The mother must have the satisfaction of being competent in helping her child to improve. The therapist must beware of demonstrating that she is a "better mother" than the child's own mother. Thus the therapeutic procedure should provide mother and child with a constructive experience, helping them to improve their mutual communication and adaptation. Both mother and child undergo a learning experience.

As can be seen, therapy does not consist of speech exercises or drills; nor can it be called a form of psychotherapy with the stuttering child alone. We like to call it the teaching and facilitating of communication between mother and child, carried through within a dynamic frame of reference. This form of mother guidance seems to work best if the therapist succeeds in rapidly establishing and maintaining a mildly positive transference in the mother. Thus regression on the part of the mother and overdependency upon the therapist are prevented (Wyatt and Herzan, 1962).

Problems of the Child

The stuttering child has experienced early in life a crucial disruption of the primary feedback chain between mother and child, which is basic for the acquisi-

---

11. See Baker (1955).
12. See Frank (1957).

tion of language. He reacts to this disruption with feelings of loss, bewilderment, and helplessness, which gradually turn into anger directed against his mother. In many instances this anger is eventually displaced upon siblings, the father, or other relatives, who are experienced as rivals for the mother's love and attention. At the same time the child becomes afraid lest his anger lead to permanent loss of the love object through rejection or abandonment. The stuttering child's early experiences are preserved symbolically in the fantasy of the search for the mother. The core problem of the stuttering child, therefore, is his aggression anxiety: anger against his mother, closely connected with the fear of losing her.

Problems of the Mother

The specific problems of the mother of a stuttering child also center around feelings of helplessness and anger. Alarmed by the conspicuous symptoms of the child's language disorder and often confused by wrong advice, the mother experiences strong feelings of helplessness. As time goes by and the child's speech does not improve, or even becomes worse, the mother begins to feel incompetent in her maternal role. At the same time the stuttering child's behavior, with its frequent alternation between possessiveness and jealous hostility, arouses feelings of reactive anger in the mother. Problems of discipline become particularly difficult to handle; the mother fears that any determined stand on her part will cause more intense stuttering in the child.

In working with the mother, the therapist provides her with some explanation of the dynamics of language development, of stuttering, and of the manner in which the mother herself became involved in the child's communication disorder. To the mother of young children the therapist demonstrates games of word matching and mutual imitation. In all cases therapist and mother together evaluate the dynamics of the family and consider the stuttering child's role in it. The therapist helps the mother understand the covert meaning of the child's behavior as an expression of his needs and anxieties. With the therapist's support the mother herself discovers times and ways in which she can be closer to the child, assure him of her understanding and willingness to help, and set the stage for satisfactory mutual interaction.

Thus the therapist teaches the mother by several means. One is through explanation and analysis of the mother's own behavior and communication patterns. Another is through demonstration of communication patterns appropriate for interaction with young children. Finally, the therapist helps the mother to understand her own feelings for the stuttering child, which are intimately connected with her ability or inability to communicate successfully.

Therapy with Young Children

In working with young children, the therapist lends herself as an object for mutual imitation and reciprocal identification. In providing corrective feedback, she actually teaches the child patterns of communication adequate for his age level. By working with the mother simultaneously, the therapist makes sure that the child will have continuous satisfactory communication experiences in his home.

Therapy with Older Children and Adolescents

Work with older children and adolescents focuses upon the disturbed relationships between the child and his parents and upon the stutterer's feelings of anger and aggression. The therapist helps the child recognize that in reality—contrary to

TABLE 5—PATTERNS OF THERAPY WITH STUTTERING CHILDREN AND THEIR PARENTS*

Therapy with Child	Therapy with Parents
Preschool Child Same Therapist for Mother and Child	
Child usually seen in mother's presence. Therapy focused upon mother; interview with father if possible. Therapist gives mother information about language learning and stuttering; explains child's need for closeness and corrective feedback, demonstrates games of mutual verbal imitation; helps mother understand and manage child's clinging, fears, and aggressiveness. Prognosis very good if mother is able to make imaginative use of parent-counseling ("Therapeutic Readiness").	
School-Age Child Same Therapist Sees Mother and Child Separately	
Play therapy. Matching of phrases and short sentences between therapist and child. Therapist uses language on child's level; helps him verbalize his angry feelings against mother, father, and siblings and cope with these feelings.	Work with mother similar to that with mother of preschool child. Occasional conferences with father or with both parents. Prolonged treatment may be necessary.
Older Child and Adolescent Divided Management: Separate Therapists See Child and Parents	
Therapy resembles more traditional psychotherapy, focused upon child's feelings toward mother, father, and siblings; analysis of defenses. Therapist explores with child communication barriers in the family.	Counseling with mother and father, or with both together; exploring of family communication. Prolonged treatment necessary.

* Reproduced by permission of *Pediatrics* (Wyatt, 1965).

his fantasies—his mother is not inaccessible. He also helps the child to realize that his anger against the mother, his siblings, or his father and other authority figures is not as dangerous as he feels it to be and can be expressed verbally without leading to catastrophic consequences.

As Wittgenstein (1953) pointed out, a child originally has no words for his feelings of anger or pain. In providing the child with words for such feelings, the adult teaches the child anger or pain behavior. Helping the child to verbalize his undifferentiated feelings, the therapist makes them accessible to the child's ego; their repression or denial is prevented, and eventually the child learns to cope with them. The sector chosen for therapy with older children consists of the difficulties in their relationships and not in their speech. Parallel to the work done with the child, the parents are assisted in handling their relationship with the stuttering child. Specific aspects of this process of parent counseling will be discussed later.

A summary of the methods of communication therapy used with children and parents is presented in Table 5.

A Theoretical Model

Goldman-Eisler, in her studies of speech analysis and mental processes (1958), developed a linguistic model for psychotherapy which, with suitable modifications, may serve to illuminate further our procedures. Goldman-Eisler described the therapeutic encounter as an exceptional form of interpersonal communication. Psychotherapy, in her words, proceeds through verbal expression of affect by the patient. Time pressure is no factor; while in a conversational situation time must be shared between the speech partners, the patient in psychotherapy is the sole possessor of the interview time. Intelligibility in logical terms is not demanded and the premium is on spontaneity. The setting of the therapeutic interview thus is favorable to a detachment from linguistic constraints and habitual verbalizations. The relative passivity of the noninterfering therapist enables the speaker to talk freely, "on his own time."

In communication therapy the conditions described by Goldman-Eisler are provided. The therapist, who is attuned to the feelings and interests of the child or his parents, listens attentively and permits his speech partner to express feelings and impulses both verbally and nonverbally. Through his behavior, the therapist provides freedom from the usual linguistic constraints. However, certain factors have been added to these conditions basic to most forms of psychotherapy and practiced with either adults or children.

In working with children with communication disorders the therapeutic interaction is further enhanced by the therapist actively helping the child to verbalize his feelings. Thus, the therapist assists the child simultaneously in coping with his impulses and wishes, and in learning to move gradually from "egocentric speech-for-oneself" to "social speech with others."

In working with parents, on the contrary, the therapist encourages the adult to overtly verbalize his "internal" speech, a form of speech which, as we know, is the adult remainder of the egocentric speech of childhood.[15] Thus, the adult, guided by the therapist, permits himself to regress to earlier and more primitive forms of communication. Having experienced this form of positive regression in their interviews with the parent counselor, the mothers and fathers of stuttering

---

15. See Chapter 5.

children gradually learn to communicate with their child on the infantile, often prelogical level of imagination and fantasy. When parents are enabled to function comfortably on a linguistic level closer to that of their stuttering child, they truly become coworkers in the therapeutic endeavor.

In the following demonstrations, taken from treatment records, this process will be illustrated.

EXAMPLES OF COMMUNICATION THERAPY[16]

Our aim in therapy was to establish a close relationship between the child and his mother. For this reason, we urged each mother to spend time alone with her child each day in a manner that was enjoyable for both of them—playing games or looking at picture books. We instructed each mother to speak to her child at his level of understanding and to match her words to his in their conversation. Such a situation provided excellent opportunities for language learning. The child received a continuous corrective feedback of his own speech, and he began to feel that his mother was listening carefully to him and was interested in his ideas.

In the case of the preschool children we worked primarily with the mothers. If the child was present, we demonstrated to the mother how to talk with the child in such a manner that an appropriate and corrective feedback would result. The following is an example of such a demonstration.

Johnny, a child of 3 years, came to see the therapist with his mother. The therapist was able to talk with Johnny while he played with a color-form set. He began to place kitchen utensils and food where he thought they should be in the toy kitchen. Carrying on a running commentary as he worked, the therapist had an opportunity to pick up his conversation and to match his words.

Johnny. Here is a cup. Goes on the table.
Therapist. The cup goes on the table.
Johnny. Coffee pot goes—goes on the stove.
Therapist. The coffee pot goes on the stove.
(Johnny picks up an ice-cream cone.)
Therapist. Where will the ice-cream cone go?
Johnny. Ice cream cone in the stove.
Therapist. In the stove?
Johnny. No, here.
Therapist. Here, in the icebox?
Johnny. Yes, here in the icebox.

Johnny and the therapist continued to play with this set for about 15 minutes. The therapist carefully matched her words with Johnny's, at the same time presenting him with a model of correct grammar and syntax. Johnny was then asked

16. Some of these examples were first quoted in the paper "Therapy with Young Children and Their Mothers," by Lois Scott, Louise Brown, and Jacqueline Harmon, presented at the 38th annual convention of the American Speech and Hearing Association, November, 1962 (see Wyatt and collaborators, 1962).

to go into the next room and play by himself. His mother remarked that he had spoken so fluently while he talked with the therapist that she did not think the therapist would believe that he stuttered. It was easy to convince this mother that careful listening to her child and speaking with him on his level provided him with the kind of comfortable language experience that was helpful to him.

As mothers spent time alone with their children in this way, they sometimes began to notice, and reported to the therapist, that their previous communication with the stuttering child had not been helpful to him. When Mrs. Smith, the mother of 4-year-old Billy, began to work with the therapist, she evaluated her usual way of speaking to her child throughout the day. She mentioned that she spoke rapidly and at an adult level of conversation, using words that Billy did not understand. She also gave many directions to him that might confuse him. She began to understand that she was doing this out of loneliness and need for adult companionship. This insight into her own needs made it possible for her to make a conscious effort to tune in to her child's level of understanding.

Another mother discovered how she enjoyed talking and playing games with her 3-year-old son, Jack. She was quick to understand how to work with him and was creative as she set up play situations which they both enjoyed. She was amused to report to the therapist how she herself regressed in play activity as well as in speech. For instance, when it was her turn to be the conductor on a train, she found herself shouting "Choo choo!" as the train came to an intersection. The mother mentioned that at first this kind of behavior had been difficult for her, but when she noticed how Jack responded with pleasure and with improvement in speech, she knew that she was doing the right thing. She remarked that he stuttered much less while she was alone with him than when she was occupied with activities around the house or with her other children.

When the mother spent time alone with the stuttering child, playing verbal games with him, she provided the child with a daily period when his speech was at its best. This kind of interaction between child and mother served a dual purpose. The mother became more aware of the child's personality and his particular needs and the child felt that he had more access to his mother. It was this kind of physical and verbal closeness that opened the way to an improved relationship between them.

The mother of 3-year-old Will reported in the course of therapy that she was shocked to find that until then she had "shut Will out" and had given him a minimum of care and attention after his brother was born. Now the mother again began to enjoy being with Will. Even though Will's hyperactive personality was a burden to her, she noticed that he added a "spark" to her family.

We found that mothers differed in their ability to carry out recommendations for setting up good language learning situations for a child. How well a mother was able to function in this area seemed to depend on her current state of mental health, family situation, and relationship with her child. Most mothers in our sample seemed desirous of helping their children and were strongly motivated to carry out our suggestions.

Mrs. B., who herself had a childhood history of emotional disturbance, found it exceedingly difficult to spend time with 6-year-old Richard, who stuttered severely. Mrs. B. complained that her son didn't talk to her when they were alone together. This made her feel very anxious. Nevertheless, she continued her conferences with the therapist and tried to help her child at home.

Richard often had complained at home and to the therapist that he was afraid to be alone in his basement playroom. His mother felt irritated by the child's fears and considered him a sissy. Also, she was interested in sports and felt frustrated because Richard could not play baseball. After several months of parent counseling, her perception of the child changed gradually and she was more able to sympathize with his fears. Spontaneously, she went with him to the basement playroom and began to play ping-pong with him, an activity he enjoyed very much. This was the particular way in which this mother was able to enjoy a common activity with her stuttering child, as well as to provide him with verbal feedback. Once she began teaching him ping-pong, she found out to her surprise that he played quite well.

Evidently, a therapist can recommend to a mother that she spend time with her child in common activities and verbal interaction, but the therapist cannot prescribe to the mother how this should be done.

We felt that mothers were able to help their children in this way because the therapist supported them. As a rule, the therapist saw a mother every two weeks. The therapist presented herself as a helping person who was willing to listen carefully and with interest to the mother as she talked about her child's personality and her everyday management of him. The therapist seldom offered advice except about ways to set up better language learning situations for the child. She helped the mother to make better use of her own resources in reaching out to the stuttering child.

The pattern of therapy with school-age children was different from that used with preschool children. The same therapist saw the mother and the child separately. The therapist tried to establish a friendly, warm relationship with the child. She played games, modeled clay, built with blocks, or shared other activities with him. When the therapist talked with the child she was careful to speak slowly, to use simple sentence structure, and to feed back to the child his own words, though sometimes in an improved pattern. This technique helped the child to feel that the therapist was close to him and wanted to know him better. Most stuttering children very quickly understood the meaning of this supportive relationship and after a short time began to trust the therapist and to confide their problems to her. Clues to a child's unconscious feelings often were found in the symbolic messages expressed in play activities. Here is an example of such symbolic expression.

The therapist had learned from Jamie's mother that he had killed a puppy. Knowing the ways in which young children communicate, the therapist did not expect Jamie to mention this incident directly to her during his therapy session. During the next session Jamie set up a picnic scene, including a police car. The therapist asked him why he needed a police car at the picnic, and he answered that the policeman could stop people if they had a fight. The therapist suggested that people sometimes get mad and fight, but usually they don't need a policeman. Jamie remarked that the people might kill each other if they were really mad, and the policeman would shoot them. The therapist explained to Jamie how everyone gets mad at times, but that it should not lead to violence. Jamie assured her that he never got mad! The therapist acted surprised. Before the hour was up, Jamie began to knock blocks down in a manner that suggested that he was very angry. The therapist asked him if he was mad and Jamie smiled as though to say: "Yes, I am." This play incident helped the therapist to know that Jamie was afraid of the consequences of showing anger: to get mad is deadly. Jamie's guilt feelings and fears and the mother's reactions to his killing the puppy had to be explored with them further in subsequent sessions.

Whatever troubled the stuttering child, he gained strength when he was able to talk about it to his therapist and when he finally could approach his mother directly about it. It was difficult for most of the stuttering children to approach their mother unless they felt sure her reaction would be accepting. The following is a case in point.

In Fred's early years, separation from his parents had been very frequent as his parents often traveled for business or pleasure. His parents continued to take frequent trips during the two years of therapy. Fred reacted strongly to these separations; he appeared extremely anxious and his stuttering became markedly worse whenever his parents went away.

On the eve of one trip he left a note for his mother saying "I hate you." He felt very bad the next day and hoped that his mother had not found the note. His mother, however, had read the note and become extremely upset about it. Both mother and child talked about this note for weeks to the therapist without talking to each other about it! The therapist suggested to the mother that Fred must feel bad for writing the note and suggested that the mother should talk to Fred about it. The mother replied that she could not do that, it had hurt her too much.

This particular barrier in communication between mother and child existed for more than two months, and much careful work by the therpist with both the mother and the child was necessary before they were able finally to talk directly to each other about the incident. The mother—who had experienced much rejection from her own mother during her childhood—gradually began to understand that her son's message had aroused in her feelings of counteraggression and anxiety. On the eve of the parents' next trip the boy wrote another note, telling his mother that he hated her and would run away. However, having worked through his feelings with his therapist, he was able also to talk to his mother about the note. His mother read the note in his presence and sat down to talk things over with him. She told him that she understood now that he was angry at her for going away. She explained to him the reasons for her trip, assured him of her continued love, and pointed out on a calendar the day when she would be back again. The boy felt much relieved and asked his mother to throw the note away, "It didn't mean anything." Following this significant conversation, the child felt less fear in talking to his mother about his own dangerous feelings, and she felt less hurt or punitive when he expressed aggressive feelings or fantasies.

Most of the cases in our research studies resembled each other insofar as the children had suffered a disruption in their relationship with their mothers. However, there was a wide variety of different family situations. In some instances, a child improved even with a minimum amount of therapy. The case of Jerry illustrates this.

Jerry was brought to our attention by the kindergarten teacher, who reported that he stuttered in the classroom. The therapist observed him several times, alone or in a group situation, but was unable to hear any unusual repetitions. An interview with the mother was arranged, and the mother revealed that Jerry's father had been a stutterer also. The mother seemed very concerned about Jerry. She mentioned that at times Jerry got violently angry, "So angry that he cannot talk and he looks as if he wanted to kill somebody," she said.

As the school year was almost over, arrangements were made with the mother to begin therapy with Jerry in the fall. The therapist observed Jerry again at the time he entered grade one, and he was stuttering quite noticeably. The mother had the usual intake interview and it was decided that the same therapist would work with the child and with his mother. As the year went on neither the child nor the mother could be seen frequently, as there was much illness in the family. Altogether, the therapist had nine conferences with the mother and the child was seen 14 times.

At the beginning of therapy Jerry was extremely shy. He did not speak unless spoken to, and he could not look into the eyes of the person he talked to. He spoke in a whisper and his speech showed frequent repetition of sounds and syllables.

In her conferences with the therapist the mother described Jerry as being completely overshadowed by his sister, who was two years old and who did everything faster and better than he. A brother, three years younger, was a great teaser and often made Jerry feel very angry and frustrated.

Jerry's mother talked with the therapist about everyday family problems. The mother was urged to spend a definite time each day alone with Jerry and to use simple patterns of speech which were fitting for his level of language development. The mother was reassured that she was able to deal with her problems and that many of her ideas and ways of handling the children were very good. As the mother talked to the therapist she gained some perspective on her children and on her relations with them.

During the fifth session with the therapist the mother mentioned that she had discussed with Jerry his fear of darkness, a problem that she had passed over lightly a week earlier. During the sixth session, which occurred during the spring, the mother mentioned that the general atmosphere in the home had improved greatly and that the competitive feelings among her children had diminished. The mother described this as "taking the pressure off the family."

Parallel to her meetings with the mother the therapist had seen Jerry also. Even though he was sick a great deal through the school year, the therapist succeeded in establishing a positive relationship with him. During his meetings with the therapist Jerry told of his fantasies and the imaginative play he indulged in when he was sick: He drew pictures, thereby working out a certain amount of anger and frustration against his parents and siblings.

His whispered speech had been a real problem, both in the classroom and in the home, and it had even made some people assume that he was not very intelligent. The therapist soon realized that he was a child of wide interests and high ability. As the year progressed his speech became more fluent and strong. There was one acute period of regression when he needed more intensive help from the therapist.

In the fall of the following year Jerry attended the second grade and he was seen for appraisal by the therapist and by the chief investigator. Both felt that Jerry's speech was excellent and that his way of expressing himself was quite advanced, compared to other children of his age. To the therapist Jerry appeared like a different child. When she called for him he could hardly wait to get out of the classroom to talk to her. He told her a great deal about his experiences during the summer. He described hikes, mountain-climbing, places visited, all with a perception and a vocabulary which were surprising for a 7-year-old child. He was full of enthusiasm and his voice was loud and rich in expressive qualities. His speech was fluent except for occasional repetitions of an initial word or phrase, a speech pattern which we considered normal for his age.

His mother also had a conference with the therapist during which she mentioned how very pleased she was with Jerry's development. The mother's main topic of conversation was Jerry's wide range of interests and his eagerness to learn. When the therapist reminded the mother of the whispering voice Jerry had used a year earlier, the mother seemed very surprised; she had forgotten it completely. When the mother left the therapist she remembered a remark made by Jerry's kindergarten teacher two years earlier. The teacher had told the mother that Jerry probably would be "slow" going through school. This had been a shock to the mother and probably it had affected her perception of the child and her approach to him.

Mothers' Reactions to Therapy

As mentioned before, the mothers differed in their readiness to become co-therapists. In general, the mothers fell into two groups, those who showed therapeutic readiness, and those who were at the time not capable of cooperating effectively with the therapist. The two groups differed markedly in their behavior during the therapeutic encounters.

The mothers in the first group were reasonably concerned about the child's stuttering; some were even bewildered or anxious at the beginning of treatment. They expressed their willingness to be of help to the child, if only they could know how to proceed. These mothers were intellectually and emotionally able to profit from explanations and demonstrations, to accept suggestions and to utilize them constructively. Once they understood the principles of therapeutic communication, they were able to use their own imaginations in setting up situations of constructive interaction with the child. They soon learned to understand and handle the child's anger without retaliating and without feeling guilty or depressed. They established a relationship of trust and confidence with the therapist, and they were willing to work through periods when the child relapsed into stuttering. Thus, such a mother rapidly became the child's primary therapist.

Mothers in the second group seemed highly irritated by the child's speech and behavior peculiarities. Their relationship to the child, as well as to the therapist, was ambivalent and inconsistent. During a conference they seemed to understand and accept the therapist's explanations and suggestions, but they followed these suggestions all too literally, often turning them into absurdities. One mother complained to the therapist: "You told me that I must *never* leave the child alone. How can I exist that way?" Thus, these mothers succeeded in proving to the therapist that her advice had been useless. Particularly striking was their behavior when they were asked to observe the therapist working with their child. While the therapist demonstrated word matching with the child in a play situation, these mothers showed their lack of attention through restlessness or yawning, or they interrupted the demonstration, talking about their own problems, reminiscing about their own childhood, or making hostile remarks about the child or other family members. They seemed to compete with the child for the therapist's attention. They wavered between excessive praise for the therapist during periods when the child's speech improved and intense hostility against her when the child had a relapse into stuttering. Through their behavior these mothers expressed symbolically that they themselves needed treatment before they would be able to act appropriately in a complementary relationship with their children.

Like Furman (1957), we found that a mother's capacity for cooperation frequently could not be assessed during the initial interview, but could be judged only after a period of working with her. The mothers of two young children, for example, seemed at first to be quite understanding, but it soon became evident that they could not deal with the specific area—need for closeness to the mother— in which their children needed help. Other mothers who appeared rigid or over-anxious at first were amazingly capable of following guidance and of cooperating effectively, often in spite of difficult home situations, after gaining an understanding of the significant factors.

CHAPTER EIGHT

Illustrations of the Therapeutic Process

Three extensive case histories, followed by commentaries, will be presented in this chapter. These three histories could be called "Variations on a Theme," the theme being the re-establishment of satisfactory communication between parent and child. The variations consist of the specific family situation and the related dynamics, which differed in each case.

In all three cases, one therapist worked with child and parents (see Table 5, p. 130). This form of therapy puts a heavy responsibility as well as an emotional burden upon the therapist which, fortunately, the therapist was able to share with the consulting psychiatrist. In the interest of descriptive clarity, the interaction between therapist and consultant and its effect upon the therapeutic process have only been touched upon in this chapter; this interaction will be discussed further in Chapter 10.

In our approach to parent-child therapy we assumed that older children would be less willing to share their therapist with the parent than would younger children, and we decided, therefore, to use "divided management" for children over 12 years of age. In the course of our work we found, however, that in some instances even somewhat younger children could be helped better if child and parent were seen separately by two different therapists. Eventually two members of our therapeutic team—M. Prentice and R. Dutton—worked primarily as parent counselors. Their experience in working with the parents of older stuttering children and the techniques which they found most helpful will be described at the end of this chapter.

TREATMENT OF A PRESCHOOL CHILD

The Case of Joe

The following case history has been reconstructed from the records written by the therapist after each therapeutic encounter.

Joe was first seen in the spring of 1958, after his mother had asked for help with his speech. I made an appointment and paid a visit at the child's home. Joe was then 4 years and 6 months old. He was a handsome, sturdy youngster, who impressed me as very lively and energetic. He received me with a paper bag over his head, shouting "Boo!" Mrs. E., his mother, was a very dainty young woman. Her small modern home, her little son, and her 14-months-old baby daughter were all kept immaculately neat and clean.

The mother reported that Joe had stuttered on and off for the last year. She seemed very much afraid that his stuttering might become worse if nothing was done about it. During my visit I did not observe any stuttering. Joe spoke with a slight interdental lisp and with frequent repetition of words or phrases in a manner which I considered to be normal for his stage of language development. I gave the mother some explanations about the nature of language development and tried to reassure her that Joe's speech was adequate for his age. Suggestions were made how mother and child could look at picture books and play games together.

Four months later, in the fall, the mother called again and reported that Joe had developed a very conspicuous stutter and that he seemed extremely frustrated and angry about it. When I observed him during my next visit, he spoke with frequent rapid repetitions and often blocked at the beginning of words. His mother reported that the day before my visit Joe had been so angry because he could not talk fluently that he had kicked the door in a fit of fury, hurting his foot.

The little boy was very friendly with me and took me into his room to show me his toys. He talked a great deal in spite of his stuttering. I told him that I could see that he had some difficulty in speaking, that this happened sometimes to children of his age who were learning to speak in long sentences, and that his mother and I would try and help him learn how to speak well.

Later, Joe went outside to play with a friend and I had an opportunity to talk to his mother alone. She seemed very anxious and upset about Joe's difficulty and mentioned that she had several sisters and brothers, all of whom had children. She exclaimed: "They all are doing very well—why should *my* child not be all right?" I pointed out to the mother that she had a very fine boy who obviously was quite well developed, both physically and mentally, and very well cared for. I explained to her that stuttering was a temporary disorder, a difficulty in learning to speak. I also pointed out Joe's possible jealousy toward his baby sister and his present exaggerated need for closeness to his mother. I suggested that when Joe had difficulty in speaking, she should not deny the existence of his difficulty, but should discuss it with him in a friendly and helpful manner. I also demonstrated to her games of reading together, word matching, and other forms of mutual imitation.

The mother was a friendly person of middle-class background. Her husband was a highly skilled craftsman who made a good income and who had built a charming little house for his family. Mrs. E. seemed somewhat compulsive in her desire to have the house neat at all times in spite of the presence of young children. She seemed overwhelmed by her little son's aggressive masculinity. With the mother's permission, I later got in touch with the family physician, who felt that the mother was tense and overanxious.

Joe and his mother were treated following Pattern I (Table 5). I met the mother every second week. When Joe and his mother came to my office two weeks later, he absolutely refused to leave his mother. He would not even stay with me in a room with the door open into the next room where his mother sat. Consequently mother and child again were seen together. Joe did not want to look at picture books but he was interested in crayons. While he drew pictures, he and I did some word matching together in the mother's presence. I repeated Joe's phrases, expanded them, and induced him at times to repeat phrases simultaneously with me. During this drawing-and-speaking situation Joe showed some playful aggression: He made a tapping noise with his foot under the table. When I acted surprised about "the mouse" under the table, he made the noise louder and louder, obviously to frighten me. We both talked about the mouse under the table and how scared I was of it. All this was done in the mother's presence; thus, it was demonstrated to her how Joe's aggression could be handled without retaliating. Finally, I declared that the game was over, as it was time for Joe and his mother to go home.

During my next home visit, two weeks later, Joe was in and out of the room, trying on his Halloween costume and showing it to me. The "blocking" had disappeared from his speech; frequently he repeated words, but with less tension than I had observed a month earlier.

Joe's mother reported that his speech had been "somewhat better." In spite of this, she seemed extremely upset and worried about Joe's speech as well as about his behavior. Again she compared her "difficult" child with the children of her relatives. I repeated my assurances that there was nothing "wrong" with Joe and that he was a boy any mother could be proud of. Mrs. E. asked whether it was advisable to send Joe to nursery school; she also reported Joe's great unwillingness to leave her. In this connection Mrs. E. mentioned Joe's difficulties in going to bed and his need to get up again and again "for a glass of water, attention, or just to say something." The therapist explained to the mother the connection between Joe's distance anxiety, his jealousy toward the little sister, and his speech disorder. The mother was asked to give Joe the opportunity for increased closeness to her for the next few months, until he had learned to speak sentences fluently. I suggested that Joe's attendance at the nursery school should be postponed until that time. The recommendation was made to leave Joe's door slightly open at night so that he could hear this parents' voices and see the light in the house before falling asleep.

The mother asked very anxiously how often I would be willing to see her. I explained to her that we would meet every second week, but that I would be available at any time if she felt she needed an additional conference. It seemed that this mother felt threatened by a boy's specific ways of growing up—by his intense bodily energy and his impulses—and that having him "close" was difficult for her to handle at that time. I discussed with her instances of Joe's "naughty" or "difficult" behavior and tried to make her realize how normal and healthy Joe actually was. His possible interest in sexual matters also was touched upon.

Two weeks later Joe came again to my office, but this time he did not mind leaving his mother in the next room. He did some drawings and he was willing to tell stories in response to pictures. Repetitive speech, but no "blocking," was observed during the session.

Later his mother joined us, while Joe was drawing, and asked in his presence: "When he goes to kindergarten next year, is he going to have a special class?" I explained to her that "special classes" were for mentally retarded children but not for boys like Joe. The mother replied: "I thought they had special classes for reading and a special class for those!" pointing to Joe. I assured her in the child's presence, that Joe's repeating of words was only a passing stage in his learning to speak, that by the time he entered kindergarten he would most likely speak quite well, and that he was a very fine boy who would do well at school. On the way out the mother mentioned: "We have done everything you said about his sleeping, we left the door open a bit when Joe wanted it. It works very well."

Soon afterward, I visited both parents in their home in the evening, when Joe was already asleep. During our conference the mother seemed much more tense and worried about the child than the father. I discussed with the parents what kind of information concerning stuttering they had had in the past, and the mother reported with some irritation that the father's mother had "threatened" Joe because of his stuttering. It was during this interview that the mother mentioned Joe's bed-wetting. The father seemed to understand quite well that Joe's growing up, his learning to go to the bathroom, and his learning to speak, were related. He also reported laughingly that his own mother had said that he had been "much worse" than Joe when he was growing up. The management of Joe's aggressive behavior, his difficulties in going to bed, and his bed-wetting were discussed with the parents. I pointed out to the parents that my role was a limited one, but that helping him with his speech at this time might also help him with his anxieties at night.

During my next home visit, two weeks later, Joe spoke quite fluently. I pointed out to the mother that his occasional repetitions of words were common among children of his age and should not be considered as symptoms of a speech difficulty. His mother reported that his speech had been very good lately and that he had had no difficulties going to bed, but that he continued to wet his bed.

During the following weeks Joe's mother continued to report that Joe spoke well. As the mother obviously wished to have Joe attend nursery school, I suggested that he should attend on a trial basis. His mother took him to school the first time; from then on he went there in the teacher's car. At that point—January, 1959—Joe seemed to be able to tolerate the separation from his mother and he seemed to enjoy going to nursery school three mornings a week. The mother, who now was relieved part of the time of Joe's aggressive energy, seemed to feel less anxious. She herself put him to bed every evening and she described to me how she and Joe were speaking together while he went to bed, in the manner I had suggested.

Toward the end of January, when I made another home visit, I observed that Joe spoke with complete fluency. We did speaking together or word-matching, using a picture book. Joe seemed to enjoy it so much that we had to go through the whole book twice. Later his mother offered me coffee and cake in the kitchen, in the presence of Joe and of his baby sister. Joe stuffed lots of food into his mouth, obviously to show off. When I got up to leave, Joe made an aggressive attack against me. He put his hands around my neck, choking me, then he tried to pull my hair. I prevented him from hurting me and said: "What an angry little boy this is! Joe is really very cross with me, but I know that Joe will not really hurt me." After that he put his arms around my legs as if he wished to hold me back. I assured him that I would come again and also that he could come to my office and play again with my toys and crayons.

My major therapeutic contribution seemed to lie in giving Joe an opportunity to displace some of his aggressive and possessive feelings from his mother onto me. During the scene in the kitchen I was able to demonstrate to his mother that one could react to such feelings reasonably, without making the child feel guilty. In addition, I was able to support his mother in her management of Joe and to help her in working through her complex feelings concerning the closeness–separation conflict in herself and in her child.

Soon afterward, Joe's mother reported by telephone that Joe spoke very well at all times and loved to go to nursery school. My conferences with the mother were then arranged on a monthly basis. During a conference in February the mother reported that Joe had had a very bad dream about a ghost in his father's clothes. He woke and screamed and his parents took him into their bed. At that time Joe may have experienced his father as another rival for his mother's love.

Joe continued to speak well. During a visit at my office in March, he appeared more quiet and controlled than he had been in the past. He expressed some aggressive fantasies in his drawings and in playing with clay. Altogether, he and his parents had had ten therapeutic sessions during a period of six months. The treatment was discontinued at that point. A recommendation was made to the parents to visit the local mental health clinic, in order to get further help with Joe's bedwetting. As the bed-wetting stopped soon after, the parents paid only three visits to the agency.

It was made clear to the mother that I would be available at any time should stuttering appear again in Joe's speech and also that I would keep an eye on Joe once he was in kindergarten.

The following September, I called the mother on Joe's first day at school. She seemed very pleased to have me call her and said: "I am all excited, I feel as if I was getting ready for a big wedding!" This mother obviously felt extremely excited about the event of her first child's going to school.[1] Asked about Joe's speech, the mother reported: "He was doing very well until three weeks ago.

---

1. Mothers' reactions to their children's first school attendance have been the object of a research study carried through by members of the Wellesley Human Relations Service, Inc. See D. C. Klein and A. Ross (1958).

He got excited about school, some kids told him how tough it will be in school, that they take their pants down in school." Before the opening of school Joe had begun to repeat words again more frequently. One day he said: "I am not talking too good today. My motor is not working good." Then his mother had explained to him that he was just learning new words, that he would be all right again, and that many children of his age talked the same way. I praised the mother for having handled the situation very well. Mrs. E. then said to me: "I am glad you called. If he stutters again as badly as he did last fall, would he still go to school or would he have to stay at home? Are you going to watch over him? Are *you* going to teach him or another teacher?" I assured her that his teacher was a very experienced, capable and friendly person who was very fond of energetic little boys and that I would be around the school and would observe him in the classroom once in a while. It was evident that this mother needed help in coping with her separation-anxiety in sending her child to school.

During the following three months I observed Joe several times in his classroom. Quite obviously he enjoyed working with the carpenter's bench and tools and building with large blocks. There was more opportunity for muscular activity and even for rough games at school than in his mother's extremely neat and orderly house. The teacher reported that Joe's speech had been normal at all times.

Joe is now a student at the junior high school. His speech remained normal, he has been an average student academically, and he has always been well-liked by his teachers and peers.[2]

TREATMENT OF SCHOOL-AGE CHILDREN

The dynamics of the treatment of school-age children and their mothers will be illustrated in the following excerpts from two cases.

The Case of Don: A Child from a Large Family

In October, 1958, Donald S. was referred by the kindergarten teacher because of his severely defective articulation. He was then 5 years, 2 months old. He was the fourth in a family of eight children, 5 boys and 3 girls. He was a good-looking boy of bright to superior intelligence.

Both of Don's parents had college degrees. Don's father had 2 sisters and his mother had 7 brothers and 1 sister. Two of the mother's brothers stuttered. Don's parents enjoyed having a large family and were very dedicated to their children. The family lived in a medium-sized house and as the mother had no domestic help, often there was a good deal of confusion in the home. The parents' relatives lived in other states, and when the mother went to the hospital to give birth to another baby, the father stayed home and took care of the children.

---

2. Further to help the reader envisage the therapeutic process, we have added a verbatim transcript of a tape-recorded interview between a therapist and the mother of a young stuttering child, to be found in Appendix XVI.

Don's birth had been full term and the mother had had a normal delivery. Don suffered from pneumonia during the first year of life and had severe allergies until he was 4 years old. He was bottle-fed and began drinking from a cup when he was $2\frac{1}{2}$ years old. He had had the usual childhood diseases but had never been hospitalized. He began to walk at 10 months. The mother did not recall when Don began to speak; she remembered, however, that he spoke later than his older brother and sisters. He was approximately 3 years old when he tried to speak in sentences. Until then he "would take somebody's hands and demonstrate through gestures what he wanted."

When Don was referred, a therapist made a visit at his home and found both parents, surrounded by four young children. Don's parents expressed great interest in helping him with his speech.

Don had weekly sessions with a speech therapist who also instructed the parents how to help him at home. As soon as Don received intensive and individualized verbal stimulation and auditory training, his articulation improved, and a year later his speech was considered normal. In first grade Don's speech remained normal.

Shortly before Don was to enter the second grade, Mrs. S. telephoned Don's former therapist and reported that Don had begun to stutter. Soon afterwards, I observed Don in the classroom. Don's second-grade teacher was a quiet, soft-spoken young woman whose teaching program was well organized. However, when she called upon Don he appeared tense, he twisted his lips and mouth trying to form words, and he spoke with repetition of initial syllables and, occasionally, with prolonged vowel sounds.

Don's previous therapist and I then visited Mrs. S. at home and learned more about the onset of Don's stuttering. Mrs. S. had had another baby and while she was away at the hospital the father again had taken care of the children. At that time the ages of the children were as follows: boy 11 years, girl 9 years 6 months, girl 8 years 6 months, Don 7 years, boy 5 years 6 months, boy 4 years, girl 2 years 6 months, girl 1 year 3 months. The new baby was a girl. Soon after the new baby came home she fell ill and lost weight, and there was considerable concern in the family about her condition. Three weeks after her birth Don appeared to have difficulty in communicating. At that time his best friend, Johnny, who lived next door, went away for two weeks. In earlier years, Don, because of his incomprehensible speech, never had had a friend outside his own family. Johnny was his first personal friend and Don had become very much attached to him. When Johnny came back from his vacation he told Don that he and his family would be leaving for good. Don seemed very much upset about this and told his mother: "I feel very sad, Johnny is going away forever!" The baby's birth and illness and Don's loss of his friend all had occurred within a few weeks. Mrs. S. felt that Don's difficulty in speaking was connected with this crisis situation.

The same therapist who had helped Don earlier with his articulation was assigned to see him again every week; she also planned to have occasional conferences with his teacher and mother. As Mrs. S. was very much occupied with the care of her baby and with illnesses in her large family, the therapist actually had only two conferences with her and one with both parents. Contact between the mother and the therapist, however, was kept up through occasional telephone calls.

The dynamics of the therapeutic interaction between Don and his therapist can be glimpsed in the following excerpts from the therapist's records. (Not all sessions will be reported here.)

September 30:
Don seemed emotionally upset when I saw him this week. He had just experienced a scene in the classroom that caused him to cry in front of his classmates. His teacher had reprimanded him sharply and asked him to stay after school. When the class was dismissed his teacher spoke gently to him; Don stopped crying and appeared to be comforted. When he met me in the hall a few seconds later, it seemed to me that he was struggling to cover up his feelings and to keep me from noticing that he had been crying.

We went to the teachers' room on another floor, and walking upstairs, Don had time to compose himself. He told me that his friend, Bryan, had stuck his tongue out at the teacher. I asked him if Bryan liked the teacher and Don said: "Yes he does, but he gets mad at her sometimes." I explained to him that we all get mad at people even if we like them.

Don stuttered only slightly during this session.

October 7:
When we sat down in the teachers' room, immediately Don asked me "Why don't you say 'What's new?' like you usually do?" He was bursting with pride because of the new jacket he was wearing. He said his older brother got a new one too. He explained that some of the children get new jackets this year and others wait until next year. This gave me an opportunity to talk with him about how we have to share lots of things in a large family, including time alone with parents. He said he was almost never alone with his mother. I asked him if he felt he would like to be alone once in a while with his mother. His answer was "Yes," but he began to fidget in his chair and look away which made me feel that he didn't want to discuss this any further.

We looked through a book together, which Don really enjoyed. We came to some animal pictures and I asked him about his friend the chipmunk who eats from his hand. Don got up from the chair and walked to the window and said, "Jim has a very bad throat infection." He seemed quite nervous. I asked him if he knew what that meant and when he said "No" I explained that Jim had a sore throat and would feel much better in a couple of days. Don didn't want to talk about the chipmunk or Jim any longer. I felt that if I could reach him without upsetting him too much, it would be valuable to talk about ambivalent feelings we have toward people we love. I mentioned that if somebody in our family is sick we feel very bad, especially if we have been mad at that person. I reassured Don that all people at times feel this way. Don seemed relieved and smiled almost in gratitude that we had talked about it.

At the mention of his mother, Don began to talk about how much he misses her when she has her babies at the hospital. He said that when Susy was born he hoped his mother could come home in one day and leave the baby there. He went into great detail about the baby's illness, and said: "My mother did come home before the baby." He said the baby was still sick when she came home and she had "green stuff" in her mouth. I told him I knew he felt badly when the baby was sick and perhaps he felt worse about it because he wished his mother didn't have to leave home to have the baby. Don next said that his mother had left him to have Ben, Jim, Ann, Michelle, and Susy.

I noted that Don said "she left me" rather than "us." He also mentioned Ben, who actually was born before him.

October 14:

Don seemed anxious to talk about his family and more than at other meetings he wanted to tell me about situations that particularly disturbed him.

He mentioned that his brother Jim's throat was better and he was back at school. Jim often "bosses" him. They share a bedroom and Jim makes him do all the errands. He makes him turn out the lights every night. "I pull up the covers and hide my eyes so Jim will think I'm asleep." I feel that Don "hides" in situations he cannot face and keeps his worries, anger, and guilt to himself. I asked him if he would try to speak up to Jim and make him take a turn with the errands. "It wouldn't do any good. He would make me do it anyway." I asked him if he ever complained about Jim to his mother and he said "Sometimes."

As we were leaving Don said: "Some of my friends think you are my mother." I told him that I do many things with him that mothers do, spend time alone chatting with him, and so on.

Don stuttered frequently during this session.

October 21:

Don was not anxious to talk with me today. He was more quiet than usual and I thought I perceived a hostile feeling toward me. I wondered if he didn't regret telling me about his feelings of anger toward his siblings and his mother during our last visits together.

Don had a library book in his hand and when I asked him about it he sat down and fumbled through the pages to find three photographs that interested him especially. The subject of the book was World War I. Don turned first to a picture of a dead child on a war-torn street. Next he turned to a picture of fighting soldiers that showed one of them dead. The third picture showed a group of children eating food rations.

After showing me these special pictures, he went carefully through the whole book and talked about each photograph. The book obviously was too difficult for a second-grade reader and I asked him if he planned to try to read it. He said he got the book for Jim. I told him that I thought it was a fine idea to get a book that Jim would like. Don let me know that he wanted to go home.

October 28:

Today Don stuttered very little. He was happy to see me and appeared very relaxed. He showed me two books he got from the bookmobile. One was his and he wanted me to hear him read one of the stories. The other book was for Jim. He talked at great lengths about his relationship with Jim. The other day Jim asked him to do an errand for him and he refused to do it until Jim gave him a model airplane. Don seemed very pleased that he had made a point with Jim. He wanted me to know that he likes Jim very much but he does not like his bossy manner. He told me that he no longer shares a bedroom with Jim but sleeps with Ben. Ben is afraid at night; he is afraid of shadows at the window and imagines people in the room. "I tell Ben it's trees that make the shadows and he shouldn't be afraid, because Jim is right across the hall."

Conference with Don's mother, October 28:

I spoke with Mrs. S. and, as always, she was extremely interested and cooperative in regard to Don's problems. I explained to her that I was trying to find what kind of things Don worried about. She said that Don had always been a worrier. She spoke of the time when he was 3 and 4 years old and had horrible nightmares and many fears. I asked her if she would try to spend time alone with Don, talking to him, especially if anyone in the family was ill.

December 2:

Today Don had some difficulty with initial sounds. He brought a book with him from the bookmobile and read part of it aloud to me and we talked about the story. Don loves to read aloud and takes pride in his ability to read. When we finished the book, he began to talk about a recent automobile accident in which four boys had been killed.

We talked about the fact that accidents usually occur when people do foolish things. I tried to explain to him that if we use our heads we can avoid many accidents. Don told me how careful he is when he rides his bike: he doesn't ride in the street, he comes in the house before dark, and so on. It seemed to me that Don was worried that accidents could happen to him.

December 9:

Don brought a library book and we looked at it together. When we finished talking about the book, he appeared to be nervous and walked around the room. He seemed to have something that he wanted to talk about. Suddenly he blurted out: "Jim's eye isn't getting any better and he may have to wear glasses forever; Ben might be getting cross-eyed too; Ann's eye is worse, my mother thinks."

I tried to reassure him, telling him that many people wear glasses from the time that they are children until they are grown up, and that this is really not a terrible handicap. Children who wear glasses have just as much fun as other children do. I told him that his mother takes the children to a very fine doctor who knows how to take care of them. We are lucky to have fine doctors to help us. Don seemed relieved and asked "We are?"

We talked at length about how sensible it would be for him to ask his mother about these things as they come up, rather than worry about them quietly. His mother may be busy, but I was sure that she would explain things to him as I did, if she knew he was worried. Sometimes when we hear adults talk about things we don't really understand, we worry unnecessarily.

I told him that I knew he loved his brothers and sisters and wanted them to be well. I stressed again that though we love our brothers and sisters we sometimes get very mad at them and perhaps this makes us feel worse when they are sick or when something goes wrong for them. Don listened very carefully each time we talked about ambivalent feelings, but did not make any comment. I think that he didn't dare take an active part in the conversation.

Conference with Don's parents at their home, December 18:

Mrs. S. mentioned that Don had frequent displays of temper. In one instance, this upset him to the point where he was not able to go to school. I tried to impress upon the parents that they should use their regular kind of discipline with Don at all times, whether he was stuttering or not. It would be harmful to him, as it would be to any child, to find that familiar boundaries were gone. They both reassured me that they were trying very hard to carry out a normal discipline with Don. Mrs. S. said that when she was a child, she and the rest of her family were frustrated a great deal because her mother felt that a brother who stuttered needed extra privileges and care. She wondered whether she was perhaps harder on Don than she would be normally.

Often I had mentioned to Don that he should try and "push" for time alone with his mother and father, and I spoke of this to his parents. I was interested to hear that Don does ask his mother—more often than she can oblige—to take him alone on errands, and the like. Mrs. S. said that this was new for Don, and that she spends time with him as often as she can without upsetting the balance of privileges in the home.

I am always impressed with the sincerity of these parents and the efforts they are making to treat all their children justly.

December 28:

Today Don told me that Jim broke his ankle and his leg is in a cast. I asked him how it happened and I thought he said: "I don't know, really, I didn't do it, I was in bed." Don spoke softly and I couldn't be sure of what he said, so I asked him to repeat. When he answered he did not include "I didn't do it." I must watch carefully in the future for an indication that he feels responsible for accidents that happen to his siblings.

January 8, 1961:

For the past three weeks Don has been speaking very well. He brought his library book with him as usual and we talked about it for a few minutes. He was not interested in talking with me and he made it clear that he was in a hurry. He planned to do Jim's paper route with his sister who was waiting at home for him. I didn't see any point in holding him there against his wishes, so our meeting was very brief. I told him that I thought it was a fine idea to help Jim with the paper route. "Oh, he pays me all right," was his reply.

January 13:

Don read to me from a book that he brought with him. I noticed that he stuttered very infrequently in conversation, but when he tried to read he had pronounced difficulty with the first sound in the first word of almost every sentence. He stuttered in reading words that were very familiar to him. In the past, Don had never stuttered while reading aloud.

Within the past month Don had been advanced to the second reading group. He loves to read and always takes books home. My experience with Don at the time when he had severe articulation problems made me feel that he is intense about doing a good job. Perhaps he is driving himself hard to keep up with his new reading group.

I talked with him for some time about how well he reads; how fine I think it is that he enjoys reading; how hard he has worked; and what a great deal he has accomplished since he started school.

January 24:

Don read aloud to me for a few minutes and had severe difficulty in starting every sentence. Since he had begun to stutter frequently while reading aloud very soon after the report cards were sent home, I discussed his report card with him today. Don said that he had seen his report card but he added, "I don't know if it was good—all right, I guess." I asked how he was marked for reading and his reply was "Oh—what does 'ability' mean?"

I had spoken with Don's mother on the telephone to try to find out what Don's report actually had been. The mother reported that Don had been marked as "not working up to his ability." Mrs. S. had stated that she and her husband were pleased with Don's report card.

I told Don that his teacher was pleased with his progress and so were his parents. Also I explained to him the meaning of the word "ability"; I told him he was a smart boy and his teacher wanted his parents to know that she expected him to be an excellent reader some day.

When we finished this conversation Don finished reading the story. He did not stutter at all. Coincidence?

January 27:

Today Don did not stutter during conversation. He read five pages of a second-grade reader rapidly and with ease.

I believe that Don had been anxious about his progress in reading because he had mis-interpreted his report card. I spoke with him again today and stated how pleased we (I, teacher, parents) were with his progress in learning to read. I mentioned again that he had accomplished a great deal since he entered school. Don seemed pleased but a little bored with this conversation. He had heard it from me last week. I notice that when Don is free of stuttering symptoms, he is impatient when he has to spend time with me. He seems to have a lively interest in people and activities and lets me know that he has more important things to do than talk to me.

February 24:

Today Don spoke well and seemed to be relaxed. He told me that his sister, Ann, had cut her foot on a sharp can that fell out of the waste basket. "Her toe was hanging off." Don made a face telling me how bad it looked. He said that his mother did not have the car so she called a neighbor and the neighbor drove Ann and his mother to the hospital.

Don thought that was very kind. He said his mother told him that there was nothing to worry about in case of an emergency because if one of the neighbors did not have a car available, she would just call the police and they would be glad to give her a ride. Mrs. S. must have been careful to reassure Don in this instance. This is the first time that Don has not stuttered when telling about one of his siblings.

Note: Mrs. S. seems to take the time to explain to Don exactly what is happening when she feels that he may not understand a situation. Perhaps Don is now better able to ask his mother about things that he does not understand, or to tell her when he feels uncomfortable. I have talked to Don and his mother in this regard. May we assume that here we have evidence of a change in the relationship between mother and child?

I also noticed in the past few weeks that Don often refers to his mother as though he were closer to her. This is a new feature in Don's conversation.

March 3:

Today Don spoke well. He was anxious to get out to play in the spring-like weather. I told him that I thought that was a fine idea. I did not want to hold him up. I mentioned to him that I noticed he did not stutter anymore. "No, not much, and I am glad," he answered.

Conference with Don's mother, March 3:

I phoned Mrs. S. today to ask her if Don was stuttering at home. She said that she mentioned to her husband last night that Don had not been stuttering lately. She added: "As a matter of fact, almost not at all." She told me that she was very pleased about the fact that Don had a "best friend" again. They seem to enjoy each other very much and have good times together. This is the first close friend Don has had since little Johnny moved away.

Note: I feel that this new friendship may be further evidence that Don is less anxious.

March 10:

I have noticed that when Don is not having difficulty with his speech he is not interested in spending time with me. Today I perceived an attitude of polite detachment from me. I feel that Don did not want to talk with me, he had other, more important things to do. I wonder if it is a good time to end therapy with Don or to continue with less frequent meetings.

Note: In conference with the psychiatric consultant it was decided that I would see Don once a month for the remainder of the school year. During a short visit at Don's school I explained this to him and he seemed pleased with the idea. I also called Mrs. S. to inform her about the change in our schedule.

April 14:

Today Don seemed embarrassed to have me waiting for him after school. He walked ahead of me so that his friends would not wonder about where he was going.

When we reached the teachers' room where we usually talk, Don relaxed and seemed friendly. I asked him about his report card. "Oh, it was good." He was very proud of his report. I asked him about reading and other subjects. "I don't know. They must be good."

When we finished our conversation about his report card, Don told me that he was in a hurry to get home so he could do Jim's paper route. Jim had a cold. I asked Don if he liked to help Jim doing the paper route and he answered, "Oh, I don't like to do it, but the girls won't do it and Ben is too little." He added that he helps Jim because Jim was good about teaching him how to play baseball. "Jim teases me a lot, but he does favors for me, too." I told him that Jim must appreciate help and that I would not keep him any longer.

Note: Here is further evidence that Don is now closer to his mother. His mother made it clear to him that his report card made her proud, without examining it with him in detail. The last time Don had a report card, he knew what was in it and misunderstood the ratings.

I think that Don is beginning to accept his ambivalent feelings toward Jim. He used to get very mad when he spoke of Jim; later he seemed guilty about his feelings for him; now he talks about this relationship in a matter-of-fact way.

Conference with Don's mother, May 3:

I spoke with Mrs. S. today to tell her that we had decided that Don did not need to see me on a regular basis any more. Don seemed to be ready to end therapy. Mrs. S. agreed with me that Don had changed a good deal. Not only had his speech improved to the point where he hardly ever hesitated, but he seemed to be at ease in many ways. He has close friends, he doesn't display a quick temper, and in general, he is "easier to live with."

May 4:

I saw Don briefly during school hours today. We went to the nurse's room to talk. He seemed happy he didn't need to see me every other Friday.

During the following year Don met the therapist occasionally in the school building. Two years later, at the time of our evaluation of treatment results, Don spoke well and his mother reported that he had never had a relapse into stuttering.

Altogether, the treatment of this case consisted of 19 sessions with Don, 2 conferences with his mother, 2 with both parents, and occasional telephone conversations with his mother. We must not forget, however, that because of Don's earlier articulation difficulty, he and his parents had already been familiar with the therapist and this may have shortened his treatment.

COMMENTARY

Don's case presents certain features with which we are already familiar. It is typical in certain aspects and atypical in others. Contrary to other cases—to be discussed in Chapter 11—Don's stuttering did not occur as a secondary reaction to the frustrations caused by his articulation difficulty. Don's stuttering has to be considered as an independent communication disorder (developmental stuttering), appearing *after* he had overcome his original difficulties in articulation of speech sounds. His stuttering began during a typical crisis situation: He had lost access to his mother because of the birth and subsequent illness of another baby; he resented the new baby and then felt guilty when the baby was sick. Thus, we find again the core problem of the stuttering child: agression-anxiety, that is, anger against the mother combined with the fear of losing her. To make things worse, Don had lost his only friend at a time when his relationship with his mother had become precarious. In Don's case—as earlier in the case of Nana—several disturbing events occurring simultaneously had contributed to a developmental crisis.

The late onset of Don's stuttering is of interest. Don was 7 years old at the time of onset, in contrast to the large majority of the children in our sample who had begun to stutter before they were 6 years old. However, Don did not talk until the age of 3. It seems justified to assume that his linguistic schemata were not as well established as those of other 7-year-old children. His frequent illnesses during the first four years of his life may have contributed to his delayed language development, at the same time making him overly dependent on his mother. When he made friends with Johnny he had for the first time in his life attempted to transfer some of his allegiances and communications from his mother and other family members to a person outside the family. Identification with his new friend may have helped Don gain a sense of identity and separate himself from his brothers and sisters. When his friend left him "forever," while at the same time his mother was inaccessible to him, his intense feelings of loss and disappointment interfered with his language processes, and regression to early repetitive speech (stuttering) resulted.

In getting help from a familiar therapist, Don found a person who spent time alone with him, communicated with him without linguistic restraints, matched her words with his, and helped him to verbalize his feelings of anger, guilt, and anxiety. While the therapist served as a temporary mother substitute for Don, she also encouraged him to communicate more often with his real mother and to take his confusions and disappointments directly to her. Parallel to her work with Don, the therapist interpreted to the mother Don's urgent need to communicate with her and the fears and inhibitions which kept him from doing so.

The themes which Don brought to his therapist centered around his resentment of his mother's frequent absences, his wish that the baby would have stayed at the hospital, and his feelings of guilt and anxiety when the baby was ill. These, in turn, led Don to express his apprehensions when one of his siblings had an illness or accident, and his ambivalent feelings toward his brother Jim. With the help of his therapist, Don talked about his brother Ben's and his own fears and nightmares. Finally, he was able to face some confusions about himself, his role in the family, his personal identity, and his own "goodness" or "badness," expressed in his worries about his report card and "ability." Most of Don's worries can be seen as a child's intense reactions to actual difficulties in his life situation. His therapist responded by helping him to verbalize his feelings and by clarifying his misunderstandings. Thus, the therapist also remained primarily reality focussed.

Don's treatment had been relatively easy and was accomplished in a short period of time. Positive factors in the child, as well as in the parents, contributed to this favorable outcome. In spite of his anger and ambivalence. Don had not yet lost his trust in his parents or in other helping adults. He easily established a positive relationship with his therapist and later was able to "push for time" with his mother, to transfer his expectancies from the therapist back to his mother, to establish a relationship with a new friend, and to give up his close relationship with the therapist when he felt sufficiently sure of his relations with his parents, with Jim, and with his new friend.

Positive factors in the family situation were the parents' sincere interest in their children, their loving relationship with them, and their desire to be just to all of them. Don's mother, in spite of her busy schedule, managed to spend time alone with Don, and she talked to him and reassured him when one of his siblings suffered an illness or accident.

In Don's case, the stuttering and the disturbance in the mother-child relationship were caused by reality situations beyond the mother's control, rather than by deep-seated interpersonal conflicts. The successful outcome of Don's therapy was due to the basic soundness of the family and the skill of the therapist. Also important was the fact that Don had received help very soon after the onset of his difficulties, before he developed advanced symptoms of communication disorder and debilitating defense mechanisms.

The frequency of language disorders in Don's family should be noted. Two of Don's younger brothers showed moderately defective articulation when they entered kindergarten. Don's mother had two stuttering brothers. However, we must remember that the mother herself grew up in a family of nine children. We have every reason to assume that similar conditions in both families—the large number of children and the lack of individual attention and feedback—may have caused similar communication disorders. We do not know the exact nature of the language disorders of Don's uncles, but we see no reason to introduce the assumption of an innate or hereditary disposition to stuttering.

The Case of Budd: Disturbance in Family Communication

One third example, the case of Budd, is in marked contrast to the case of Don. The nature of the mother-child relationship and the dynamics of the treatment process in each case differ considerably.

HISTORY

Budd and his mother, Mrs. R., were referred to the research project by a pediatrician. Budd was then 6 years 2 months old. He had two younger brothers, George, 4 years, and Mark, 1 year. Budd lived in a neighboring town and attended a private kindergarten.

I paid a visit to Budd's home and met the intelligent, young mother with her three handsome, strong, and healthy looking little boys. The small house was very neat and clean and the mother seemed determined to run her home and her family in an efficient manner. Though Budd spoke with considerable stuttering (Rating 5-6)[3] he was very friendly, showed the visitor his toys, and talked a good deal.

Both parents were present at the intake interview. The father was an engineer and also took evening courses to earn a college degree. The mother had attended junior college. The father reported that he had "stuttered" for about a year during his early childhood. He remembered that he had "repeated words"; his mother had told him that his "stuttering" had disappeared gradually. The father had an older sister, and the mother had an older brother and an older sister. The R. family frequently visited the father's parents, who lived nearby, and also spent summer vacations in the grandparents' beach house.

The mother's pregnancy and delivery had been normal. Budd was breast fed for six and a half months. The mother described Budd as being "different from his brothers from the very beginning." He screamed very much and got angry easily. He stood up at 5 months and began to walk at 10 months. Generally he was in

---

3. See Appendix II.

good health, but had frequent, painful ear infections. His hearing was normal. Budd always had been extremely active and was easily frustrated "when he could not do something." He had rocked in bed at night and had banged his head against his crib during his early years.

Budd began to speak at 22 months, at the time when his younger brother George was born. Budd, who was then a "very tense child," stayed with the mother's parents while the mother was in the hospital. Returning home the mother was surprised to find that Budd had learned many new words. Soon afterward, the family moved to another house in the same town. A boy next door spoke with very poor articulation. The mother reported that she was afraid "Budd would speak like the boy next door" and that she corrected Budd's speech a great deal at that time. Soon after the move Budd began to stutter. He was then 2 years 9 months old.

Budd had resisted toilet training strongly but his mother persisted in her efforts to train him. Her attempts at toilet training coincided with the beginning of his stuttering. The mother remarked in this connection: "I do not have much patience, I can get very mad."

Budd's stuttering had fluctuated; at times it seemed to disappear, at other times it got "very bad." When the parents tried to correct him, his speech got worse. "In the beginning he repeated words, then syllables and whole sentences. Then he began having difficulty with breathing—he stiffened and held his breath. Sometimes he exclaimed 'Hey!' and after that he could speak." The parents described Budd as a very tense child "who screams and screeches and stiffens." At the same time they stressed that Budd was "really a very gentle, serious child and basically a very sweet kid."

In the fall of 1962, at the age of 5 years, Budd had entered kindergarten. He loved school, was not at all shy, and talked a great deal during "show and tell" time.

Budd's case was evaluated and a therapist was assigned to work with mother and child. It was felt that both parents were intelligent, well-meaning people who tried hard to provide a good home for their children. However, the prediction was made that this would be a difficult case because of the mother's apparent rigidity and Budd's marked tension and advanced symptoms of communication difficulty.

THE TREATMENT PROCESS

The prediction turned out to be correct. The treatment process extended over 24 months, an unusually long period for a young child. Altogether the therapist had 2 therapeutic encounters with mother and child, 53 with the child alone, 35 with the mother alone, and 2 with mother and father together.

The therapist's first meeting with mother and child, April 1963, was a difficult one. The therapist wrote the following report about it.

Mrs. R. came today with Budd. I played and talked with him to demonstrate to the mother how to provide the child with corrective feedback. I offered Budd a play kit,[4] but he was reluctant to take toys out of the box. He looked at them with interest but waited for permission to touch them. Finally, he started to make a fence with blocks and then said he didn't want to do that. He took the animals out of the box and stood them up. All the animals were close together and he said they were all friendly. Then Budd placed trees and flowers around on the "farm." He did not at any time show an interest in the people. I asked him if he could use the people and he answered "No." When he finished with the toys, he carefully put them back in the kit. He spoke frequently as he played. Once he repeated one of my phrases in the same manner that I had repeated his words to him.

Mrs. R. sat at the table while we sat on the floor. Each time I looked in her direction, she was looking out of the window with her back to us. When I finished with Budd and sat down at the table, Mrs. R. immediately said: "Am I supposed to interrupt him when he speaks, the way you do?" Mrs. R. then directed some conversation toward Budd. She asked him to tell me about his new rabbit. She asked Budd several questions. Budd had more difficulty speaking as he answered these questions than he did while he played with the toys. Mrs. R. was upset that I did not hear Budd stutter very much and remarked that she knew that I interrupted him before he stuttered. She wanted to demonstrate his difficulties to me by engaging in this question–answer conversation. I told Mrs. R. that children always have less difficulty speaking when they play with toys. I did not want to continue talking to Mrs. R. in Budd's presence.

Note:

Mrs. R. seems to feel hostile about my work with Budd. I do not believe I interrupted him as he talked. It must be difficult for this mother to be shown how to talk with her child.

COMMENTARY

In the course of our work we learned that it was unwise to give a mother demonstrations of therapeutic communication patterns during the first meeting with her and her child. Many mothers were not able to benefit from such early demonstrations. It is preferable to have one or two meetings with the mother alone and one or two with the child alone before seeing them together. During the first individual conference the mother, as well as the child, gets to know the therapist and begins to understand the meaning of the therapeutic situation. Once the nature of communication therapy has been understood by the mother, she begins to perceive the difference between corrective feedback and word matching, on the one hand, and interrupting the child, on the other.

THE FIRST THREE MONTHS OF THERAPY

During the spring, the therapist met primarily with the mother, trying to help her to become aware of her own manner of communicating with Budd. Several important themes emerged during these sessions. The mother confessed that she had been extremely irritated with Budd's stuttering symptoms. Often she had told him not to talk to her because she could not stand his stuttering. She

---

4. G. von Staabs, Sceno Test (1952). The kit contains building blocks, a family of bendable dolls, including babies and grandparents, and small toys in the shape of cars and trains, household objects, trees and flowers, and domestic and wild animals. The material can be used either for play therapy or as a projective test.

felt that she had tried hard to do a good job with her children and that Budd, through his stuttering symptoms, demonstrated that she was an incompetent mother. "My husband and I love our children, we do get along with each other, we do not have big problems—but Budd's stuttering shows everybody that something is wrong in our family!" The mother dreaded mealtimes in particular, when Budd in his father's presence talked and stuttered a great deal. She said: "I sit on the edge of my chair waiting for him to have difficulty."

With the help and reassurance of the therapist, Mrs. R. gradually became more tolerant of Budd's symptoms. In May she reported that she was "no longer afraid of Budd's stuttering. When he begins to tell me something I sit down and give him my full attention." Gradually the mother began to listen to Budd and to spend some time alone with him every day, sharing his interests and matching words with him occasionally. The mother reported: "I now feel much less upset about Budd's stuttering because I am now doing something about it." The fact that Budd's speech improved at that time further relieved the mother's anxieties.

However, it was not easy for this mother to change her manner of relationship to her child. When the therapist asked the mother, early in June, whether she still spent time alone with Budd, the mother replied: "He does not like to spend time to sit with me, he would rather be outside." The therapist suggested that a time might be found which was more convenient for Budd, but Mrs. R. responded: "Budd thinks it is silly for me to sit and look at books and talk to him." Asked what they talked about, the mother reported she asked Budd directly what was bothering him. It was only after her own relationship with the therapist was more fully established that the mother began to listen to her son patiently and let him introduce the topics of their conversations.

At the same time, Mrs. R. tried sincerely to change her approach to Budd. Earlier in therapy she had described the recurring domestic battles between her and Budd, and had stated: "He should know that I will never change my mind!" Now she began to wonder whether her manner of controlling Budd's behavior was appropriate.

The therapist reported:

Mrs. R. mentioned that the other night her husband had told her she was hard on Budd, he wished they would not have so many clashes. Mrs. R. thinks that she has been trying consciously to have fewer scenes with Budd. She feels that when she and Budd "get into a bind" with each other they are each trying to win a point. She wondered whether sometimes she did not give orders to Budd just because she wanted to see if he would mind her or put up a fight. I told Mrs. R. that she seemed to be examining her motives for "getting into binds" with Budd. Without blaming either her or the child I suggested that in situations like this it was easier for the parent to initiate changes than for the child. I said that I understood how difficult it was to cope with a stubborn, aggressive child. Mrs. R. said quickly: "I need to change and I am trying."

THERAPY DURING THE SCHOOL YEAR 1963–64

Mrs. R. telephoned the therapist early in September, asking for an interview before she "blew her stack." She reported that at times Budd was so blocked that he would turn around in circles before he was able to get a word out. The therapist saw Mrs. R. on the following day. She learned that during the summer vacation mother and child had not been as "relaxed" as the mother had hoped. The maternal grandfather, who was particularly fond of Budd, had reprimanded her for having so many clashes with Budd. She described several of these clashes to the therapist, stressing that Budd antagonized her so much that she finally "blew up." During August, when Budd's father joined the family for two weeks, Budd was sent to a day camp. The mother felt that "It was good for the whole family that Budd was not at home during the day. George really came out this summer. He had a chance to shine!" Budd's father had objected to sending Budd to camp, but Mrs. R. felt that she needed "a quiet vacation." The camp director had observed that "It was obvious that Budd needed a lot of affection." This remark had upset Mrs. R. very much.

The therapist then asked the mother whether she was still spending some time with Budd, now that they were all at home again. Mrs. R. reported that Budd usually was "not interested" in spending time with her, got very mad when he could not talk, and told his mother how mad he was.

It was obvious that Budd and his mother were again in a severe "bind"— as the mother so aptly called it. The therapist told the mother that from now on the treatment would include Budd. Budd had already asked his mother whether he could see the therapist and get help. The therapist reported:

In my conference with Mrs. R. I explained to her again the nature of corrective feedback, and pointed out to her that this kind of communication was different from the usual conversations with a child of Budd's age, that it was a technique of communicating which we found most helpful with stuttering children, and that it was something that I could teach her to use with her child at home.

After the next session the therapist reported:

Mrs. R. joined Budd and me to observe how I use corrective feedback in conversation with Budd. I put out some crayons and paper for Budd to use. He didn't want to draw a picture. I asked him what his dog looked like. He began to describe the dog to me as I drew the picture. Budd was careful to test crayons on a piece of scrap paper before handing them to me. Next Budd drew a picture of his rabbit. He was cautious as he did this and asked his mother occasionally how to make a part of the body. Budd said his dog doesn't like the rabbit, he tried to bite him. I asked why the dog disliked the rabbit and he said he didn't know.

Next we looked at a book together. At one point in the story, the little elephant was frightened and unhappy and the illustrations clearly showed his feelings. I asked Budd how he thought the elephant felt and he answered that he did not know.

Mrs. R. seemed to pay careful attention to what was going on. This was quite different from the last time she observed me with Budd.

This session was used to show Budd and his mother that expressions of unhappiness and of negative feelings are not necessarily a deterrent to communication.

On October 1 Budd and the therapist met again, and the therapist reported:

Today Budd used the *Staabs* kit again.[5] He carefully took the blocks and animals out of the box. He looked over the people—picked them up and put them down without commenting. He chose not to use the people. I asked him why and he said he didn't need them.

Budd set up three play yards with the blocks. These areas were separated by fences. He put the animals in these yards. He mixed up the animals—did not separate them according to species. I asked him if they all get along, the fox and chickens, for example. He said that they do. The animals whispered secrets to each other. Budd would not tell me what they were saying. I told him that I thought it was all right for them to have secrets. One of the two foxes was a "bad fox." He scared all the other animals. Budd isolated the fox. The dog tried to tell the fox to be good. The fox escaped one night. The goose ran to tell the monkey, in charge of all animals. The monkey put the fox back in isolation. I asked Budd how the fox felt all alone. Budd said he didn't know. Again the fox escaped when the monkey was asleep. He went to scare the other animals. The horse trampled him. The monkey again was called by the goose. The monkey was very mad and made angry noises as he brought the fox back to his cage. I asked Budd if this fox was always bad. Budd said that he was. I asked him about the other fox in the next yard. Budd said the other fox was always good. I mentioned that this was unusual; I would think the bad fox might be good some of the time and the good fox be bad some of the time. Budd thought about this and answered that it was not that way with these foxes. Budd repeated again the escape of the fox. When the fox was safely locked behind the fence, Budd decided he was through playing.

Budd carefully put each piece back in the kit. Everything had to go where he thought it belonged and where it fit the best. While he was putting things away, a child was hollering on the playground outside. Budd said that the child was being "too noisy." I asked Budd if it wasn't all right to be noisy on a playground. He did not answer me. A few minutes later Budd dropped a block (on purpose) and made a face. He wanted me to know that he did not like the sharp noise. I told him it was perfectly all right for him to drop the block and make a noise, it did not disturb anyone.

Note:

Budd seems to see things in black and white. The good and bad fox; the quiet and the noisy; the correct and incorrect way to put toys away. All this makes me think that Budd's own standards of right and wrong are clear-cut. He seems so definite in these matters that there doesn't seem to be a chance for compromise. I think he was showing me the good and bad in himself.

During the course of the school year the therapist saw Budd once a week, while the mother came for conferences every two weeks. Budd then was attending the first grade at the local public school. In working with the mother and the child, the therapist had the opportunity of observing the similarities in their personality structures as well as in the themes they both presented. Gradually the therapist began to understand better the nature of the conflicts and "binds" between this mother and her child.

Mrs. R. had a conference with Budd's teacher and learned that Budd was doing very well in school and was in the top reading group. His teacher was pleased to hear that "Something was done for Budd's stuttering." Mrs. R. mentioned to the therapist that she was not astonished to hear that Budd stuttered at school; Budd did not like new situations, new things, new clothes, or meeting new

---

5. G. von Staabs, Sceno Test, *op. cit.*

people. She felt that getting started in new situations was difficult for Budd, but once she had forced him into it, he seemed to have a good time.

Mrs. R. also expressed her resentment at her husband's being away from home so much because of his work and his classes. She said that she sometimes got very mad at her husband and "clams up." She stressed that she did not like noise and would do anything to avoid a scene with her husband. When the therapist asked whether Mr. R. knew when his wife was angry with him, Mrs. R. replied that her husband could tell that she was angry when she was quiet. She added: "Maybe if I could scream at my husband, I wouldn't scream at the children so much!" The therapist asked whether she ever discussed her worries with her husband, and Mrs. R. replied that she never talked to him about them.

Mrs. R. then revealed that two of her close relatives had had bad marriages ending in divorce. There had been much "screaming and yelling" in the homes of these relatives, and this had upset her very much. She desired so much to have a perfect marriage and to bring up her children well.

In discussing mealtime situations in her home, Mrs. R. complained that Budd's eating habits were bad, he "chomps on his food and makes more noise than necessary. I don't like noise." She often sent Budd away from the table when he was noisy. On such occasions Budd used to have temper tantrums and would stay in his room for half an hour before returning to the family. In October, Mrs. R. reported that she now tried to explain to Budd why she did not like his behavior, and she assured him that she loved him even though she disapproved of his manners. She was happy that Budd now seemed less upset; when he was sent away from the table he returned to the room peacefully after a few minutes. The mother felt that she scolded the children less than she used to do, and also that she "spoke out to her husband more," telling him more often when things annoyed her.

In his sessions with the therapist, Budd showed many signs of rigidity and denial of feelings. For a long time he refused to have anything to do with the people in the play kit. He refused to reveal his own feelings, even indirectly by telling how the "good" and "bad" animals felt. When his therapist continued to ask him how the animals felt, he became angry at her and told her to stop talking. At some point in therapy he even developed a signal to keep the therapist from talking about things which he disliked: he looked straight at her and raised his hand, which meant "Stop talking!" Toward the end of October his therapist reported:

Budd made a large fence with the blocks from the *Staabs* kit. He put all the animals in together, except the monkeys who were outside the fence as usual. Budd did more talking than playing today.

The animals were friendly and got along well together. The monkeys fed them and gave them water. Budd picked up a racing car and pushed it carefully around the edge of the table. The racing car began to knock down the fence. Budd said the car was mad at the animals. He would not say why. The fox got mad and bit the car twice. One of the trees kept getting knocked down by Budd's sleeve as he pushed the car. Obviously he was annoyed by this and I asked him if that made him mad. Budd became annoyed with me—he does not like to discuss feelings—and said that he does not like to come to see me. I asked him why.

Budd said he would much rather be outside playing with his friends. I told him I did not blame him, what we did together was not play. I asked him if he noticed that it was more like work. He said that he did. I told him that it was not easy to talk about feelings. I explained that this kind of work would be of help to him and might cause his speech to improve.

I asked Budd how things were going in school. He said three children in his class did not mind the teacher. I asked Budd if the teacher hollered at them. He said that she did. He had a new workbook and he missed some of the words. I asked him if the teacher got mad at him. He said that she did not as she knew the work was hard. I asked him if it made him mad and he told me that it did make him mad, as he would like to know all the words. I explained to him that he couldn't know all the words yet. Wasn't it all right to make a mistake? Budd seemed annoyed at this suggestion and answered that he didn't like to make mistakes.

Note:

Budd is better able to say that the animals and people (including himself) get mad.

He seems to have much less difficulty with his speech. The change has been gradual. He now takes deep breaths less frequently. While he is playing with the toys his comments are fluent.

In November, Mrs. R. reported that her husband would go out of the state for a few months on business. He had promised to telephone every night and to come home for weekends as often as possible. She was afraid that she would feel lonely when her husband was away and she alone had the responsibility for the three little boys. She seemed very much upset and depressed about this threatening change in her life.

In spite of her depressed mood, Mrs. R. continued to try hard to avoid clashes with Budd. Describing Budd's refusal to eat squash, she said in an amused manner: "Budd is as stubborn as I!" The therapist continued to recommend that Mrs. R. should talk things over with Budd, trying to understand his reasoning as well as explaining hers to him.

On December 5, Mrs. R. asked the therapist, for the first time, what she and Budd were doing during their therapeutic sessions. The therapist reported:

I told her we use toys and games as a way to talk about feelings. "I try to help Budd to talk about his feelings and to urge him to talk to his parents about many things." I reminded Mrs. R. that my job was to help Budd understand that it was all right to express feelings, but the biggest job was hers. She was the most important person to Budd and it was important that he felt free to talk to her. Mrs. R. quickly said that the system seemed to work. She now felt "well informed." Budd now told her everything that went on in school. She thought that she was careful to tell Budd her reasons for expecting him to obey her. She found him more cooperative.

I asked Mrs. R. how Budd felt about his father's work in Maine. Mrs. R. said that she didn't think it bothered him. She had noticed when the father had come home the first weekend, the little children ran to him, but Budd stood back and waited for his father to approach him. I asked Mrs. R. to explain to Budd what kind of work his father was doing while he was away from home.

In December, for the first time, Budd did not avoid people in his play session. He chose puppets to play with, in particular the witch, the pirate, and Santa Claus, and acted out a big fight between them. All the puppets apparently were quite mad at each other but—as usual—Budd would not explain why they were fighting or what they were mad about. While the puppets were fighting Budd made loud, angry noises with his mouth. It was a way of testing the therapist, finding out whether it was dangerous to make angry noises; it also was a way of keeping the therapist from talking.

Budd and his mother seemed cheerful before Christmas, looking forward to having the father home for the holidays. However, in her first meeting after Christmas the mother again seemed in a very bad mood, and announced: "Everything is horrible!" Budd's speech was bad again and he had been disagreeable and jealous of his brothers. The mother also complained about all the work and the rushing around before the holidays, when her husband had not been at home to help her. She felt tired and tense and mentioned that her patience was very low.

The therapist stated that she was not surprised to hear that Budd had more difficulty communicating during the Christmas vacation, as many stuttering children had increased difficulties or relapses into stuttering at that time. Mothers were busier than usual and it was more difficult for a child to have access to the mother. The therapist understood that this had been a very difficult week for Mrs. R., particularly as she did not have the accustomed help from her husband.

Mrs. R. reported that her husband had asked her what she and Budd were doing with the therapist. She had told him that it was a great help for her to have somebody to talk to who was interested in her child, it helped her "to blow off steam." Her husband had expressed his interest in meeting with the therapist. A conference with both parents was arranged for later in January.

During January Budd continued to show more aggression during his play sessions. He also was more aggressive at home, in particular with his younger brother George. Mrs. R. complained to the therapist, asking: "What is he trying to do to me?" The therapist explained that children who are in therapy often begin to act up a little at home, as they try out different ways of expressing themselves. Mrs. R. then described the following incident: Budd was in the bathtub and he shouted that he wanted a towel. Mrs. R. told him to wait a minute, as she was busy with the other children. Budd kept screaming for a towel. His father was busy downstairs and shouted to Budd to be quiet, he would get him a towel in a minute. Budd kept screaming. Mr. R. ended up by spanking Budd and putting him to bed, without allowing Budd to read to him. Later, Mrs. R. went into Budd's room to talk with him. She told him that he must know why his father spanked him. "He is teaching you—you have a lot to learn and he is trying to help you." Budd said he would never read to his father again or show him any school papers. She said that she knew he was mad at his father at the moment, but maybe he wouldn't be mad the next day. The next morning Budd showed his father a school paper. Mr. R. smiled and said that he had thought Budd would not show him any more papers. Budd hugged his father (a very unusual thing) and said he had only been mad last night. Mrs. R. said her husband was thrilled that Budd hugged him.

The therapist wrote in her record:

I was thrilled too. This is the first real sign of change in all three—father, mother, and child. I told Mrs. R. that it seemed to me there was in this story evidence of a great deal of progress. Mrs. R. looked puzzled. I pointed out to her that Budd had talked to her about his anger; she had explained the father's motive in spanking him so that he understood; Budd was able to tell his father the next morning that he was only mad for a while; and his father was pleased with the hug and was not punitive about Budd's angry feelings. I told Mrs. R. that even though Budd's speech was still poor and his behavior was frustrating, when things like this occurred it meant that Budd was making progress.

Mrs. R. agreed. "That was nice, wasn't it?" she added.

A week later Mrs. R. complained to the therapist that her house was a mess, that George was repeating words a lot—was he beginning to stutter?—that Mark had poor articulation, and at times she felt overwhelmed trying to do a good job raising three boys. The therapist agreed with Mrs. R. that it was not easy and complimented her for trying so hard to help Budd. Mrs. R. was close to tears as she replied: "I really do care." She was happy to report that her husband soon would be home again. She mentioned that she was so excited at the thought of his return that she had had a headache all week.

Budd's speech improved gradually. During his sessions with the therapist he often showed two sides of his personality, the violent and the quiet. Often he began a session with violent play, acting out fights with the puppets which he called devils, father, mother, or pirates. After this acting-out period he would put the puppets away and read with the therapist, or write words he knew. Thus, at times he put the therapist in the role of the ambivalently loved mother, and at other times in the role of a supportive teacher. In March he talked fluently at school; at home and in his therapy sessions his speech was fluent most of the time, but occasionally he held his breath before he began to speak. The therapist wondered whether this breath-holding was another way in which Budd tried to control his feelings, and also to control the person with whom he was speaking.

Mrs. R. had become more understanding and skillful in her attempts at spending time with Budd. Once when Budd read to her he stuttered somewhat and she was so upset about it that she told him she did not like his stuttering. Budd got visibly mad and refused to read any more. The next day when his mother asked him to read to her, he answered that he would not read as it would only make her mad. Mrs. R. apologized for being impatient the day before. She explained to him that she was very proud of his reading and loved to hear him read. Budd then read to her and afterward, mother and child talked a long time together about school, play, and all sorts of things. Mrs. R. happily told the therapist how much she had enjoyed the conversation; it had really been a rewarding experience. She began to see that Budd could be good company! The following evening Budd read to his father and when he had finished he said to him: "All right, let's talk now." Mr. R. was delighted with Budd's initiative and told his wife about it.

In March, Mrs. R. told the therapist that a "wonderful thing" had happened with Budd the night before. He and his brothers had been wrestling and carrying on after supper and after several warnings her husband finally sent them to bed at 6:30. Half an hour later Budd came down and asked his mother to come up-stairs and "talk this over" with him. His mother was very pleased to find out how much her bedtime talks with Budd meant to him.

In April, Budd played a game with the therapist and through most of the hour he talked freely with her about his younger brother George. At the end of the session Budd asked the therapist whether she had noticed anything: "I did not tell you to stop talking today!" Apparently, Budd had become less anxious about hearing his therapist talk about feelings, and expressing his own feelings in words. *The act of speaking, which had been an instrument of ambivalence and hostility in his clashes with his parents, had now become a medium to establish friendly and trusting relationships with people.*

However, Budd's rigidity and his fear of new situations still existed. On two occasions the room in which he usually met the therapist was unavailable and he had to have his session in another room. Each time he was angry about the change and seemed to blame the therapist for it. Once when the therapist was a few minutes late, he was exceedingly angry at her, but was not afraid of expressing his anger openly. It appeared that new situations still aroused in him a good deal of anxiety.

Budd and his mother continued their therapy sessions for another six months. Budd had become much more able and willing to talk with the therapist, rather than to express himself primarily through play. He liked to talk about school; he still disliked it if the teacher "hollered or yelled", and he still seemed to be afraid of the teacher's anger. He still had symptoms of mild to moderate stutter-ing which were most evident when he read aloud. The therapist spent considerable time reading aloud with Budd, often "reading together." Budd began to show a sense of humor about his fears and at times he talked laughingly about his teacher's, his mother's, or the therapist's anger. He seemed less worried about making mistakes. He tried to help his brother get used to school, and was surprised when George did not seem to need any assistance. Budd remarked wistfully to his thera-pist: "Everything is easier for George!" Although Budd now discussed many of his daily experiences with the therapist, he still decided when and how much he would talk about a certain topic; he still needed to control his sessions.

As the year went on, Mrs. R. reported fewer clashes or "binds" between her and Budd. They often disagreed on something, but she no longer felt the previous rage against him and the strong desire to "win" every time. Mr. R., who no longer attended classes, spent more time with his sons. Often he had long chats with the three boys, in which they planned how they could cooperate with their mother instead of fighting her. This kind of support from the father obviously was very gratifying to the mother.

In April, 1965, Budd himself wanted to terminate his treatment. He wanted to play outside after school instead of seeing the therapist. He was very outspoken about this, and broke into tears when he talked to his therapist about it. When the therapist told him that they had had many good times together and that she had enjoyed seeing him, he stopped crying and talked and played for the remainder of the hour. Mrs. R., in her next meeting with the therapist, supported Budd's wish; she felt that Budd had a right to make this decision. At the same time she herself wanted to keep up her relationship with the therapist a little longer.

The termination of Budd's therapy was discussed with the psychiatric consultant. The therapist felt that Budd had made great progress in his behavior; that he was better able to cope with his feelings and found it easier to establish relationships with others. He still showed occasional symptoms of mild to moderate stuttering. The consultant recommended terminating the treatment; she suggested that over a period of weeks Budd might further integrate the gains he had made and might give up his symptoms.

In the fall of 1965, Mrs. R. reported that Budd had, indeed, become symptom free during the summer.

Budd's father had changed his job and his new firm had sent him to the West Coast for advanced technical training. The whole family had spent the summer in California, and they had had "a marvelous time." Budd had decided to take swimming lessons. He swam well and he and his family were proud of his new accomplishment. Budd seemed to have lost his fear of new situations and he thoroughly enjoyed all the new sights and activities which California offered. The family had to live in a motel, but though they shared cramped quarters, they all seemed to enjoy each other and quarrels were at a minimum.

Back in their own home, Mrs. R. wrote to the project director: "When a child is as unhappy as Budd was, it affects the whole family. We certainly were in a turmoil—but we are not any more. . . . Budd's and my therapy has been invaluable for all of us. I have learned so much about Budd and myself. I always felt that we were a close family and now I know that we are and will be. . . . We all thank you so much for your help and interest—it is most difficult to want to help your child and not to know how to accomplish it. . . . I hope that you too have gained some knowledge in working with Budd and that this in turn will help other children. . . ."

COMMENTARY

Budd's case demonstrates certain essential features of the psycholinguistic syndrome of stuttering. Budd's communication difficulty had its onset during a "critical period" in language development, "a period of maximum susceptibility to developmental modifiers" (Garrard and Richmond, 1963). Compulsive repetitions first began to appear in Budd's speech when he was 30–31 months old, seven months after the birth of his brother George, but only a few weeks after his family moved to a new home. It coincided with the mother's insistence upon toilet training and her corrections of Budd's speech, based on her fear that he might speak "like the boy next door." This period of time, during which the mother gave birth to a new child, had to move, and attempted unsuccessfully to train her older child, can well be regarded as a crisis in the R. family, which in turn led to a crisis in Budd's development. Again—as in the cases of Nana and Don—we find that the disruption of language learning began at a point in time when several stressful factors impinged upon a young child; a child, moreover, who had been described as congenitally tense and easily frustrated.

Individual differences in children's primary reactions to environmental stress have been described by a number of investigators (Pulver, 1959; Chess, Thomas, and Birch, 1959; Birch, Thomas, Chess, and Hertzig, 1962; Thomas, Birch, Chess, and Hertzig (undated); see also Eichorn, 1963). Thomas, Birch, Chess, and Hertzig pointed out that children's organismic characteristics, combined with their primary reaction patterns, may significantly influence the mother-child relationship. The same maternal approach may have a different impact on babies with different reaction characteristics, while babies with differing reaction patterns may influence the mother's response in varying ways. The care of infants with more intense, negative response patterns causes more work and effort and is less gratifying for the mother, who, in turn, may develop reactions of tension and rejection of the infant.

One of the striking features in the case of Budd is the similarity in reaction patterns between mother and child, which was further elaborated in the similarity of their neurotic fears and defenses. In their overt behavior both appeared to be tense, rigid, stubborn, angry, and anxious. Both also were intelligent, attractive people, with a strong need to master and control their environment. Both showed a strong desire to get out of their incapacitating "bind." Both had difficulty in controlling their aggressive and destructive impulses. The anxiety caused by these impulses, threatening to overwhelm the ego, was reflected in the mother's fears of noise ("yelling and screaming"), of "blowing up," and that she might destroy her marriage if she expressed her anger toward her husband. Anxiety was also reflected in Budd's parallel fears of noise and of anger in the teacher, the therapist, his parents, and himself; in his avoidance of talking about his feelings; and in his need to control the therapist, lest she increase his aggression-anxiety.

Therapy with this child and his mother differed in many ways from the treatment of Don and his mother. As mentioned earlier, the disruption in Don's relationship with his mother was caused by reality situations beyond the mother's control. In Budd's case the disruption was more severe, indicative of an intense conflict between mother and child. The differing dynamics of the two cases affected treatment techniques and the length of time necessary for successful therapy. Both Don and his mother developed a positive relationship with the therapist, and the content of the therapy sessions was primarily reality oriented. Both Budd and his mother had highly ambivalent attitudes toward the therapist and much of the therapy had to be carried out in an atmosphere of negative transference. The strong tendency toward denial or avoidance of feelings in both child and mother caused them to present their problems and worries mostly in an indirect or symbolic form, particularly during the first year of treatment. This displacement was demonstrated in Budd's play with animals and blocks and his avoidance of people and in the mother's complaints about noise, her misperception of the therapist's demonstrations, and her difficulties in carrying out the therapist's recommendations.

The specific dynamics of the personalities and relationships made Budd's case much more difficult than Don's for the therapist. It should be stressed, however, that the salient features observed in the case of Budd can be found again and again in the treatment of stuttering children and their parents. Evidently, *the treatment of children with severe stuttering, which means with severe disturbances in the areas of relationships and communication, calls for unusual skill in the therapist.* Trying to intervene in such situations of severe interpersonal conflict also is a very stressful experience for the therapist. The support and advice given by a mental health consultant are indispensable for the therapist, who must be helped to cope with her own feelings of frustration and anxiety, which are unavoidable in the course of the therapeutic process.

Of great interest in this and similar cases are two additional features: the communication barrier in the family and the role of the father in family dynamics.

We have reason to assume that Budd's mother was angry at her husband, who had to be away from the home a great deal and thus did not give his wife the help she needed and desired in bringing up three lively little boys. Her fear of "blowing up" and of destroying her marriage through her anger, caused her to bottle up her feelings, thus setting up a barrier in her communications with her husband. In this connection we remember that Budd's play animals were whispering "secrets" to each other, indicating Budd's feelings that open communication was noisy and might be dangerous. Mrs. R.'s repression of her anger at her husband led to a displacement of her negative feelings upon her children, in particular upon Budd, who thus became the family scapegoat. Mrs. R. herself became aware of this when she exclaimed: "Maybe, if I could scream at my husband, I wouldn't scream at the children so much!"[6]

Such barriers, or outright taboos, in the communication between parents or between parents and children were found frequently in our sample of stuttering children and their families. In two of our cases the disturbance in communication was so extensive that father and mother no longer talked to each other, but used the children to deliver messages between them. Thus, the treatment of the stuttering child, in some instances, may have to include not only the child and his mother but also the father and—at least indirectly—other members of the family as well.

The core of the disturbances in such cases seems to lie in a communication of negative messages, first between the mother and the child and later involving others. Sensing the disruption in the family network of communication reinforces the stuttering child's fear of communicating and contributes to his growing conviction that communication is dangerous and may lead to violence and destruction. The role of the therapist, thus, can be seen as that of a helping person who inserts himself into the network. Through his example, his listening, providing of corrective feedback, teaching, and interpretations, he demonstrates to the members of the family the possibilities and benefits of mutually adaptive communication. This

---

6. The dynamics of using a child as symbolic representative of the parent's repressed feelings have been particularly well described by H. E. Richter in *Eltern, Kind und Neurose*, 1962 (*Parents, Child, and Neurosis*).

must eventually supersede the debilitating patterns of mutually interfering communication existing between family members.

The role of the father in the family communication system is of great importance. The behavior of Budd's father can be considered typical of many fathers of stuttering children. R. L. Douglass, of California State College, has aptly described the behavior of these fathers as an attempt to be uninvolved, to remain outside the "battleground," the protracted conflict between the stuttering child and his mother.[7] As the father withdraws from his stuttering child, the child loses a potential ally and, in the case of boys, a model for appropriate sex behavior. In our work with older stuttering children we commonly observed a marked paucity in the communication between father and child. With boys, we saw an inability to assume a masculine role. This, in turn, led to marked passivity in many older stuttering boys, which at times was broken by sudden outbursts of rage and violence.

Because of the marked preponderance of male stutterers and the psychodynamics of the stuttering syndrome in boys during the latency years and during adolescence, we found it advantageous to employ male therapists for the treatment of older stuttering boys. Young stuttering children may experience the female therapist partly as a substitute mother and partly as a helping teacher; similarly, older stuttering boys will relate to the male therapist as a father substitute, as an older brother, and at times as a helping teacher or counselor. In trying to communicate with a male therapist, the stuttering boy learns to try out new and more comfortable patterns of communication, to reach out for and eventually to communicate with his distant or seemingly inaccessible father, and eventually to communicate successfully with other male authority figures, previously dreaded. As his fear of communication diminishes under the guidance of his therapist, *the stuttering boy finally will take the initiative in communicating with his father.*

The change from passivity to initiative was well illustrated in Budd's case. First we saw his "standing by," waiting for his father to approach him when he came home for Christmas vacation; later, his spontaneous hugging of his father, making peace with him after a fight; finally, we saw his invitation to his father: "Now, let's talk!" This invitation obviously delighted his father.

COUNSELING THE PARENTS OF OLDER STUTTERING CHILDREN

In Budd's case direct counseling of the father was kept at a minimum. It was the father himself who wanted to learn more about what was going on in the mother's and the child's therapy sessions. Earlier the father had made unsuccessful attempts to intervene in the continued "binds" between his wife and Budd. Later, he reacted positively to the improved relationship between them and to Budd's direct approach to "talk together." At this point, the father became a partner in the

---

7. Personal communication, 1964.

therapeutic process. Thus, the trend toward "mutually interfering communication" was reversed early in the history of the R. family and "mutually adaptive communication" was established.

In the families of older stuttering children we often find disruption, or even disintegration, of family communication, and extensive family counseling may be necessary to reorganize the family communication system. In our project, a parent counselor of either sex was assigned to attempt this restructuring process with the parents, while a male therapist worked with the stuttering boy.

Parent Counseling[8]

A close working relationship between parent and counselor develops in the course of this particular type of treatment. Parents discover that the relationship built up during their counseling sessions is in itself a sort of laboratory where they can try out new ways of looking at things and can plan new ways to be constructive in handling problems at home. They find that it does help them to talk freely about genuine but frequently distressing feelings. Eventually they experience the deep satisfaction that comes from coping with human difficulties in a mature and responsible way.

The atmosphere of the sessions is encouraging and supportive. The parent does most of the talking. The counselor points out themes, clarifies feelings, and helps the parent understand how emotions influence the ways in which we act. On occasion, the counselor suggests changes in the parents' approach to child-rearing. The counseling process, then, is based on expressions of feeling by the parents and active involvement by the counselor.

Very few of the parents in our sample were seeking help for themselves, and almost none anticipated the extent of involvement that was expected of them. Therefore, it was necessary to motivate them by explaining how counseling could help them in helping their children.

A sound counseling relationship requires mutual trust and respect. In the early phase meetings should be frequent enough to permit the counselor to get acquainted with the parents, to show his interest in their concerns and his acceptance of their feelings about them. For this reason, parent counseling usually began with one session a week, to be followed by one session every two weeks, once a working relationship between parent and counselor had been established. All mothers of older stuttering children in our sample came for individual counseling sessions. In addition, fathers were seen as often as possible and, in many instances, the counselor also saw both parents together.

Gradually the parents gained insight into their child's personality dynamics and emotional needs, and also into their own reactions to the child's symptom and

8. The following section is based upon a paper, "Counseling the Parents of Older Stuttering Children," presented by Ronald F. Dutton at the 38th Annual Convention of the American Speech and Hearing Association, New York, N.Y., November 1962 (see Wyatt and Collaborators, 1962).

behavior. Parents came to see the importance of the emotional atmosphere in the home, the nature of the relationship with the spouse, and the opening-up of outlets for bottled-up anger in both themselves and their stuttering child. Sometimes, a mother learned to see her children more clearly, as people with differing competencies, emotional needs, and levels of maturity. One parent was delighted to discover: "Suddenly, the kids have become real people!"

Many parents desired information about specific approaches to discipline. Some asked for marriage counseling. A few seemed to benefit from learning about rational decision-making.

During the counseling process, long-standing emotional barriers to effective action had to be cleared away. Such barriers were (1) denial of problems, (2) rigidity, (3) anticipatory worrying, and (4) lack of faith and trust in other members of the family. When the problems seemed overwhelming, we heard statements like this: "Lots of times I feel like a little girl, but then I know I ought to get more responsible." This particular mother did become more responsible; after 17 sessions she made a different statement: "I like the new me."

Frequently we found that a child's progress in therapy was slowed down because one or both parents, quite unknowingly, were using the child to satisfy their own emotional needs. Some of these parents' needs could be met through the counseling relationship itself. Other needs were satisfied more wholesomely as better relationships were developed with the spouse, with relatives, and with adult friends.

Parents needed help in three areas: (1) better handling of the child's expressions of feelings; (2) better family relationships; and (3) better communication with the child. Purely intellectual understanding had to be translated into conviction and drive leading to improvements in the home. Sometimes a great deal of change was needed when the home atmosphere was chilly. For example, much of the warm, free-and-easy atmosphere had disappeared from the home of a mother who stated in a matter-of-fact way: "I act towards the children just as I act towards company."

When children began to express their feelings and fantasies at home, most of these parents tended to feel punitive or retaliative. Whether or not the parents kept such reactions to themselves, they felt guilty and depressed. One of the primary purposes of counseling was to let the parents see for themselves how the counselor accepted the parents' genuine feelings and handled discussion of sensitive matters. From this experience, the parents learned new ways to react when their children confronted them with their feelings, thus acting toward their children in the way their counselor acted towards them.

In some cases we had to resolve major breakdowns in family communication, when cooperation was at a standstill and parents were living together for long periods without saying a single word to each other. We intervened in these crisis situations, bringing about a frank discussion to "clear the air" of smoldering irritations, misunderstandings, and resentments. Such crisis-intervention had an unexpected by-product. The tremendous relief felt by the parent who had until then been less involved in counseling—usually the father—acted as a lever to bring him into the treatment program with full cooperation.

Our efforts to help the parents enjoy a relaxed and natural relationship with their child, within which he could express feelings and communicate well, focused on what we came to call the "Time-for-Johnny Campaign." Each parent was recruited for that campaign.

Just as mothers of younger children were urged to spend time with them individually, so too, parents of older stutterers were advised to find time every day when they could sit down alone with the child and have an informal chat about his activities, his wishes, his concerns, or whatever he felt like talking about. It was impressed on the parents that this period of time together should not be used for a speech lesson or any form of tutoring; rather, it should be given to a free-flowing conversation in which the child and his interests came first. Most often, these chats took place just before the child's bedtime, but sometimes they followed help with homework or joint work on another project.

The parents received several ground rules to follow in carrying out the Time-for-Johnny Campaign. These rules were (1) give the child your full and undivided attention; (2) make clear to him your eagerness really to understand whatever he is trying to put into words; (3) let him set the course, don't probe; (4) help him straighten out any misunderstandings or worries he may have; and (5) give particularly close attention and sympathetic attention to things he says that may seem trivial, inconsequential, or silly. The latter may be the things the child has been hesitant to express for fear of getting a cold shoulder.

Toward the end of the counseling process, the counselor's role changed considerably. As the parent became more effective, the counselor functioned more as an interested but somewhat less involved consultant. Problems in improving family communication were dealt with as they came up, but this was handled on a less frequent schedule, perhaps with a session every month or so.

We found that as the parent achieved more satisfying relationships, the child also built relationships more easily. In one case, we could see clearly how the parent's progress had a direct effect on the child's adjustment, when the mother reported: "I've made quite a shift this year. I used to discourage the children's friendships, but I see now from what I'm doing myself that it's better to make ties and sink roots. I am trying to help them now to get along better with their friends."

The termination of counseling was prepared for well ahead of time. Gains were highlighted in a brief review, and parents were given specific suggestions about how to handle a potential crisis. A crisis might develop if the formerly stuttering child found himself in a situation involving a major change, such as the inaccessibility of a person because of unexpected absence, illness, or death. To some children, changes such as moving or entering a new school might mean a crisis. At such times, the former stutterer would need particular attention and support and should be given a prompt chance to express his feelings in words. The parents were also urged to refer the child for a checkup if a relapse into stuttering should occur, or to get in touch with their counselor should they feel the need of further help for themselves.

After the parent counseling process had run its course it ended much as it had begun, on a hopeful note. The parent was graduated with assurance that he would be able to cope with future problems, to consolidate wholesome relationships, and to meet the child's emotional needs effectively.

It is important to remember that this type of parent counseling ran parallel in time with intensive treatment for the child. This form of joint treatment requires unusually close collaboration between the team of therapists working with members of a family. The child's therapist and the parent counselor have to keep informed on a session-by-session basis about the problems and themes with which each worker is dealing. Time and again, the two therapists may be able to attack a difficulty from both sides, working together to bring parent and child closer to each other.

The collaboration between the two workers included joint planning of treatment strategies and joint progress evaluation. The two therapists also saw the psychiatric consultant together for supervision. We believe that this close collaboration is essential for the successful treatment of older stuttering children.[9]

---

9. As this book goes to press, a paper has come to my attention in which a combination of techniques has been described which were used successfully in the treatment of an older stuttering boy (Ruderman and Selesnick, 1968). The treatment patterns resemble our own techniques, though with some modifications. The authors, a female social worker and a male psychiatrist, working at the Cedars-Sinai Medical Center in Los Angeles, California, used "multiple avenues of approach" to the treatment of a 10-year-old boy. Over a period of 2 years and 10 months the boy was seen in individual psychotherapy by the female social worker, who also saw the parents once a week. In addition, at particular times, the therapist met with the whole family—the boy, his sister, and his parents—and she also conducted auxiliary sessions with the boy and his father and the boy and his sister. Furthermore, in an unusual procedure, the male psychiatric consultant met directly with the patient and his therapist "at highly significant moments" during the treatment period. Thus, although the boy worked with a female therapist, the particular modifications of the treatment process—joint sessions with his father and with the male consultant—made it possible for him to develop a male identification and eventually to accept the male role.

CHAPTER NINE

Treatment Results

Any form of therapy, independent of its theoretical foundations, can be judged only through an evaluation of the results obtained. Parallel to our therapeutic activities we worked on developing a methodology which would enable us to identify significant variables, to collect and analyze data, and to evaluate the treatment results. Eventually, during the spring and summer of 1964, we assessed the results of the treatment of 28 stuttering children (See Wyatt, 1964a).

TREATMENT OF TWENTY-EIGHT STUTTERING CHILDREN

Termination of Treatment

Whenever a therapist, or a team of child therapist and parent counselor, recommended termination of treatment, this recommendation was discussed in a conference with the chief investigator and the consulting psychiatrist. Once termination was agreed upon, the frequency of the sessions with child and parents was reduced before actual termination. In 15 cases termination was carried out in this manner prior to the spring of 1963, while treatment with 10 children was continued during the school year 1963–64; these cases were terminated in May, 1964, when the research project came to an end. In two cases termination was decided by events beyond the therapist's control: in case 4 the child's family moved to another state, and in case 17 the child died of meningitis.

The Evaluation Form

A form was developed which permitted the analysis of variables in the following areas:

1. Age of child at onset of stuttering.

2. Age of child at beginning of therapy.
3. Change in therapists.
4. Time spent in therapy with mother and child, with child alone, with mother alone, with father alone, and with father and mother, as well as total number of therapeutic encounters.
5. Complexity of problem, additional problems.
6. Ratings before and after therapy in the areas of severity of stuttering, social effectiveness of family, and mother's cooperation and therapeutic readiness.[1]
7. Role of significant adults other than parents.
8. Additional variables:
   a. Characteristics of child and of parents which contributed to child's improvement.
   b. Characteristics of child and of parents which worked against improvement.
   c. Factors in the child's life situation during treatment which contributed to improvement and factors which worked against improvement.

Each case was evaluated by the therapist—or by the therapist and parent counselor, in the case of older children—and by two independent raters. The evaluation was done independently by each evaluator and the ratings then were discussed in a joint session in which the raters reached a consensus. Items on which no consensus could be reached were excluded from tabulation. The ratings established were tabulated and statistical comparisons were worked out for certain variables.

Criteria for Improvement

As mentioned before, severity of stuttering was rated from a score of 7 ("infrequent, severe stuttering") to a score of 1 ("normal speech, appropriate for the child's age"). Ratings in each case were based on observations made by the therapist plus two other observers, such as a parent, a teacher, or the chief investigator. Two types of change can be represented on the scale (Appendix V): A movement from 7 toward 1 indicates improvement in speech, while a movement in the opposite direction indicates aggravation of the symptom.

In analyzing the data it became evident that the steps on the rating scales were not equidistant. Thus, an improvement indicated in a move from 7 to 4 cannot be called equivalent to the improvement indicated in a move from 4 to 1. In the first case, the child has moved from frequent, severe stuttering to infrequent, moderate stuttering. While this indicates improvement in his speech, he still must be considered a stutterer. In the second case the movement of 3 steps indicates that the child has acquired normal speech, appropriate for his age. As normal, or nearly normal speech must be the ultimate aim of therapy, it was decided that all children with a terminal rating of 2 or 1 would be listed as "improved".

---

1. See Appendixes IV, Rating Scales, and V, Ratings before and after therapy.

In addition, children who had started treatment with a rating of 7 and who had moved as far as a rating of 3, at the time of evaluation also were listed as improved.

Using the above criteria of improvement, the following speech ratings were established at the time of the evaluation.

	Rating	Cases
	1	10
	2	11
Movement from 7 to 3		1
Improved		22
Movement from 7 to 4		1
„ „ 5 to 4		2
„ „ 5 to 3		2
„ „ 5 to 6		1
Unimproved		6

Age of Child at Onset of Stuttering

Information concerning this variable was available in 25 cases. According to parental reports, the onset of stuttering occurred before the age of 6 years in 21 cases, and after the age of 6 years in 4 cases. The difference is significant at the .001 level ($\chi^2 = 22.88$).

These findings agree with those of our pilot study, 1958–59, and with our theoretical assumption that stuttering in most cases presents a deviation in language learning. They also support our hypothesis of a critical period for the onset of stuttering (age 3 to 6).[2]

Change in Therapists

Twenty children were treated by one therapist only, while 4 children had 2 therapists in succession. Of the 20 seen by 1 therapist, 15 improved, while of the 4 seen by 2 therapists, 3 improved. If a change of therapist was necessary it occurred as a rule at the beginning of the new school year; thus the separation from the original therapist was already somewhat removed in time when the new therapist took over. Because of the low threshold for separation anxiety which we had observed in stuttering children, the children were always prepared for the change ahead of time. Of the 4 children who experienced change in therapists, 3 reacted with mild, temporary difficulties, while 1 (unimproved) reacted with severe and prolonged difficulty.

---

2. See also Penfield and Roberts (1959).

Of the 27 mothers—1 the mother of 2 cases—20 worked with 1 therapist or parent counselor, 4 worked with 2 in succession, and 3 worked with 3 counselors successively. While several mothers expressed regret at losing the original therapist, no mother showed strong resistance to the change.

Age of Child at Beginning of Treatment and Time Needed for Successful Therapy

It was our hypothesis that children whose treatment began before they were 7 years of age would show marked improvement or return to normal speech after a significantly smaller number of therapeutic encounters than children whose treatment began after they were 7 years of age. In our previous study, this hypothesis had been confirmed at the 1 per cent level of significance (Wyatt, 1959).

Of the 28 children in the present study, 22 were listed as improved and 6 as unimproved. Of the 22 improved children, 12 were under 7 years of age at the beginning of treatment and 10 were over 7 years of age. The number of therapeutic encounters for the improved cases ranged from 3 to 91, and the total time elapsed in the course of treatment ranged from 3 months to 26 months.

Table 6 presents a comparison between younger and older improved cases with regard to number of therapeutic encounters and total time elapsed.

TABLE 6—COMPARISON BETWEEN YOUNGER AND OLDER IMPROVED CASES

Over 7 Years at Beginning of Treatment			Under 7 Years at Beginning of Treatment		
Case No.	No. of Sessions	Time in Months	Case No.	No. of Sessions	Time in Months
4	79	13	2	88	24
5	78	15	12	55	26
6	72	15	15	36	13
8	64	19	17	27	19
9	62	14	20	23	11
10	59	25	21	12	8
11	56	15	23	9	8
16	32	12	24	5	5
19	25	20	25	5	7
22	10	7	26	3	3
			27	3	5
			28	3	6

N = 10
No. of Sessions = 537
Median = 60.5
No. of Months = 155
Median = 15

N = 12
No. of Sessions = 269
Median = 10.5
No. of Months = 135
Median = 8

Application of the Mann–Whitney Test, for two samples (Moses, 1952), yielded the following results:

1. Number of treatment sessions—$U = 20$, $p < .01$ (1 tail). The median number of treatment sessions is greater for the older group (over 7).

2. Months of treatment—$U = 32.5$, $p < .05$ (1 tail). The median number of months of treatment is greater for the older group (over 7).

Thus, there is a significant difference between the two groups, both in time elapsed and in number of therapeutic encounters. As in the pilot study, our hypothesis was confirmed: *Therapy with stuttering children under 7 years of age is more economical in time and expense than therapy for stuttering children over 7 years of age.*

Duration of Stuttering Before Referral for Treatment

An analysis was made concerning the amount of time between parents' first awareness of the child's stuttering and his referral for treatment.

It was our assumption that therapy with stuttering children and their mothers should be initiated as soon as possible after the onset of stuttering, before the child has developed secondary or advanced symptoms. The hypothesis to be tested was: Children who were referred for therapy less than 3 years after onset of stuttering should show less severe symptoms (ratings 3, 4) than children who were referred more than 3 years after onset. The time of onset was established in 24 cases. Of these, 14 had been referred less than 3 years after onset, while 10 were referred 3 to 7 years after onset. Table 7 shows the relationship between the time elapsed between onset and referral, and the severity of stuttering at the time of referral.

TABLE 7—TIME ELAPSED VERSUS SEVERITY OF STUTTERING

Less Than 3 Years Elapsed Between Onset and Referral

Severity of Stuttering	No.
High (ratings 5, 6, 7)	6
Low (ratings 3, 4)	8
Total	14

More Than 3 Years Elapsed Between Onset and Referral

Severity of Stuttering	No.
High (ratings 5, 6, 7)	8
Low (ratings 3, 4)	2
Total	10

There is no difference between the groups. χ^2 with Yates Correction = 1.9. We must conclude that the severity of stuttering observed at the time of referral was independent of the time elapsed between onset of stuttering and the time of referral. However, the number of cases is very small and the power of the test would be minimal.

Ratings Before and After Therapy

In addition to the rating scale I, Severity of Stuttering, the following rating scales were developed: II, Social Effectiveness of Child's Family; III, Mother's Cooperation and Therapeutic Readiness. (See Appendixes IV and V.)

Appendix VI shows the number of therapeutic sessions for each case, the age of each child at the beginning of treatment, the severity of stuttering at the beginning and end of treatment, the family's social effectiveness at the beginning and end of treatment, and the mother's therapeutic readiness at the beginning and end of treatment.

Actually the steps on Scales II and III—like those on I—were not equidistant. On the Social Effectiveness Scale (II) scores 5, 4, and 3 indicate an essentially unfavorable environment, while 2 and 1 indicate a favorable one. On the Scale of Mother's Therapeutic Readiness, (III), scores 4 and 3 are close to each other, as are 2 and 1. A change from 3 to 2 in social effectiveness thus indicates a significant, positive change in the child's environment. Similarly, a change from 3 to 2 on the scale of the Mother's Therapeutic Readiness indicates a significant, positive change in the mother's behavior and in her insight into the child's difficulties.

For the purpose of data analysis, the ratings on Scales II and III were, therefore, divided into high and low. Correlations were investigated between the number of treatment sessions up to termination and the initial ratings in each case concerning severity of stuttering, the family's effectiveness, and the mother's therapeutic readiness.

The following hypotheses were formulated:

1. Children whose rating in severity of stuttering is low at the beginning of treatment (ratings 3 or 4), will acquire normal speech with significantly fewer therapy sessions than children whose rating is high (ratings 5, 6, or 7).

2. Children whose families rate high in social effectiveness at the beginning of treatment (ratings 1 or 2), will acquire normal speech with significantly fewer therapy sessions than children whose families rate low in social effectiveness (ratings 3, 4, or 5).

3. Children whose mothers rate high in therapeutic readiness at the beginning of treatment (ratings 1 or 2) will acquire normal speech with significantly fewer therapy sessions than children whose mothers rate low in therapeutic readiness (ratings 3 or 4).

These hypotheses were tested statistically. Comparisons were made for (a) all cases, improved and unimproved, and (b) improved cases only. Cases with number of sessions greater than the median and those with number of sessions fewer than the median were compared with regard to severity of stuttering, family's social effectiveness, and mother's therapeutic readiness, all rated at the beginning of treatment. The statistical results are presented in Appendix VII.

In comparing improved cases only, no significant difference was found with regard to severity of stuttering, family's social effectiveness, or mother's therapeutic readiness, all at beginning of treatment.

However, when all cases were compared as to number of treatment sessions, the following differences resulted:

1. Children whose rating in severity of stuttering was low at the beginning of therapy (ratings 3, 4) tended to be seen for fewer sessions than children whose ratings were high (ratings 5, 6, 7) (χ^2, Yates Correction = 7.15, $p < .01$).

2. Children whose ratings in family's social effectiveness were high at the beginning of treatment (ratings 2, 1) tended to be seen for fewer sessions than children whose ratings were low (ratings 3, 4, 5) (χ^2, Yates Correction = 7.00, $p < .01$).

3. There was no difference between the groups with regard to mother's therapeutic readiness at the beginning of treatment.

Additional Problems

Of the children treated in this study 11 were monosymptomatic, with stuttering the only cause for referral. Seventeen had a variety of additional problems: difficulty with school work, underachievement (6); bed-wetting (5); extreme shyness (4); restless behavior in the classroom, difficulty in concentrating, compulsive talking (3); sleeping disturbance (2); extreme stubbornness (2); speaking in a whisper (1); asthma (1); lisp (1).

Speech improved in 10 monosymptomatic children and did not improve in 1. Twelve children with additional difficulties improved while 5 did not improve. There was no significant difference between the groups.

Prognosis for Success of Treatment

Our statistical findings should be pertinent for the prognosis of future cases to be treated with the methods described here. Apparently, the prognosis will depend upon the age of the child, severity of stuttering at the time of referral and—last but not least—the degree of social effectiveness or social pathology in the child's family.

The mother's therapeutic readiness at the beginning of therapy appeared to be of less importance than the other three factors mentioned above.

Additional Variables Reported by Therapists

A tabulation of the characteristics of the parents which either contributed to the child's improvement or worked against it showed that these characteristics had been represented already in the rating scales for family's social effectiveness and mother's therapeutic readiness.

The variables representing characteristics of the child and of the child's life situation during treatment which either contributed to his improvement or worked against it were tabulated, and are reported in Appendixes VIII and IX.[3]

A FOLLOW-UP STUDY

In the spring of 1964 we also attempted to contact the mothers of 25 children who had been treated prior to 1960. The time elapsed between the termination of therapy and the follow-up study ranged from 3 years to 11 years. The majority of the cases had been treated during the pilot study 1958–59. One case had been seen in 1961 during the second research study, but the family had moved to another state before termination of therapy. Three cases, seen 10 and 11 years earlier, had been treated with a form of mother-child therapy which was, at that time, tentative and experimental but basically not dissimilar from the patterns of therapy worked out more systematically during the later research studies.

It seemed worthwhile to find out how these former stutterers had developed over the years. We asked these principal questions: Did the children who improved with this form of treatment remain free of stuttering symptoms or did they relapse into stuttering? Did the unimproved children improve later, and if so, did they improve spontaneously or with the help of some other treatment technique?

A semi-structured interview was conducted with each available mother. The topics covered were: child's present address; child's school and grade; status of the family; child's present speech as perceived by the parent; child's relapse into stuttering; any further treatment the child might have received; what form of treatment (such as conventional speech therapy, psychotherapy, or counseling) did the child receive; what person or institution provided the treatment; result of further treatment; any difficulties, scholastic, social or otherwise, developed by the child since the original therapy; child's present relationship to peers, siblings, and parents. Finally, the informant was asked what aspect of the original therapy had seemed to her most important and most helpful, and what recommendations she might want to make to improve future services for stuttering children and their parents.

A letter was sent to the 23 mothers of 24 children, in which the purpose of the follow-up study was explained and the mothers' cooperation was solicited. The letter then was followed by a telephone call, during which an appointment was made with each mother who was willing to ccoperate. Parents who had moved out of town were invited to telephone at the expense of the research grant.

Eventually 20 mothers of 21 children were reached. Of these, 18 mothers reacted in a cooperative fashion, while 2 were unwilling to cooperate. One of these

---

3. In our analysis of variables we were stimulated by the Psychotherapy Research Project of The Menninger Foundation, in particular by the following publications: Luborsky, Fabian, Hall, Ticho, and Ticho (1958); and Sargent, Modlin, Faris, and Voth (1958).

2 finally gave some information cursorily over the telephone, while the other was so suspicious of the purpose of the follow-up interview that information about her child had to be obtained from the child's teachers and school records. Finally, in one case, information was received from the child's present psychotherapist.

The informants for the 22 cases were: mothers, 19 cases; school personnel, 1 case; psychotherapist, 1 case. In no instance was a child observed directly.

Information was gained through home visits in 14 cases, by telephone in 6 cases, through school personnel in 1 case, and in an interview with a psychotherapist in 1 case.

Status of Children at Time of Therapy

The age range of the children was the following:

Under 7 Years at Beginning of Therapy

Years	No.
3–4	1
4–5	5
5–6	10
Total	16

Over 7 Years at Beginning of Therapy

Years	No.
7–8	1
8–9	2
9–10	2
14–15	1
Total	6

It was our hypothesis that children who had been treated successfully before they were 7 years old should be less liable to relapse into stuttering than children who had been treated successfully after they were 7 years old.

Original Treatment Results

Of the 16 children under 7 years old at beginning of therapy, 11 had improved and 2 had not improved; 3 had moved out of town before termination of therapy, after mother and child had met the therapist from 4 to 11 times.

Of the 6 children who were over 7 years old at the beginning of therapy, 4 had improved and 2 had not improved.

The findings concerning each child are presented in Appendix X. A summary of these findings is presented in Tables 8 and 9.

TABLE 8—RESULTS OF FOLLOW-UP: PRESENT SPEECH OF CHILDREN TREATED

	Under 7 Years at Original Referral Present Speech		
Original Treatment Results	No Stuttering	Mild—Moderate Stuttering	Severe Stuttering
+N = 11	9	2	0
—N = 2	0	1	1
Moved Before Termination: N = 3	2	0	1

	Over 7 Years at Original Referral Present Speech		
Original Treatment Results	No Stuttering	Mild—Moderate Stuttering	Severe Stuttering
+N = 4	2	2	0
—N = 2	0	1	1

TABLE 9—RESULTS OF FOLLOW-UP: FURTHER TREATMENT

Under 7 Years at Original Referral		
Original Treatment Results	Further Treatment	
+N = 11	No further treatment	9
	Individual counseling, public school	2
—N = 2	Psychoanalysis	1
	Psychotherapy, mother supported by social case worker	1
Moved Before Termination: N = 3	No further treatment	2
	Conventional speech therapy, public school and rehabilitation clinic	1

Over 7 Years at Original Referral		
Original Treatment Results	Further Treatment	
+N = 4	No further treatment	2
	Psychiatric therapy	1
—N = 2	Individual counseling, public school	1
	No further treatment	1
	Psychotherapy and parent counseling	1

New difficulties which had developed since the time of therapy were reported for 11 cases.

Great difficulty in learning to read	3
Poor school work	5
Incident of school phobia	1
Brief periods of bed wetting	1
"Not happy at college" during freshman year	1

School achievement was called satisfactory or excellent in 11 cases. Regardless of speech, excellent reading was mentioned in 3 cases. One little girl maintained her excellent speech despite the fact that two years after therapy she had to spend two months in a hospital being treated for a bone tumor.

Reports concerning relationships to peers, siblings, and parents were unrevealing. Apparently a single interview with a strange interviewer did not induce mothers to reveal significant material in these areas.

The following numbers of mothers considered the following aspects of therapy as most important:

Mother appreciated therapist's suggestions on how to handle the child, how to take time to read and talk with him, how to slow down and use simple vocabulary in talking with him.	6
Mother learned to understand her part in the problem of stuttering and in its treatment.	4
Therapy changed the family's attitude toward stuttering child.	3
Mother realized that she should not nag or correct the child all the time.	2
Mother began to see that she had treated the child as "older than he was," or made him "grow up too fast."	2
Mother felt that during therapy the child had learned that he was "not alone with his problems," that there were people interested in helping him.	1
Work with therapist helped the Mother to understand the child's relationship with his sister; made mother devote more time alone to the stuttering child.	1
Mother realized that her working and leaving the child with a nervous grandmother was undesirable. After moving and spending much time with the child, excellent speech improvement was seen.	1

Mothers made the following recommendations for future treatment of stuttering children:

Early, preschool treatment was recommended. Parents, teachers, and nursery school teachers should be made aware of the importance of early treatment, schools should establish services for preschool stuttering children, and notices should be sent out to parents before the child entered kindergarten, bringing available services to the parents' attention.[4]   7

Availability of more follow-up conferences with parents after termination of the child's treatment was requested.   5

Psychoanalysis or psychiatric therapy considered essential for the treatment of stutterers.   2

More counseling sessions were wanted by the mother herself.   1

It was regretted that the family had to move; "If the treatment had continued, the child would be all right now."   1

Several mothers did not comment or make recommendations.

CONCLUSIONS AND EVALUATION

Clinical Analysis

On the basis of the data derived from all our studies, the following clinical findings can be presented.

CHILDREN WITH MILD STUTTERING SYMPTOMS

Frequent but mild symptoms of stuttering (rating 3) were observed in many young children. These children repeated initial sounds and syllables, but no "secondary symptoms" such as prolongation of vowel sounds, blocking, or tic-like accompanying movements, were observed. Whenever a child with such initial symptoms was referred, suggestions were made to the mother as to how to provide corrective feedback in a climate of affectionate closeness. No further treatment was attempted. In several cases such minimum intervention was sufficient

---

4. All of these recommendations have become regular policy of the Wellesley Public Schools. Classroom teachers, local physicians, public health nurses, and nursery-school teachers are informed of available services, and the importance of early identification of children with communication disorders is stressed.

and the child developed normal speech within the school year. Such cases were not included in our research report.

Two cases reported in the follow-up study fell into this category, one of preschool, the other of kindergarten age. In each case the child was observed twice and two conferences were held with each mother before the families moved out of town. The family situation in one case was very satisfactory; in the other family situation improved markedly after the move, when the mother was able to stop working outside the home. During the follow-up interviews, both mothers reported that their children had developed normal speech within a few months and no relapse into stuttering had occurred in either case, within periods of 3 and 6 years respectively.

In another instance, a 5-year-old girl with mild to moderate stuttering of 1 year's duration was seen twice with her mother, and one meeting was held with the mother alone. The child's speech became normal within a 4-month period, and no relapse was reported at the follow-up interview, 11 years later.

Mild, initial stuttering was also observed in two children between 2 and 3 years of age (Cases 27, 28, Appendix VI). In one case the parents, in the other, the grandmother, showed concern about the sudden appearance of frequent repetitions in the emerging speech of these children. In both cases three meetings were held with the parents during a 6-month period, and the parents were instructed to use corrective feedback in a particulary slow manner, using simple, short phrases and sentences only. After 4 months in one case and 6 months in the other, the children were able to express themselves fluently in short phrases or sentences, and treatment was discontinued.

These results seem to indicate that, under favorable circumstances, a brief period of crisis intervention can be sufficient to help a child in acquiring normal speech. Favorable conditions were: the early age, the relatively mild symptomatology, and the absence of additional problems in the children; the social adequacy of the families; and the mothers' low anxiety level together with their intelligent and imaginative participation in the treatment process.

To our surprise we also found four older boys with frequent mild stuttering, without secondary symptoms. In two 7-year-old boys stuttering was the only presenting symptom. These children needed 10 and 29 treatment sessions, respectively, to develop normal speech. Two boys of 10 and 11 years presented severe learning difficulties in addition to frequent mild stuttering of long standing. Severe family conflicts and difficulties were found in the background of both children. In these cases the problem of stuttering was actually minor, but parents and children needed extensive therapeutic help in coping with severely stressful family situations.

While in these four cases the initial stuttering symptoms had remained almost unchanged over the years, a different developmental pattern was observed in Case 8. The boy repeatedly had been referred by successive teachers because of his mild but frequent stuttering. Each time the parents had declined our offers of treatment. In grade 5 the boy experienced serious academic difficulties. He developed a symptom of compulsive throat clearing and his speech became worse rapidly. When the parents finally asked for therapeutic assistance, the boy's stuttering had reached the frequent, severe stage (rating 7). During the treatment sessions both mother and child demonstrated severe anxiety. Forty sessions with the child, 13 with the mother, and 2 with both parents were necessary to help the child achieve normal speech. Because of his anxieties concerning school success, which apparently had triggered off his severe stuttering, a school counselor worked with him twice monthly in a part tutorial, part therapeutic relationship. The boy's school work improved and his speech remained normal.

Thus, it appears that some children with originally mild symptoms of stuttering react to increasing home or school pressures with increasing severity of stuttering, while others show no change in the original symptom but develop symptoms in other areas, such as behavior or learning difficulties. So far, we do not know what factors determine the choice of symptoms.

YOUNG CHILDREN WITH SEVERE STUTTERING SYMPTOMS

A different type of syndrome was found in the cases of young children with severe stuttering symptoms (Cases 2, 12, 14, 17, 20, 23). All were boys between 3 and 7 years of age who received severity ratings of 5 or 7 at the beginning of treatment. The primary characteristic of these children was their stubbornness. The children exhibited intensive anger and rage directed against their mothers or against both parents, and often also against their therapists. Four of these children showed no additional symptoms, one was restless and treated animals cruelly, and the youngest one had difficulty with bowel control. Four of the mothers reacted to their children with great irritation and counteraggression. One mother was a very shy, withdrawn person who had to work evenings to add to the family income. Another had a very large family, in which the stuttering child was in a middle position. In therapy, these boys produced many of the classical fantasies of stuttering children—of being lost, homeless, or excluded—which were reported in Chapter 6. All of them had begun to stutter during the critical period between 3 and 6 years of age. All had reacted to their early symptoms with intense frustration, followed by intensive anger directed against the mother, who was perceived as inaccessible and unhelpful, and who gradually became devaluated as a love object. All of these children exhibited severe separation anxiety. They reacted with relapses into stuttering when the therapist proposed termination of treatment. In all cases, mother and child were seen by the same therapist and, at times, the therapist found the work with the mothers as difficult as that with the child. In all cases, except one, normal speech was established at the time this study was terminated.

UNIMPROVED CASES

As reported earlier, six children had not improved significantly at the time the study had to be terminated (Cases 1, 2, 7, 13, 14, and 18). As can be seen from Appendix VI, five of these cases had low ratings in family's social effectiveness at the beginning of treatment, and little or no change occurred during the period of therapy. The ratings represented severe and prolonged disruptions of family life caused by marital discord, death, severe or chronic illness in the family, or temporary absence of the father.

Case 18 was not representative of the group. This child was seen during the final months of the study only. At the time of termination a positive therapeutic relationship had developed between therapist and child, but the mother had maintained a distant attitude toward the therapist. "Divided management," or separate therapists for parent and child, would have been the method of choice if the treatment of this case had continued.

In Case 14, the case of Budd, the child's speech was rated as unimproved at the time of our treatment evaluation. As reported earlier, another year of treatment with mother and child led to great improvement in the child's speech and behavior, as well as in the family situation.

Cases 1, 3, 7, and 13 demonstrate that the *prognosis for the treatment of older stuttering children is relatively poor if there is severe family pathology*, or if the family is exposed to unusual and long-lasting situational stress.

In summary, all our clinical as well as statistical findings confirm our assumption that *stuttering originates as a disruption in parent-child communication, occurring on the psychological level, calling for a psychologically oriented approach to therapy*.

Modification of the Original Hypothesis

At the time of the pilot study (Wyatt, 1958) it had been the primary hypothesis that the onset of stuttering in a child was causally connected with actual separation between mother and child, occurring during a critical period in language development. This hypothesis had to be modified. From our findings during the second research study (Wyatt, 1964a), we came to the conclusion that actual mother-child separation was a possible but not a necessary condition for the beginning of stuttering. At our present state of knowledge, we assume that the core event connected with the onset of stuttering in young children is an unexpected disruption of a well-established speech chain between the young child and his mother, or mother substitute. This frustrates the child's expectancies to receive corrective feedback from his mother and causes him to experience anxiety and anger with regard to her. Such a disruption may be caused by a variety of circumstances which may interfere with the highly specific mother-child network of communication. We found that the mother's actual physical absence or her temporary inaccessability, caused by illness, moving, or other circumstances, frequently were connected with such disruptions of mother-child communication, but they were not the only causes.

Comparison with Flosdorf's Study

Peter Flosdorf, a clinical psychologist in Wuerzburg, Germany, carried out an extensive clinical study of stuttering children (Flosdorf, 1960). Comparing his findings and interpretations with those derived from our studies, we found similarities and differences which are of interest.

The samples of the Wellesley and the Wuerzburg studies differ markedly from each other. In the course of our two research projects we examined and treated 48 stuttering children, ranging in age from 3 years 6 months to 16 years. All children came from American middle-class families—lower to upper middle-class—and all parents had a fair amount of education, ranging from high school to graduate school. Flosdorf examined 131 stuttering children; 101 were referred by the public schools and by a child guidance clinic in Wuerzburg and 30 were referred by a child guidance clinic in the neighboring town of Kulmbach. The ages of the children at the time of examination were not reported, but in reading Flosdorf's paper one gains the impression that his study comprised children from beginning school age through adolescence. The paper contains a number of brief case histories. Fathers mentioned ranged from army officers, teachers, and business-men, to factory workers, artisans, and farmers. In general, it appears that a large number of Flosdorf's cases came from working-class families.

One would expect that the role of the fathers in these German families, the role relationships between the parents, and the patterns of family communication differed from those prevailing in middle-class American families. In our cases, the mothers, as a rule, had a focal and often dominating position with the children, while the fathers—most of whom commuted to work or traveled frequently—played a marginal role in the care of the children. Fathers in our cases often were described as being less tense and concerned than the mothers or as somewhat distant from their children and withdrawn from the conflict between the stuttering child and his mother.

In Flosdorf's case descriptions, most of the fathers emerge as the powerful and dominating centre of the family, sometimes dreaded because of their harshness or even brutality in disciplining the children. In his inquiries, Flosdorf evidently was more interested in the father-son relationship than in the early relationship between the young child and his mother, which we found so revealing. Flosdorf's specific interest in the father-son interaction may have been influenced by the more dominating role of the father in the German family; it also suggests that Flosdorf worked mostly with older stuttering children. As reported earlier, we also found that older stuttering boys showed a tendency to displace their aggression-anxiety from the mother upon the father and upon other male authority figures; thus, the conflict between the older stuttering boy and his father may overshadow the earlier one between the young stuttering child and his mother.

In spite of the differences between the samples and the different interests of the investigators, there are several important areas of agreement. Each child in Flos-dorf's study, as in ours, had a comprehensive diagnostic examination, including psychological testing, history taking, and evaluation of the family situation. Home visits also were made in most cases. Flosdorf's findings concerning the onset of stuttering agree with ours. He reports that 67 per cent of the children in his sample began to stutter between age 3 and 4; 30 per cent between, 6 and 7; and 3 per cent between 9 and 12. In agreement with Busemann (1927, 1953) and Wiesenhuetter (1955, 1958) Flosdorf interprets the beginning of stuttering in childhood as a "developmental crisis," coincident with the "early phase of stubbornness" (*Trotz-alter*). He stresses that stuttering is not a speech disorder per se, but rather is a difficulty the child experiences in establishing verbal contact with others, particularly with adults. In a number of Flosdorf's case histories the onset of stuttering was related to traumatic situations. The young child experienced exposure to threat or to actual attack by an adult, in the absence of the mother, unable to flee and get help from the mother.[5] This material resembles our findings concerning the intense distance-anxiety observed in young stuttering children.

Flosdorf further assumes that the communication of children afraid of verbal contact with others may deteriorate in situations in which new interpersonal contacts have to be established; hence, the flare-up of stuttering among children entering school, and again—though in a small number of cases—during early adolescence.

Discussing the stuttering boy's personality development, Flosdorf mentions the strong tendency in older boys to repress hostility or anger, their increasing passivity, their difficulty in incorporating the paternal image, and their "dependent goodness" (*gefuegige Bravheit*) in overt behavior. These observations agree with our findings, as reported earlier.

Flosdorf stresses the fact that stuttering is not a speech disorder but a difficulty in communicating with others, a disturbance in that form of speech only which is directed at a partner; in short, a disturbance in the essential human encounter between the "I" and the "You."

Flosdorf's comments concerning the spontaneous disappearance of stuttering also are worth mentioning. He observed that, in some cases and under favorable life circumstances, stuttering may disappear gradually without specific treatment. Such circumstances may be: success in school learning or in sports, or other accomplishments leading to acceptance by one's peers; the attainment of vocational or professional competence; or a happy marriage and the gaining of authority as the father of one's own children. All of these experiences may strengthen the ego of the stuttering adolescent or young adult and decrease his feelings of self-doubt and guilt. Having obtained confirmation of the worth of his own self, he may then be increasingly able to enter into successful communication with others.[6]

Flosdorf's discussion of therapy unfortunately is brief. Apparently Flosdorf practices psychotherapy with stuttering children, but the parents seem only marginally included in the therapeutic process. Flosdorf mentions that the therapist

---

5. Flosdorf states: (*Das Kind) fuehlt sich der Bedrohung ganz allein ausgeliefert, ohne die Naehe der Mutter und die Moeglichkeit einer Flucht.* "The child feels all alone in being exposed to a threat, without the mother being near and without a chance to escape" (p. 134).

6. Flosdorf's assumptions agree with the findings of Joseph G. Sheehan in "Spontaneous recovery from stuttering" (1966). In September, 1964, Sheehan examined all incoming students at the University of California, Berkeley, and divided his samples into three groups: (1) recovered stutterers; (2) active or present stutterers; (3) normal controls. Sheehan found that four out of five former stutterers in his sample had recovered spontaneously. The recovered stutterers attributed their spontaneous recovery to a variety of factors, among them "strengthening approach behavior ('going ahead anyway'), and building up self-esteem."

may speak or read with the child, holding the child's hand or putting his arm around the child's shoulder in a supportive gesture. This bodily contact helps the stuttering child experience "mutually identifying communication"; speaking with the therapist thus becomes a "common monologue" rather than being a "dialogue with the other," which the stuttering child dreads. Though Flosdorf's conceptualization differs from ours, we feel that this therapeutic approach resembles our methods of word matching and providing corrective feedback in a setting of mutual closeness, including bodily closeness, with the stuttering child. While Flosdorf recommends this approach be used by the therapist, the child's mother or father apparently are not being trained to use a similar form of communication with the child at home.

The "model" of Flosdorf's treatment of older stuttering boys is derived from psychoanalytic psychotherapy and from educational therapy (*Heilpaedagogik*). Flosdorf recommends intensive psychotherapy with individual stuttering boys, to be carried out by a male therapist; this is supplemented by assisting the child to participate successfully in the activities of a youth organization. Speech drills are counterindicated. Regrettably, the paper contains no treatment results.

Obviously, there are important points of agreement between Flosdorf's and our investigations. The differences lie in three areas:

1. Flosdorf applied the principles and concepts of developmental, social, and clinical psychology to his analysis of the dynamics of stuttering. We feel that, in addition to psychological principles, a fuller understanding of the process of language learning in early childhood is necessary to comprehend this particular disorder which interferes with both the social and the language development of the child.

2. An interactional approach to the study of language development induced us to perceive the child's overt language behavior as a component within a system of communication. If we adopt Chase's definition (Chase, 1965a and b), that a system is "a collection of components which function together to perform a general function," we realize that a disturbance in one of the components—the child—will effect the general functioning of the family as a social and communication system. Our therapy, then, is system-oriented rather than component-oriented.

3. In our research we have demonstrated that a system-oriented form of therapy is highly promising, particularly if the therapeutic intervention occurs early in the life of the child, before the network of family communication has become seriously disrupted.

CHAPTER TEN

Administration of Treatment Programs

ROLE AND TRAINING OF THE THERAPIST

From the preceding chapters it should be evident that the treatment of stuttering children and their parents calls for professional workers with advanced training in psychodynamics, interviewing, counseling, and psychotherapy with children and adolescents. In addition, these workers should be familiar with theories of child development and of psycholinguistics, and with the specific character of communication disorders in children. The training of speech therapists, in this country as well as in most European countries, so far, has not included training in the theory and techniques of counseling and psychotherapy, nor can such techniques be taught adequately through lecture courses only. Training through supervised casework, which has been found indispensable in the education of psychiatrists, social workers, and clinical psychologists, should be made available for speech therapists who wish to work with stuttering children.

Sheehan (1965, 1966) has demonstrated that stutterers who received speech therapy, chiefly in the public schools, had a lower rate of recovery from stuttering than stutterers who received no treatment. Sheehan pointed to the "sheer irrelevance" of the techniques and practices used by most speech therapists presently working with stuttering children. At the same time, he is aware of the fact that the public school speech therapist is in a strategic position to bring help to the young stuttering child and his family. We also agree with Sheehan in his observation that public school speech therapists are eager to help the stuttering child and "hungry for knowledge of the means to do so" (Sheehan 1965, p. 5).

So far, the clinical aspects of the role of the school speech therapist have not been understood clearly, and faculty members in training centers for speech therapists have been reluctant to develop interdepartmental training programs in counseling and therapy. In some instances, practicing speech therapists, eager to

190

render more effective service to children, have been ahead of the graduate schools in establishing contact with other professions. Speech therapists in some of the more advanced public school systems have asked for and have entered into close cooperation with consulting psychiatrists, psychologists, school social workers, human relations consultants, or other mental health workers. They have been able to move from the traditional role of speech teacher—with all its limitations—to that of a professional consultant, member of a team of helping professions working within a school setting.

The potential scope of speech therapy was well delineated in *The British Journal of Disorders of Communication*, whose first issue appeared in April, 1966. We quote from the editorial:

> During the last twenty years it has become increasingly apparent that the scope of speech therapy is wider than was initially conceived, and that we are concerned with that aspect of human behaviour which enables one individual to maintain communication with another. . . .
> The understanding of disorders of communication in children and adults, developmental or acquired, must be based on knowledge of the normal. The study of audiology, psychology, linguistics, phonetics, neuroanatomy and physiology is basic to the understanding of normal verbal communication. Again, much information concerning normal verbal behaviour has been gained through study of its disorders, whether due to anatomical, neurological or emotional causes, and reactions to treatment. In addition to the application of such knowledge in the rehabilitation of individuals, change in thought and growth of knowledge occurs through competent clinical observation and long-term follow-up, whilst much has also been gained through clinical associations with those in other professions such as medicine, surgery, teaching, psychology and dentistry. 1966 (Vol. 1, No. 1, pp. 1–2.)

The principles and methods of supervised training in counseling and psychotherapy have been discussed widely by members of the mental health professions and were succinctly presented in a Symposium, "Qualifications for Psychotherapists," organized by the American Orthopsychiatric Association in 1954. (See Welsh, *et. al*, 1956; also *Trends in Orthopsychiatric Therapy*, 1948; Feldman, Spotnitz, and Nagelberg, 1953; *Therapeutic Play Techniques*, 1955; and Ekstein and Wallerstein, 1958).

Contributors to the Symposium expressed their conviction that the techniques of counseling and psychotherapy could be utilized in some form by all helping professions, but that only trained workers should practice them, under conditions which safeguard the welfare of the patients. Competent supervision during the period of training of communication therapists, and consultation for more experienced workers, will safeguard the welfare of the stuttering child and his parents. At the same time it will help to reduce the anxieties of the therapist, who is exposed to his clients' intense emotions.

The task of providing psychological help for others, be they children or adults, puts the therapist in situations of unusual stress. The communication therapist, like other counselors or psychotherapists, has to learn the proper strategies for managing his cases, he has to acquire the special skill necessary to understand the meaning of emotional expression in symbolic form, and he has to develop a kind of tolerance that will permit him to remain objective even in situations that are taxing emotionally. The therapist learns to use his own person as a tool within the therapeutic process. Such learning is emotional as well as intellectual in nature, and the supervisor or mental health consultant supports and guides the learner in this process of self-development. This type of learning is highly personal and can not be derived from books or pamphlets; it occurs gradually within the process of human interaction between the therapist and the consultant.

SUPERVISION AND CONSULTATION OF THERAPISTS

In our research projects, supervision of therapists of various professional backgrounds was carried out both individually and in small groups. Dr. Helen M. Herzan, the psychiatric consultant, described her supervisory experience in the paper, which follows.[1]

Even though I feel very much a part of the research group, I hasten to say that the therapists and parent counselors were the ones who carried out the work and my involvement, though very real, has been but an indirect one.

The image that comes to mind is that of a driving instructor sitting next to the actual driver in a car equipped with dual controls. The instructor lends his experience to build a sense of security in the new driver. His knowledge of the road to be traveled, his ability to size up the distances to be covered within given time and space limits, serves as a guiding post. It is an occasion for learning how to pick up clues and signals not only under ordinary road conditions, but also in circumstances where unexpected or sudden changes in course become imperative.

All analogies have their shortcomings and this one seems to break down at probably more than one point. I would like to come back to the earlier statement about the supervisor's "indirect" involvement and elaborate on it. If the driving of the car is in some ways comparable to the procedure whereby therapists in the school system see stuttering children and their parents in closed interview situations, the supervisor or consultant, unlike the driving instructor, does not sit in or next to the therapist during these sessions.

It follows, therefore, that the supervisor has to rely on the written or verbal accounts presented to him by the actual therapists. In other words, he obtains a report of the therapeutic events which is once removed, bearing the colorings of the therapists' personality and therapeutic strivings.

The therapist, in treating the child or his parents, establishes a meaningful relationship which works both ways. The child, after having successfully overcome his initial reservations about treatment, comes to like his therapist and the time spent with him. Likewise, the therapist grows fond of the child entrusted to his care and in his ardent desire to "cure" him has a readiness to see him cured, even though this may not be borne out by the reality situation. All those working with stutterers know that after a while we "get used to" or even "do not hear anymore" what, by someone's else's standards, would still qualify as stuttering.

In order to obtain a more-or-less objective report with only minimal distortions from his supervisees, the supervisor is expected to establish a good working relationship with the

---

1. The paper "Consultation and Supervision" was presented originally before the 38th annual convention of the American Speech and Hearing Association, New York City, November, 1962 (See Wyatt and Collaborators, 1962).

therapists, based on mutual trust and respect. This means that the worker should be able to say to himself: "Maybe this time I missed the boat or did something the wrong way, but the supervisor will not think less of me, he may even help me out of this fix and I can learn something and thus benefit by the whole experience." The supervisor, in turn, must at all times be accepting of the people he works with. He supports and enhances their innate intuitive power and previously acquired skills, however, without indulging their mistakes.

The therapist and his supervisors have a common goal, namely the welfare of the child and his family entrusted into the former's care. Professionals such as speech therapists, teachers, or even educational psychologists do not, as a rule, receive formal training in their respective curricula toward this kind of treatment procedure. However, their educational background, their familiarity with a variety of children through their teaching experience, and their knowledge and tolerance of speech disorders enable them to offer a healthy relationship to children.

Often the establishment of a meaningful relationship with stuttering children is extremely difficult. The therapist, in spite of his best intentions and efforts to help the child, may get only a mumbled, cluttered response or no response at all. The child may be destructive. He may act younger than his chronological age. All this can be disappointing, baffling, and taxing to the therapist.

Having to work concommitently both with the child and his parents, most frequently with the mother, can make matters even more complicated in terms of the therapist's double identification. The therapist's role here is not to take sides, but to remain an interested and supportive figure to both child and parents. This does not mean that the therapist may not be more inclined towards one or the other—usually toward the child. Awareness of such preference is gained in the supervisory session. Once this is made conscious, coping with it becomes less of a problem.

Essentially the work with the parents consists of: (1) obtaining further information about past developmental issues and important recent happenings in the child's and the family's life; (2) offering a meaningful, supportive, and clarifying relationship to the parents who feel concerned or guilty, and who sometimes deny their child's speech and behavior difficulties. Parents must understand that sometimes a child's behavior may even become worse during the beginning phase of treatment; (3) helping the parent by imparting new insights concerning the child's symptoms, and thus promoting changes in parental attitudes conducive to further unimpaired emotional growth and maturation in the child.

Throughout the supervisory sessions the main focus remains on the child. It is the supervisor's role to help the therapist toward: (1) the patient acceptance of the child; (2) the understanding of the meaning of speech and behavioral manifestations; (3) the setting of limits; and (4) the establishment of a therapeutic alliance.

In describing the child's productions to the supervisor, the therapist sometimes directly, sometimes by inferences, reveals his own emotional response of frustration, annoyance, or even anger in the face of the child's behavior.

Looking at the therapeutic material in the company of interested and informed listeners —such as the supervisor and the other coworkers participating in group supervision—puts the whole current issue into a new perspective. One learns that even mature, grown-up professionals can feel angry at times, even though they usually don't act upon it. This insight enables the therapist to be more tolerant toward an angry child, which circumstance helps the therapeutic process further along.

The understanding of the meaning of speech and behaviorial manifestations comes from a double source: (1) a thorough knowledge of the child's past history, particularly his painful experiences; (2) information about the current real events of his everyday life.

Through information obtained directly from the parents or via the parent counselor, one has a "reality check" on the actual happenings, in contrast to the possibly distorted version expressed in the child's productions and fantasies in the play sessions. It is the supervisor's role to point out the correlation between the chid's past experiences and his present attitudes, in the therapeutic situation. The child's behavior is a repeat performance of earlier difficulties or breakdowns in communication with close family members.

The therapeutic role presupposes permissiveness. The child is encouraged to act and talk spontaneously. Yet this situation can get out of hand, and in order to protect the child from undue anxiety and consequent guilt, one can gently but firmly set limits to extreme behavior. Rather than encourage regressive behavior, the therapist makes a continuous appeal to that part of the child's personality that wants to overcome the difficulties and weaknesses. This is what we call the "therapeutic alliance."

The importance of patient listening cannot be emphasized enough. The less experienced therapist runs the danger of "out-talking" the child or interpreting too early or too frequently in the course of treatment. Parallel to the word matching, there is an emotional tuning in with the child. Once this is established, the therapist becomes more and more sensitive to picking up clues and main themes, as well as moods and affects.

The supervisor stresses the value of the regularity of contact, the being on time for appointments, and the necessity to prepare the child ahead of time in case cancellation of an appointment should be unavoidable. This means to the child that the therapist cares, that he respects the child, that he takes the commitment to the child and his parents seriously. The therapist then is in a position to expect the same in return. The therapeutic give-and-take brings about a corrective emotional experience through which the child patient comes to modify his behavior and abandon his symptom.

The therapist, at times, runs the risk of getting overinvolved with his child patient. He may feel sorry for him and would like to pamper him. The supervisor intervenes at this juncture, pointing out to the therapist the nature of his role and his original commitment to the child.

Since painful separations at crucial developmental stages occur so frequently in the history of stuttering children, special attention is given to carefully planned termination. In our research project it always was a joint decision of the chief investigator, the therapist, and the supervisor as to when and how to terminate treatment.

Generally the "open-door" policy, with or without scheduled follow-up interviews at regular intervals with both children and their parents, helps to attenuate the sense of loss that inevitably accompanies the cessation of treatment. The improved child carries with him the memory of a valuable relationship, and whatever he may have learned in treatment is now part of his own mental equipment.

A last word about the technique and structuring of supervision. In our project we used considerable flexibility and some experimentation with the grouping of therapists. In the first year of our joint work we resorted to the method of group consultation and had weekly sessions, each lasting a little less than two hours. At the time, it was felt that the group was too large and too heterogenous for the supervisory work to proceed at its optimum. Occasional individual consultations were needed for discussion of specific or unforeseen therapeutic problems and to draw out the less outspoken members of the group and give them a chance to talk.

Soon, however, the disadvantages of this became obvious: the group wondered about those "favoured ones" who had access to individual consultation. For all these reasons, as the next clinical year began, we broke down the large group into two smaller groups. We felt that the work proceeded more efficiently with better case coverage.

In summary, I have attempted to describe very briefly the nature and process of consultation and supervision. I tried to give an impression of the purpose of supervision and demonstrate how it works. I hope I conveyed the idea that it is primarily aimed at giving the therapists more security, as well as a sense of shared responsibility in handling the psychological problems of families seeking their help. Supervision gives the therapists an opportunity for learning and for better understanding of the therapeutic problems with which they have to deal. Most importantly, it broadens the scope of their emotional freedom to interact in a helpful way with the individuals entrusted to their care.

As to the consultant, he has much to gain through this opportunity of studying the variety of cases brought to him by the therapists. He admires and learns from the intuitive and often ingenious ways used by the therapists. It is gratifying also for the consultant to witness evidence of real professional growth in his supervisees.

ADMINISTRATIVE PROBLEMS

If communication therapy with child and parents is carried out in a clinical setting, the patterns of therapy described will agree with already established clinical practices. The practice of communication therapy in school systems, however, asks for serious administrative considerations and innovations. In Chapter 16, we proposed a more effective use of professional personnel in the service of children with communication disorders. Here we wish only to draw attention to the fact that even excellently trained speech therapists, who have access to mental health consultation, will not be able to work successfully with stuttering children unless school administrators are informed about the nature of the disorder and appreciate the specific character of the treatment process.

Both individualized approach and flexibility of schedule are important aspects of the process of communication therapy, particularly in working with younger children. In our project, as soon as a child's speech and behavior had improved sufficiently, responsibility for further therapeutic communication was left primarily with the child's mother, and conferences with the therapist were scheduled at longer and longer intervals. However, if and when a child went through an acute phase of stuttering, or had a sudden relapse after several weeks or months of normal speech, the event was treated as a crisis in the child's interpersonal relationships and therapeutic conferences with the child and the mother then were scheduled close together for some time, until the therapist was satisfied that the crisis had been worked through in a constructive manner. Flexibility of scheduling and intensified treatment during periods of acute crisis turned out to be valuable therapeutic tools. Because of our continued work with Wellesley teachers, and their understanding of therapeutic principles, classroom teachers often referred a child because of a relapse into stuttering.

It is evident that individualized and flexible therapy for child and mother cannot be provided under the traditional speech therapy services now existing in most public schools. If the therapist has the role and status of a remedial teacher, who has to work exclusively with heterogeneous groups of children at a specified time and in a specified place, she will not have the opportunity to contribute to a competent diagnostic evaluation of these children, nor can she possibly carry out a meaningful, professional program of relationship therapy. It is only when the therapist has the role and status of a professional consultant, that she is granted the freedom of adapting her program to the varying conditions and needs of the children in her care.

If therapy is carried out within a school system, thought should be given also to the setting in which the therapeutic encounter occurs. Preschool children can be seen in a centrally located office which can be furnished as a playroom. It is most helpful to have a place available where toys, finger paints, chalk and crayons, papers, picture books, puppets, a play kit, and perhaps a sandbox can be stored for use during play sessions. Therapists who work with older children in different school buildings can use play material from this playroom. With present conditions of overcrowding, much ingenuity may be needed to find a proper room which will permit the privacy and security that the stuttering child needs in order to feel comfortable during his meetings with the therapist. Older stuttering children— like Budd—often are compulsive and may react negatively to unexpected changes in the treatment setting. Kindergarten children, who still have a more fluid perception of time and space, may be less aware of the place of therapy, once they have established a trusting relationship with the therapist. The exception will be very timid children who may dread or even refuse to leave the familiar kindergarten room. The sensitive therapist will choose to stay in the kindergarten room during her initial visits, giving the timid child an opportunity to get acquainted with the therapist before following her to another room.

The teacher's attitude towards the therapist and her work will have also a subtle but significant effect upon the progress of therapy. Teachers like to be partners in any school-centered enterprise involving a child in their care. If the therapist neglects to include the teacher in the therapeutic team, the teacher may, consciously or unconsciously, interfere with the relationship developing between child and therapist. The teacher may "forget" to remind the child of his appointment with the therapist, or she may remind him in a conspicuous, embarrassing manner; she may not release the child from instruction to meet the therapist; she may receive him with a critical remark when he returns to his classroom. The stuttering child spends many hours daily in the presence of his teacher; the teacher can become a most helpful partner in the therapeutic process, provided the therapist helps the teacher to understand her role in this process.

In our own attempts at treating stuttering children within a school system, we found that certain limitations of our services were necessary. Children who have to live in a severely disturbed family, or children who exhibit symptoms of severe, pervasive anxiety should be referred to clinical facilities, if at all possible. The management of children with such extreme difficulties would be inadvisable and may even be impossible in most school settings. The advice of a consulting psychiatrist as to possible referral is of particular importance in such cases.

It should be said, finally, that not everybody—regardless of professional training and background—will be inclined or talented to work with stuttering children. Teachers of young children often have to a high degree the qualities necessary for this kind of work; their verbal interaction patterns with children are simple and unambiguous and they do not feel threatened by the impulsivity and aggressiveness of young children. With competent supervision, such teachers can become successful lay-therapists. On the other hand, not every competent speech therapist or school psychologist may feel equipped for or inclined to expose herself to the emotionally taxing encounters with stuttering children and their parents.

Being aware of this they should feel free to refer stuttering children and their families to a clinical treatment facility.

SUMMARY

We have demonstrated that a psychodynamically oriented program of therapy with stuttering children and their parents can be carried out successfully within the framework of a school system, provided certain conditions are met. (1) The therapy program must be administered in such a manner that individual therapy and flexibility of scheduling are possible. (2) The therapist working with children and parents should have regular consultations with a qualified psychiatrist or with another competent mental health consultant. Speech therapists with insufficient training in counseling and psychotherapy should not attempt to carry out the treatment described here, unless they work under expert supervision. (3) The therapy program will have a better chance to succeed if it can be integrated with other existing diagnostic and mental health services within the school system or within the community, and if school administrators and classroom teachers understand the nature of the therapeutic process and can become partners in the therapeutic program.

CHAPTER ELEVEN

Group B: Children with Severely Defective Articulation

After our extensive discussion of the treatment of stuttering children, let us now turn to the other subgroups identified in our project. As reported in Chapter 7, Table 3, 24 of the 62 children in our research project stuttered. The remaining children fell into three diagnostic categories: (1) 18 spoke with severely defective articulation but had no other speech or language deficiency; (2) 11 showed symptoms of severely defective articulation and stuttering; (3) and 9 showed multiple symptoms indicating difficulties of varying degrees of severity in the areas of motor, perceptual, and language development. Our observations concerning the children in these three categories will be presented in this and the following chapters. The methods of language training which we employed in working with these children were experimental in character and no formal evaluation of treatment results was attempted.

THE LEARNING OF ARTICULATION

In recent years linguists and speech therapists have become increasingly interested in the developmental processes underlying the learning of articulation in childhood. British investigators presented a number of stimulating ideas on the subject in a recent publication, *Signs Signals and Symbols* (Mason, 1963).[1] M. E. Morley stated: "Articulation is an acquired motor skill developed gradually in early childhood through repeated sensory-motor experiences, at conscious and subconscious levels, involving constant interplay between the receptor and effector functions. . . . The exact processes by which this function of human behavior is achieved are still mainly unknown" (Morley, 1959). L. P. Parker stressed the fact that we do not

---

1. See in particular the papers by Fry, van Thal, Hartley, Grady, and Parker.

know how these processes occur, and yet for the purpose of treatment we are forced to make assumptions regarding disorders which are supposed to result from a delay or a breakdown in these unknown processes (Parker, 1963).

Fry (1963), in an analysis of coding and decoding in speech, pointed out that English, like other natural languages, is a hierarchical system consisting of several levels and organized in such a way that units which function on one level combine to form the units on the next level above. The units on the lowest level are the *phonemes* which combine together to form the *morphemes*, which have grammatical functions; these joined together form *words*, which have semantic or lexical function; and words, finally, combine to form *sentences*. The English phonemic repertory contains about 40 items. Children, as a rule, at the age of 5 to 7 years have learned the complete phonemic system of their native language. Individual speakers do not add to their phonetic repertory, within their native language, once they have learned to talk.

R. A. Chase (1963) described the infant's learning of complex sound patterns in the following paragraph.

The developmental vocalization in the human also demonstrates the initial appearance of poorly-regulated, simple motor patterns which become shaped through progressive stages into the complex, sensitively controlled patterns of articulation which characterize adult speech (McCarthy, 1946; Miller, 1961). Initially the infant demonstrates cries which are fairly uniform in spectral content . . . but which become differentiated in subclasses during the first few months of life. Spontaneous repetition of sounds follows, first with respect to vowel sounds, then followed by an increasing number of consonant sounds. At about the age of 9 or 10 months, the infant begins to imitate more complex sounds which he hears others make. It is probably at this stage that the infant begins to consolidate the complex acoustic and proprioceptive sensory feedback patterns associated with the complex sounds of the spoken language. The repetition of complex sounds which the infant hears is probably critical in the organization of patterns of neural activity which will serve as standards for the control of adult vocalization patterns. The final stage of the acquisition of speech is characterized by the ability to produce at will the complete repertoire of sound complexes corresponding to spoken language. The development of speech from this point consists of progressive refinement and expanded capability of the semantic functions of language (Chase, 1963, 23–24).

R. Jakobson (1941) described the child's learning of phonemic discrimination and production, as summarized by Velten (1943, p. 282): "A child does not acquire a phoneme system by random selection or by taking it over ready-made from the language of the adults, but by proceeding step by step, from the greatest possible phonemic distinction to smaller and smaller differentiations." Thus, according to Jakobson's theory, a child should first be able to hear the gross differences between vowels and consonants, so that words which are simple combinations of consonant-vowel, or consonant-vowel-consonant, or consonant-vowel-consonant-vowel would be the easiest to perceive and to articulate correctly. Susan Ervin-Trip (1966) remarked, however, that, so far, no systematic study of the learning of phonemic discrimination by English-speaking children has been carried out, to test Jakobson's theory.[2]

In general, auditory perceptual development in children has received less attention than other aspects of development. A. H. Kidd and R. M. Kidd, in a recent survey of "the development of auditory perception in children" (Kidd and Kidd, 1966), stated that investigators have tended to concentrate on research in the detection of auditory handicaps, rather than on the development of auditory perception and the learning of auditory discrimination in general. It appears probable "that perception in each auditory dimension develops with the interaction of auditory experience and maturity" (*ibid.*, p. 115).

SEVERELY DEFECTIVE ARTICULATION IN THE ABSENCE OF HEARING LOSS

In determining whether or not the articulation of a child in our sample should be considered as "severely defective," relative to his age, we used the data presented in Table 10 as a guide.

TABLE 10—AGES AT WHICH 75 PER CENT OF CHILDREN TESTED PRODUCED CORRECTLY SPECIFIC CONSONANT SOUNDS*

Sounds Produced	Age Correctly Produced
m, n, ng, p, f, h, w, y, k, b, d, g (in go)	3–3.5 years
t, sh, ch, v, l, zh (in pleasure), r, s, th (in think), th (in there)	4–6.5 years
z (in zoo) j, hw (in where)	4.5–7.5 years

* From studies by Wellman (1963) Poole (1943), and Templin (1957).

Our definition of "severely defective articulation" can be found in Appendix II. The age and sex distribution of the children in this group has been presented in Chapter 7, Tables 4 and 5.

The children, whose hearing was normal, had acquired a sizable vocabulary of meaningful words and also had learned the use of simple syntax and grammar, but their articulation was so defective that their spontaneous speech was incomprehensible to an outside observer. For example, Susy, age 4 years 8 months, in meeting the observer visiting at her home around Halloween, asked her: "Doo-oo-ee-my-mah?" The meaning of her question was: "Do you see my mask?" Peter, age 5 years, urged his mother: "Daw-me-a-dah!" a request which not even she could understand. After considerable guessing on the part of the adults present it became clear that Peter meant: "Draw me a desk!" These children omitted most consonants except those learned by the majority of children during their third year. (See Table 10, above). Other children in this group, in addition to omitting

2. For further discussion of the learning of the phonological system see Jakobson and Halle (1956), and Ervin-Tripp (1966, pp. 65–69).

sounds, also used sound substitutions, distortions, or alliterations, or reversed the order of sounds in words, thus saying, for instance, *turtain*, *kurkain*, or *turkain* for curtain; *gog* or *god* for dog; *hopsical* for hospital. Evidently these children exhibited a marked linguistic deficit.

The reader may remember that in Chapter 1, we came across two children with similar deficiencies in articulation. Nicky, the "chocolate syrup boy," showed symptoms of severely defective articulation combined with a limited vocabulary and immature sentence structure. Ann, whose mother "overloaded the system," also had not acquired the phonemic repertory adequate for her age, but she had learned the use of an adequate vocabulary and sentence structure.

Careful case studies and observations of mother-child interaction revealed that in the majority of cases environmental conditions had been responsible for the low rate of phonemic learning in these children. These conditions were: (1) The children had experienced infrequent, therefore insufficient verbal stimulation in early childhood; or (2) the verbal stimulation, though frequent, had been inappropriate (as in the case of Ann); or (3) the mother was inadequate as a speech model. Sometimes two of these conditions coexisted, as in the case of Billy, whose mother spoke with a very soft voice and blurred articulation. In addition, she had given Billy a minimum of corrective feedback because of her preoccupation and overwork in caring for a large family.

In a statistical analysis of our data (see Chapter 14) we found that a significant number of children with severe articulation problems came from large families; that they were either middle or last children; and that in many families with several young children close in age more than one child showed a deficit in language development.

These findings confirmed our hypotheses that mothers of large families—particularly of families with several young children close in age—have less time and energy available to provide verbal stimulation and feedback for their children than mothers of small families; and that mothers, as a rule, spend more time in verbal interaction with their first child than with the following children.

Therapeutic Approach

The therapy used with these children with severely defective articulation consisted of providing them with frequent and appropriate verbal stimulation and corrective feedback. In view of our basic assumptions concerning the role of the mother as the child's primary speech model, it seemed natural to enlist the mothers as primary providers of verbal stimulation. It is important to stress that we did not instruct these mothers to do exercises with their child, or to practice simple isolated sounds. Instead mothers, and often fathers, were instructed how to "lessen the child's linguistic load." Simple communication patterns to be used with young children were demonstrated to individual parents. The emphasis was put on the parents' use of a simple vocabulary, a slow rate of speech, and careful articulation. Parents were urged not to correct the child's speech in life situations when the child tried to express his needs or wants, but rather to set aside a period of time daily for the playing of word and listening games with the child, using simple picture books, toys, crayons, and other interesting but not confusing stimuli. Parents were reminded of the characteristic stages in children's language learning and were encouraged to begin the child's training with the labeling or naming of objects, activities, and pictures. This was followed by expansion—though not over-expansion—of phrases, word matching with the child, and repeated speaking together of jingles and nursery rhymes. Finally came reading or telling of simple stories to the child. After demonstration of these training procedures, some mothers exclaimed: "Of course! This is exactly what I used to do with my first child!" They added wistfully: "But then I had a lot of time."

A word should be said about the choice of pictures to be used for the purpose of therapeutic communication. Pictures should be simple in outline and clear in color. Parents are encouraged to make their own inexpensive picture books with the help of the child, cutting out simple colorful illustrations from catalogues or magazines and pasting them on cardboard. The word or the phrase used with each picture should be written underneath it, so that several adults who may take turns looking at the pictures with the child, will use the same words, thus providing the child with frequent, repeated auditory input of the same sequence of sounds. In the beginning short, preferably one-syllable words should be chosen, consisting of the consonant-vowel-consonant sequence mentioned by Jakobson (*op. cit*). In choosing words and pictures, parents must remember that in English spelling the two printed letters *ou* in *soup* or *house*, or the two letters *lk* in *walk*, stand only for one speech sound. Words to be practiced early may be, for instance, *bed, soup, cap, cat, man, dog, run, go, sit, walk, house*. Words containing consonant clusters, such as *stove, drive, speak, slow, sprinkle*, should be avoided until the child's articulation of single sounds has improved. As the child's speech becomes more comprehensible, the adult will present the child also with short phrases such as: *a big dog, here is a big dog, the boy can jump, he can run, he goes to bed, see the white cat*, and so on. Whenever the child spontaneously repeats a word or phrase the adult acknowledges this with a sign of pleasure. If the child repeats correctly—or nearly so—he is rewarded by the adult's big smile and a word of praise; if the child repeats incorrectly the adult simply proceeds to the next picture, knowing well that eventually, after much exposure to the same word in varying contexts, the child will be able to repeat the word correctly. *At no time is the child asked to practice single sounds or to repeat difficult sounds over and over again.*

It is evident that in this type of training the child receives continued reinforcement or reward for correct responses through the adult's praise and acknowledgement of words spoken correctly. The child is presented with small increments of learning, beginning with simple consonant-vowel combinations and gradually proceding to somewhat longer and more complex units. These verbal play sessions should not, as a rule, last longer than 15 minutes, but should be a daily occurrence. Many parents soon develop variations on the theme, playing similar verbal games with the child at other occasions, such as when dressing the child, riding in the car, or at bedtime.

Some parents in our sample were unaware of the rapid rate of their own speech, a feature which made them inappropriate as speech models for their child. With such parents the following demonstration was found helpful. The parents were told to repeat after the therapist, as best they could, a sentence in a foreign language, even though they might not understand the words used. The therapist would say for instance: "*Wo ist denn der Aschenbecher?*" meaning approximately: "Now, where is the ashtray?" This short sentence was spoken in a natural speech melody but at a high rate of speed, making it sound somewhat like "*Woisdennderáschenbecher?*"

Many parents reacted to this demonstration with bewilderment, stating that they could not repeat anything. Others repeated a few jumbled syllables, but succeeded in reproducing the speech melody of the original sentence. Very few parents were able to repeat the whole sentence with some degree of phonetic accuracy. When the therapist asked the parents why they had had such difficulty in repeating, most of them pointed out that they had heard the sentence only once and that the interviewer had spoken so fast that the words had run into each other. The therapist was then in a position to point out to the parents that their own manner of speaking English might have a similar effect upon a young child learning his first language. Pointing to an ashtray, the therapist then pronounced the word "*Á-schen-bé-cher*" slowly and with clear articulation, and most parents succeeded in repeating it correctly. Some parents had difficulty in discriminating between the two similar sounds *sch* (*sh*) and German *ch*, a sound which resembles the initial *h* in English *huge*. Their repetition sounded like a*sh*enbes*h*er or a*sh*enbek-ker. Only after repeated trials did the parents discriminate between the two sounds. It was pointed out to them that their young child also had difficulties in perceiving the difference between similar sounds and needed repeated practice and corrective feedback to learn the necessary perceptual-motor differentiation.

With the help of this simple experiment, which, of course, can be carried out in any language, it was possible to promote the parents' understanding of the learning of sound patterns in early childhood. It was stressed that parents should not attempt to correct specific sounds in the child's speech, but rather should serve as good speech models for the child, using connected speech, albeit in a manner and on a level appropriate for the child's age and limited phonetic skill.

It is obvious that this type of therapeutic communication is nothing but a replica of the type of speech used intuitively by most parents of young children and also by many good nursery and kindergarten teachers. We presented examples of it in our descriptions of the communication of the little boy and his grandmother in the London taxicab (Chapter 1) and between the kindergarten teacher and the stuttering little girl (Chapter 7.) The reader may remember also my teaching of words and phrases to Debby in the hospital (Chapter 2) and the manner in which my efforts were reinforced by some of the nurses and even by some of the older children.

Most parents participating in our program succeeded well in adopting the simple principles described here. Thus they functioned as primary speech-stimulators for their child, and professional time was kept at a minimum. Usually fathers were seen during the initial interview only. Child and mother met with the professional therapist approximately once a month. With some parents even two or three meetings were sufficient for them to work successfully with their child. The results of this procedure, as a rule, were very satisfactory; the articulation of the children improved gradually, and in some cases, rapidly.

In the majority of mothers in our sample we found no evidence of "deviant attitudes" towards the child, such as overprotection or rejection, as claimed by some investigators. What the child needed was not a better mother, but simply a better speech model. Some mothers, however, were unable to participate in this program because of overwork in the home or a part-time job which left them little time to communicate with the child. A few others were found unskillful when they tried to participate. The reason for this inability was either limited understanding, or a type of rigidity which made a mother hesitate to "regress" to the child's level of communication. In such cases nursery school or kindergarten teachers, grandmothers, or in one case a volunteering neighbor were instructed how to act as speech models for a particular child. In all cases the professional therapist acted primarily as a resource person and the actual work of improving the child's communicative skills was delegated to a lay therapist.

Finally, we would like to mention how the children in this category succeeded in learning to read. We had expected that children who received appropriate training in the perception, discrimination and articulation of speech sounds prior to first grade would have no difficulty in learning to read, in spite of their original difficulty in articulation. Thirteen of the 18 children in this category continued in the Wellesley Schools and we were able to follow their progress in reading. As expected, none of the children had any serious difficulty in learning to read. By the end of the first grade, 4 children of superior to highly superior intelligence (I.Q. scores 120 to 140), had been placed into the highest reading group; 5 children of bright to superior intelligence (I.Q. scores 109 to 122) were in the middle group; and 4 children of average intelligence (I.Q. scores 98 to 101) were in the low group.

SEVERELY DEFECTIVE ARTICULATION AND SECONDARY STUTTERING

Thirty-eight children were referred to our research project because of severely defective articulation; 18 of these spoke with defective articulation but showed no other deficiencies or signs of delayed maturation, while 11 presented symptoms of defective articulation and stuttering. In most instances parents reported that the child's speech had been "hard to understand" from the very beginning, while the stuttering usually had appeared later, as a secondary symptom. It seemed that at some point in their development these children had reacted strongly to the experience of not being understood by their parents and by other adults. In early childhood, while their vocabulary had been small and their needs circumscribed, the mothers has been able to guess from context the meaning of their messages. Actually, the mother, and often the brothers and sisters of the child in question, had learned the child's specialized code and were able to translate it into commonly accepted language. As the child became older, however, and his world enlarged, the parents and other adults no longer were able to do this.

These children constantly experienced breaks in the communication chain between adult and child, and frequently were given answers to their questions which must have seemed meaningless to them and unrelated to their needs. In despair, the children often began to stamp their feet, to repeat their incomprehensible words over and over again, and at times to give up and walk away, thus completely breaking off communication.

The following may serve as illustration (Wyatt, 1959). A mother of twins was observed in her home. She was looking at a picture book with 4-year-old Steve and Tom, both sturdy, energetic little boys. The twins were leaning against their mother's body, one on each side of her. Though both spoke with severely defective articulation, they were most eager to communicate. The following is an excerpt of the conversation between mother and children.

Steve. How do de ho-do go? (How does the hoptoad grow?)
Tom (repeats). How do de ho-do go?
(The mother, who had just shown them a picture of a hoptoad, explained in adult language and sentence structure how the hoptoad grows. Then she turned to the next picture.)
Steve. How do da-ying go? (How does that thing grow?)
Mother (unable to understand). What?
Steve (getting angry). Da ying . . da ying . . . (stamps his foot, shouts) DA-YING—how do . . how do . . how do . . how do da-ying go?
Mother (beginning to understand). Oh that! That is a prehistoric lizard!

This mother, a bright young woman, who was very fond of her children, provided preverbal communication in the form of body-closeness, but she used an adult vocabulary which was remote from the twins' developmental level. She did not provide corrective feedback on the phonetic level. There was little if any mutual imitation or word matching between mother and children. However, a good deal of mutual imitation occurred between the twins, reinforcing their inaccurate speech patterns.

Steve, the more intense of the two children, had reacted with increasing anger to the frustrations he experienced in communicating. A month before the odserver's visit symptoms of secondary or reactive stuttering had appeared in Steve's speech.

In the majority of cases our therapeutic instructions resembled those used with mothers of children in the previous group. Mothers were advised to tell their child explicitly that they were unable to understand him but that they would teach him how to say words so that he could be understood by everybody. Thus the child experienced his mother as helpful and understanding, and his basic trust in her was reestablished. The improvement in some cases was rapid and even dramatic. As soon as the mother initiated frequent games of word matching of the kind described earlier, the child's articulation and communication improved, and the symptoms of stuttering disappeared.

However, in some instances a child already had developed such intense feelings of frustration, mistrust, and rage, that he would no longer listen to the simple words and phrases presented to him by his mother or by a therapist. The most outstanding example of such behavior was Chris, a 6-year-old boy attending kindergarten. His teacher referred him to the speech therapist and he was included in our research study. Chris made it clear that he hated his teacher, he hated school, and he hated the therapist. He refused flatly to match words with his therapist or with his mother. As his demands and accusations were more often than not incomprehensible to the therapist, she turned to play therapy, using crayons, clay, and puppets to give Chris an opportunity for nonverbal communication. Also she interpreted to him in simple sentences the feelings he expressed through his play and his behavior. More than a year of weekly sessions with Chris and intensive work with his mother were necessary before Chris was ready to listen with sustained attention to the therapist and to begin imitating her articulation patterns. Chris, who was a bright, attractive, and imaginative child, finally became quite attached to his therapist and his articulation and stuttering improved concurrently. Simultaneously, the therapist succeeded in encouraging his very quiet and timid mother to verbalize her feelings and to relate to Chris more on a verbal than a nonverbal level. In the third year of the study Chris' articulation was almost normal and his speech had become completely fluent. However, when the therapist tried to prepare him for termination of treatment, again he became extremely angry at the therapist and his stuttering reappeared. Termination with Chris—as with most stuttering children—had to be a process of some duration, during which the child had to learn that many other adults were around whom he could trust and who were willing and able to play "the language game" according to rules he could understand and accept. Stuttering children had to find out that the disappearance of the therapist from their lives was not tantamount to a breakdown of their vital communication patterns.

Three other children, in addition to Chris, showed symptoms of severely defective articulation and of severe stuttering. As stuttering appeared to be their most disturbing disorder, the patterns of therapy used with stuttering children were applied and the results of their treatment were evaluated in the manner described in Chapter 9. The data concerning these four cases were included in the tabulation appearing in Appendix VI.

CHAPTER TWELVE

Group C: Children with Multiple Motor-Perceptual and Language Disabilities, I

THE WELLESLEY PROJECT[1]

The Sample

The children described in the previous chapter responded positively to verbal stimulation. We also encountered other children, referred for apparently similar articulation difficulties who either seemed unable to listen with sustained attention or had great difficulty remembering sounds in their correct sequences. Extensive study and testing of these slow responders revealed delayed and irregular maturation, not only in auditory discrimination and articulation of speech sounds, but also in other areas of motor-perceptual skills. The poor results on motor-perceptual tests, together with the poor response to training and the slow rate of improvement observed in these children, suggested that they experienced communication difficulties on the neurophysiological level.

It was found that the children in this group showed three or more of the following symptoms: defective articulation; stuttering or cluttering;[2] difficulties in word finding, in sentence building, in rhythms, in gross or fine motor co-ordination, in writing and drawing. Among children in the primary grades in this category, severe difficulties in learning to read or spell were evident also. Some of the children were unusually clumsy, while others exhibited hyperactive behavior. Almost all of them had difficulties in attention and concentration.[3]

---

1. I am indebted to the following for contributions to this section: Mr. Alton Reynolds, school principal; Mrs. Barbara Johnson, teacher of the tutorial class; Mrs. Harriet Stanton and Dr. Newton von Sander, school psychologists.

2. Cluttering is defined here as the propulsive impulse to speak, expressed in increasing acceleration of speech, leading to irregular, nonpredictable distortion and omission of consonant sounds and occasionally to rapid repetition of syllables. (After Seeman and Novak, 1963.)

3. For a definition of terms see Appendix II.

TABLE 11—DIAGNOSTIC PROFILE*
Children with Multiple Motor, Perceptual, and Language Disorders

No.	Age Observed	Clumsy	Hyper-active	Clut-tering	Stut-tering	Articu-lation	Word Find-ing	Sentence Building	Rhythm	Draw-ing	Writ-ing	Spell-ing	Read-ing	I.Q. Range	Additional Information
						Difficulties in									
1 x	4—8	+				++	++	++	+	++	++	++	++	Average	Neurological examination negative
2	4—6		+	+	+	+		+		++	++	++		Very Superior	
3	5—6				++	++			+	+				Average	Temporary hearing difficulty
4 x	5—10	++			+	++			+	++	++	++	++	Superior	Neurological examination negative, temporary hearing difficulty
5	6—10					++	+	++				+	+	Average	
6 y	7—10		+		+	+				+	+		+	Average	
7	7—11	+				++	+	++		+	+	++	++	High Average	
8	7—8	++		+		+			+	++	++			High Average	Neurological finding: mild pseudo bulbar dysarthria
9	9—10	++	++	++		+	++	++	++	+				Superior	
10 y	9—12	++	++	+	+	+		++	+	++	++	+	+	Very Superior	
11	9—10		++	++		+	++	++	++	+				High Average	
12	9—10	+			++	+		+			+			Superior	
13	11—12		+	+		+		+		+	+	+	++	Average	

* Moderate = +   Severe = ++   x = Are brothers   y = Are brothers

Nine children with such multiple difficulties were included in our research study (see Wyatt, 1964); four additional cases came to our attention between 1963 and 1965. All children were boys. Their ages ranged from 4 years to 11 years 6 months, and their intelligence, from average to superior. Two sets of brothers were included in the sample. Three children underwent neurological examinations; two had had periods of temporary hearing difficulty during early childhood.

The distribution of symptoms observed and their degree of severity varied widely. A diagnostic profile of the 13 children is presented in Table 11.

Table 11 shows that 12 possible symptoms or types of difficulty were identified, and that three or more of these symptoms were evident in each case, though in varying degrees of severity. The degree of severity reported for each case was not determined through precise measurements, but was based upon global ratings made by several observers working with the child. It must also be remembered that symptomatology changes with the age of the child. Cases 1 and 4, Table 11, will illustrate this. As can be seen, the entries refer to observations made over a period of four and a half years. An observer who would have met these two children at the time of their entering kindergarten would have noticed their marked difficulties in speech and in motor coordination, indicated on the left half of the table. An observer who met them only after they were 8 years old would have been most impressed by their severe difficulty in learning to read and write, indicated on the right side of the table. At that later stage in their life history, the most incapacitating difficulty of the two brothers was their "dyslexia," while their difficulties in speech, in holding a pencil, and in drawing, which were so marked at an earlier age, had improved from severe to moderate or even to mild.

Diagnostic Assessment and Training

Extensive information about each case was needed for the assessment of the children in this group. Each diagnostic evaluation was based upon (a) the child's medical and developmental history; (b) observations and tests of the child's behavior and skills; and (c) exploration of the family situation, including analysis of communication patterns prevailing in the family, and incidence of communication disorders among family members. A summary of the information sought for our Clinical Inventory can be found in Appendix XI.

The following tests were found helpful in our assessment of children in this group. The second column lists aspects of behavior about which the test provided information. (For test references see Appendix XI).

1. Goodenough Draw-a-Man Test (Goodenough, 1954)

   General intellectual ability, fine motor coordination, self-image.

2. Bender Gestalt Test for Young Children (Koppitz, 1964)

   Fine motor coordination, spatial orientation, perception, possible signs of neurological dysfunction.

3. Developmental Articulation Test (Hejna, 1955)	Consonant articulation in single words, blends excluded.
4. Peabody Picture Vocabulary Test (Dunn, 1959)	Vocabulary, comprehension of words.
5. Auditory Discrimination Test (Wepman, 1958)	Recognition of fine differences between phonemes.
6. Wechsler Intelligence Scale for Children (WISC) (Wechsler, 1949)	General intellectual ability, difference between verbal and performance scores.
	Item Picture Completion: visual perception.
	Item Picture Arrangement: child is asked to tell in his own words the picture story he arranged; his response shows his skill in word finding and sentence building. Tendency to deterioration of articulation during contextual speech.
7. Tell A Simple Story (Three Bears, Red Riding Hood, etc.) If the child cannot tell a story spontaneously, the examiner tells the child a simple story and asks him to retell it.	Child's use of language in connected speech: articulation, vocabulary, sentence structure, word variety; organization of thought, memory for significant detail.
8. Informal Rhythm Test	Ability to receive and process auditory information in temporal sequence, independently of ability to understand and use words.
9. Informal Tests of Gross Motor Coordination, Skipping, Hopping[4]	Observation of possible maturational lag in motor performance.
10. Projective Tests: Mother-Child Relationship Test (see Chapter 6 and Appendix I) or Children's Apperception Test, CAT (Bellak and Bellak, 1949)	Child's imagination, feelings, anxieties, perception of relationships, self-perception. Also contextual speech, ability in word finding and sentence building.

Because of the complexity and variability of the symptoms present in each individual case, diagnostic assessment had to be an ongoing process, carried out

---

4. Tests 7, 8, 9, were adopted following consultation with Mrs. K. de Hirsch.

simultaneously with therapeutic and remedial work. Early hypotheses had to be reformulated in the light of new observations, and therapeutic techniques had to be adapted to each child in view of his needs and his response to therapy. Assessment and education of the children was carried out by an interprofessional team of pediatrician, psychologist, speech therapist, classroom teacher, reading tutor, and physical education teacher.

In planning our training program we consulted Bender (1958), Bryant (1962, 1964, 1965), Cruickshank et. al. (1961), de Hirsch (1957, 1961), Denhoff and Robinault (1960), Fernald (1943), Frostig and Horne (1964), Kephart (1962), Strauss and Lehtinen (1947), and Strauss and Kephart (1955). Our method of lessening the linguistic load proved helpful in the speech training of the children in this group; it had to be complemented by techniques for the training of visual perception, hand-eye coordination, rhythm, and gross and fine motor coordination. For the children with severe reading difficulties a program of individual tutoring was set up, which led to the establishment of a special tutorial class for children with multiple learning disorders.

THE CASE OF GEORGE

Our gradually increasing understanding of the diagnostic, instructional, and administrative problems involved in educating children with multiple and severe learning difficulties will be illustrated in a report of the history of one of these children, whom we will call George.

George was first seen at the age of 5 years 6 months, shortly before entering kindergarten. At that time he was referred by his pediatrician because of his severely defective articulation. During the intake interview it was learned that George's parents were both college graduates. Several members of George's family had moderate or severe hearing problems, and one of his male cousins had a history of delayed language development and severe reading difficulty.

The mother's pregnancy had been normal with a small amount of bleeding during the seventh month. Following a Caesarian birth, George—who weighed 8 pounds 5 ounces—had spent 24 hours in an incubator. George was bottle fed and had always been a good eater. At the time we first met him he was somewhat overweight. George had had three bad colds during the first year of life. He began to walk and uttered his first words at approximately 13 months. His articulation of speech sounds had always been quite poor and it had been difficult to understand his speech. He had been bowel-trained at the age of 2 years, but he still wet himself occasionally during the day.

George had entered a private nursery school at the age of 3 years 10 months. According to his mother's reports, George had always liked school. His teacher had described him as a friendly and cooperative child who, however, was somewhat restless and tense. During the second year in nursery school he appeared to have increasing difficulty in communicating with his teacher and classmates. His teacher had felt that George was "emotionally disturbed" and had discussed this with his mother; however, it was discovered that George had fluid in both ears and that his hearing was slightly impaired. His tonsils and adenoids were removed when he was 4 years 11 months and his hearing improved markedly, but no improvement in his speech was observed. He was referred then for speech therapy.

Following the intake interview, George's mother was instructed in how to assist him in his speech development. However, she had to attend to pressing family affairs, which left her but little time and energy for helping him with his speech. When George entered kindergarten a speech therapist was assigned to work intensively with him.

The teacher and the therapist agreed that George was an intelligent, sensitive, and cooperative little boy, but his progress in the learning of speech was very slow. He had severe difficulty in auditory discrimination of speech sounds and in remembering sequences of sounds. The therapist also observed that George was very clumsy in his motions and slow in climbing stairs. He also had difficulty in catching a ball, repeating rhythmic patterns, hopping and skipping, and using a pencil. In addition to his poor articulation occasionally he seemed to search for a word and had difficulty recalling it. When asked to speak in front of a group, George found it difficult to express his ideas fluently in sentences; symptoms of hesitancy and later of marked stuttering appeared in his speech.

At the age of 6 years 1 month he was examined by a school psychologist.

From Psychologist's Report   Age 6 years 1 month

George was referred because he seems to be restless and to have a short attention span. He is awkward in the use of his body. He suffers from severely defective articulation and received speech therapy.

The examiner observed George in the classroom for half an hour before testing him. During this time he played very well with a group of boys, making a fort out of large blocks. His speech was quite understandable although there were occasional but not consistent mispronunciations and substitutions of sounds. He is an oversized, poorly coordinated boy, who walks with a rather odd gait. Although somewhat reluctant to accompany the examiner, he did so without any fuss, but began to stutter quite severely. The stuttering lasted while he walked down the hall, talking to the examiner about his friends, his home, and so forth. While taking the test the stuttering disappeared almost entirely and although an occasional word was unintelligible, the examiner had no difficulty in understanding his speech.

The examiner gave Form-LM of the Revised Stanford-Binet with the following results:

Mental Age	6 years, 4 months
Chronological Age	6 years, 1 month
I.Q.	105

George passed all tests at the 5-year level, although he was just barely able to copy the square. At 6 years he was successful on the Vocabulary, Similarities, Opposite Analogies, and Mutilated Picture items. His ability to count was rather inconsistent. At 7 years he passed the Similarities, Comprehension, and Repeating Digits items. He was wholly unable to copy the diamond. His only success at 8 years was the Vocabulary item.

The examiner also asked George to draw a man, which he did after a fashion. It was clear that he had great difficulty in using a pencil and he was quite unable to communicate his ideas with it.

Summary: George is a boy of at least average intelligence. He has extremely poor motor coordination and it is difficult for him to handle a pencil as well as he would like. He is unable to convey his ideas through the medium of drawing. His speech is not too difficult to understand, except when he is stuttering. This latter symptom seems to trouble him most when he feels anxious.

A diagnostic assessment was carried out jointly by George's pediatrician, his teacher, a school psychologist, and a speech therapist, and a diagnosis of motor-perceptual and language disorder was made. George was seen twice weekly by the speech therapist, who, in addition to training him in auditory discrimination and articulation, also did motor, perceptual, and rhythmic exercises with him. She taught him how to play ball, use chalk and heavy crayons, work with puzzles, and practice rhythmic patterns. A number of exercises recommended by Kephart (1960) were included in this training. The therapist had frequent conferences with George's mother and his teacher. As George felt more secure in the kindergarten, his articulation gradually improved, his speech became quite comprehensible, and the symptoms of secondary stuttering disappeared. George's parents spent much time talking and reading to him, practices which were reflected in George's advanced vocabulary. However, when George attempted to express himself in a more complex and extensive statement, frequent repetitions of initial syllables appeared in his speech and his articulation deteriorated. Thus, at that point, his speech showed more the characteristics of cluttering than of stuttering.

When George was 7 years old his hearing was tested again by an audiologist and was found to be normal. He also had a neurological examination. No specific signs of brain damage were found, except for the deficiencies in his motor, perceptual, and language behavior, already described.

Because of his size and age, and also because of his speech improvement, George was promoted to first grade. It soon became apparent, however, that George was unable to learn reading. In January of the following year, his first-grade teacher reported:

From Teacher's Report   Age 7 years 2 months

George is a very polite and friendly boy who is well liked by the other children and appears eager to do well. He is one of the oldest children in the group; he is very large and is awkward in bodily movements; and he appears to be definitely left-handed.

His speech has improved and he can produce speech sounds correctly but in conversation he reverts to faulty speech patterns. His handwriting has improved, but his written work is untidy and often incomplete, with reversals in both letters and numbers and confusion in left-to-right progression.

George gives every indication that he is interested in reading but he is experiencing extreme frustration and continued failure in this area, in spite of varied techniques and an unusual amount of small-group instruction.

George has not acquired sight vocabulary except for a very few words. This continued failure is a cause for concern both for the teacher and the child.

It should be mentioned here that the child, the teacher, and the parents experienced not only concern but increasing frustration and anxiety in view of George's desperate and almost entirely unsuccessful attempts to master even the very beginnings of reading. George's predicament was discussed in joint sessions with his teacher, the reading consultant, the speech therapist, the pediatrician, and members of the school administration. In agreement with his parents arrangements were made to have George tutored individually.

From then on through the first and second grades, George worked daily for one and one-half hours with a highly trained, very imaginative, and talented tutor. For the remainder of the day he was assigned to a regular classroom where he continued to associate with his agemates and friends. Excerpts from a report by the tutor, written when George was 8 years 6 months old, will demonstrate some of the methods used by the tutor, as well as George's reactions to her efforts.

From Tutor's Report   Age 8 years 7 months

It is difficult to evaluate George's progress in terms of an average second grader as there is such a gap between his general knowledge and creative ability, and his basic language skills. Although he is just beginning to read on a first grade level, he is able to understand what he is doing and works with an increasing amount of assurance.

One of my most difficult tasks has been to reduce George's almost unbearable tension when faced with work in the language area. He is now able to concentrate on work centered on reading, writing, and spelling for at least an hour. His other activities, designed to develop muscular control and better directional orientation, have permitted casual conversation, which has led to incidental correction of speech errors. I made a special effort to have George use his excellent creative abilities as well as his strong powers of observation and memory. For example: George is very much interested in airplanes, so he has spent a good deal of time folding paper planes. At first this was a relaxing game, but he soon started dividing them into squadrons, redesigning them and keeping records of their performances, and learning about relative sizes, shapes, etc. This was useful as a reinforcement for number facts, and especially useful in stressing accuracy.

George's oral work is far superior to his written work. He speaks quite clearly now, and I find a highly significant improvement in his reading and spelling skills as he becomes able to appreciate the differences between the speech sounds. Blends are still difficult for him and I will do no formal work with them until he is thoroughly secure in his knowledge of single consonants.

The fact that George is now able to retain simple auditory and visual patterns makes me feel confident that we can build a firm base from which he will be able to operate. However, he should be exposed to knowledge commensurate with his abilities in other areas. It seems to me that he understands mathematical principles, even if he is unable to read the problems. He seems to understand the work in social studies, even though he has not been able to do the reading or written work. Science and mathematics are most interesting to him, and he has no trouble integrating his fairly wide general knowledge.

It is impossible at this point to predict how long it will take George to "catch up." We have had cooperation from all concerned, and have accomplished the absolutely essential goal of reducing tension and reestablishing George's self-confidence. It was a severe blow to his pride to be unable to learn to read in the first grade, and the fact that he has stuck to this tutorial program without protest is indicative of his determination to cope with the situation. He enjoys school and always looks forward to rejoining his class. His parents have been cooperative and understanding, which has helped George tremendously.

TUTORIAL PROCEDURES

PROBLEMS ENCOUNTERED	METHODS USED	PRESENT STATUS
I. Reading A. Nonreader. B. Tense to point of exhaustion when trying to read.	Capitalized on a few words (fewer than 10) remembered from last year to keep up some activity in reading. Wrote stories in notebook to be read. Made a "Go fish" game from a pre-primer word list. Matched words visually, also using auditory and kinesthetic clues. Spelling while looking at word. Some writing. Almost no organized reading other than on worksheets I developed as we've gone along. Have used phonovisual workbooks[5] with partial success, but found too great a weakness in the auditory-articulatory area and decided to concentrate more on visual and kinesthetic approach.	Basic pre-primer vocabulary fairly well established, though resistance to reading has been high. *Here We Go* from the Alice and Jerry Books proved successful and George is now working well in this Harper and Row pre-primer series (O'Donnell, *et. al*, 1957). His tension increases markedly when reading, and he becomes very tired. This is lessening as confidence increases. Has no problem matching words visually, though he may not be able to read them. Is able in most cases to identify a printed word if I say it, or spell it.
II. Letters A. Did not know alphabet. B. Could not name most letters.	This has required endless hours of drill—have used the Alphabet Song as basis for learning letters as he seemed able to remember it. The magnetic letters are arranged alphabetically, as is his file box of words. We've used sandpaper letters and exercises, blackboard copying, magnetic letters, writing, tracing, coloring, any possible mnemonic clues, Jr. Scrabble, cutting letters from magazines, also phonovisual workbooks (*op. cit.*), a fishing game based on this, along with regular drill with the Gillingham cards[6] (naming	Knowledge of alphabet seems secure and letters can be named or written as needed. Can identify most by phonetic clues, but is still unable to tie them together to make words. This is beginning to come, though it will, I'm afraid, require the same slow and thorough procedures used in mastering the alphabet.

5. Montgomery and Coughlan (1953); Stubbings, Haverly, Gaynes, and Montgomery (1953).
6. Gillingham and Stillman (1966).

Tutorial Procedures—*continued*

PROBLEMS ENCOUNTERED	METHODS USED	PRESENT STATUS
	letters only). Phonetic clues have been worked in incidentally, but I felt George would make more progress if we established the names and forms of the letters before the sounds.	

III. Spelling
  A. Unable to spell.
  B. Letters making up words meant nothing.
	Tried at first to establish a knowledge of phonics through use of phonovisual workbooks and chart. However, even though George learned names of letters, he was unable to establish relationship with sound. A combination of Gillingham Simultaneous Oral Spelling (*op. cit.*) and Fernald tracing techniques[7] seems to be producing results. We are developing a file box with words George will use for writing.	George can write a word if I spell it, and he is able to copy from the blackboard. He is learning to copy groups of letters, or a whole syllable, after looking at sample. Can spell a few words from memory and is almost ready to start on simple sentences.

IV. Handwriting
  A. Able to copy, but unable to read material copied, or identify letters.
  B. Reversals common, both letters and numbers.
  C. Very tense, tires easily when writing.
	Used sandpaper letters, pegboard to establish left-right orientation. Used blackboard, copying, tracing. Very low pressure, casual writing work, few writing papers. Mostly blackboard work because of tension.	Have just begun more organized writing and spelling. Less tense on familiar ground, but an error will cause reversals and tension to point of inability to function. Handwriting more relaxed, apt to be sloppy, something I overlook.

V. Extreme tension in relation to school work.
  A. Short attention span.
  B. Fear of failure.
	Very low-pressure teaching sessions. At first George was unable to work for more than 10 minutes, but this has been increased gradually without discussion. Much use of games	We now spend approximately 1¼ hours on work specifically connected with language. We do much more concentrated work, with 10–15 min. spent on each project. This varies

7. Fernald (1943).

Tutorial Procedures—*continued*

PROBLEMS ENCOUNTERED	METHODS USED	PRESENT STATUS
C. Resistance to reading and writing. D. Uncertainty in following directions.	and highly informal ways of dealing with material in attempt to overcome fear of failure. No planned work program because each session depends on what pupil is able to take—health, fatigue, home factors always a consideration. Worksheets designed by me, as so much reinforcement has been necessary. Simple directions given orally.	daily as I find that George's level of tolerance varies.
VI. General lack of left-right orientation, clumsiness, uncertainty about colors, inability to tell time.	Pegboard, coloring, many worksheets, informal games, throwing and catching a ball, drawing pictures, daily time-checks.	Can follow directions on pegboard, knows basic colors, and can read names. Great improvement in handling ball—progressed from being unable to catch large playground ball to catching tennis ball. Still not sure of left and right. Can tell positions of hands on clock, but cannot tell time.

George continued to receive individual tutorial help during the second and third grade. He made slow but consistent progress in the language areas, but he became increasingly tense and unhappy during the hours he spent in the regular classroom. Although his second-grade teacher had done her best to keep George occupied and make him feel an active and accepted member of the group, his third-grade teacher was very critical of his presence in her classroom. George spent much of his time inactive, feeling isolated from his classmates. At that point other children with similar deficiencies had been identified by the school psychologists, in cooperation with teachers and physicians. With the sanction of the school administration, a special tutorial class for children with motor-perceptual and language disabilities was established. George's tutor agreed to become the teacher of this experimental class.

The general atmosphere and the specific structure of this tutorial class have had a highly beneficial effect upon George, who no longer has to spend most of his days in situations where the experience of failure is inevitable.

George has continued to make steady progress. He now benefits from a well-organized program, alternating between special class training in the language arts and participation in selected activities, such as science, mathematics, and physical education, which he shares with his agemates in regular classrooms. The special classroom is large and uncluttered, and the furniture and equipment can be rearranged easily to permit a flexible type of small-group instruction. Although George evidently enjoys his participation in regular classroom activities, he likes to return to his tutor and to the special classroom which serves to protect him against overstimulation and fatigue.

In kindergarten and first grade George had worked regularly with a speech therapist who helped him in learning auditory discrimination and articulation of speech sounds. Once George began working with the special tutor, the services of the speech therapist were discontinued and the tutor continued George's speech training in an informal manner, providing him with verbal feedback and correcting his articulatory errors whenever this seemed appropriate. Thus his speech training formed an integral part of his overall training in motor, perceptual, and communication skills. Now, at the age of 10 years, George's articulation has become satisfactory; he has learned to speak, read, and write all the letters of the alphabet; and he is beginning to connect speech sounds (phonemes) with letters (graphemes). However, in situations of fatigue or stress, he still makes occasional errors in articulation and he also has difficulty in connected speech, showing symptoms of cluttering or stuttering.[8] It was decided, therefore, that his former speech therapist would work again with him regularly, assisting him in his use of connected speech and, in particular, helping him prepare oral reports on a variety of subjects, which he presents in the regular fifth grade class to which he has been assigned.

Recently George was tested again by two school psychologists; some of their observations are summarized here.

From Psychologist's Report, I   Age 9 years 11 months

As usual, George was friendly and quite willing to accompany the examiner, whom he knows fairly well. At the beginning of the interview he stuttered again slightly, but soon was speaking fluently. His attention was well controlled and obviously he was eager to do things well.

Tests given were:

Wechsler Intelligence Scale for Children (WISC)
Bender Gestalt Test for Young Children
Goodenough Draw-a-Man Test

Results on the WISC were:

Verbal Scale I.Q.   115
Performance Scale I.Q.   120
Full Scale I.Q.   119

Scores on the Information and Comprehension items of the Verbal Scale were average; all other verbal scores were superior. On the Arithmetic item George did many of his calculations aloud, but even then it was impossible to follow his mental processes. He was

8. The problem of differential diagnosis concerning these two disorders will be taken up in Chapter 14.

able to complete successfully two of the most difficult items which children are expected to read for themselves, but which had to be read to him. He was able to keep the information in mind and come out with the correct answers. Performance test scores with the exception of Coding, were superior. On some of the Performance tests, when faced with an unfamiliar or difficult situation, he responded in a disorganized manner, resorting to random trial and error methods, rather than approaching the situation by studying it carefully.

On the Bender Gestalt Test for Young Children George scored at the 7-year-level. The results reflected his motor-perceptual difficulties. He was aware of his difficulties and was quite critical of what he had done. At the end of the formal test he was asked to redraw the three designs he felt he had done most poorly. His second performance on all was better than the first. The one design with which he had most trouble because of his inability to keep it from falling apart, he reproduced correctly on the second trial, inserting guidelines to keep it together. While all of George's errors were, to some extent, suggestive of brain damage, none of them was of the sort found only in brain-damaged children (Koppitz, 1964).

When asked to draw a man George explained in detail that his "best people" took him a long time—a day or two—to draw. He was encouraged to do the best he could in a short time, but even with some urging on the examiner's part to work more quickly, he spent about one-half hour over his drawing. He received a mental age score of 8 years 6 months on it. He was unable to carry out his original plan of drawing a profile consistently, the trunk being shown full face. There were other respects, too, in which he had difficulty in portraying a person, particularly in placing the limbs in relation to the trunk. He blacked in his whole drawing with innumerable fine pencil lines.

Summary: George tested at the high average to superior level. His problems were most conspicuous in relation to the reproduction of designs, as in the Bender Gestalt Test. On his figure drawing he appeared to be more obsessional than he was in other situations.

From Psychologist's Report, II   Age 10 years

George was most friendly and outgoing throughout the testing period. Occasionally he stuttered but much of the time he spoke fluently.

Tests given were:

> Goldstein-Scheerer Tests of Abstract and Concrete Thinking (1966 edition)
>> Color Form Sorting Test
>> Stick Test
> Perceptual Survey Rating Scale (Kephart, 1960)

George completed the Color Form Sorting Test with ease. First he sorted the objects according to their geometric shapes. When asked to verbalize what he was doing, he said he had put the triangles, circles, and squares together. When asked to sort the objects in another way, he changed their spatial relationships. When he was asked to sort them differently again, he proposed to do it according to color. He did this quickly, with a minimal amount of effort.

On the Goldstein-Scheerer Stick Test George was careful to copy exactly from the model. Only on one of the more complicated designs did he make a slight error, this being in the spacing of the sticks. His reproduction of the designs from memory was nearly as accurate. On only one occasion did he fail to take into consideration the different size of the sticks used. He rotated his reproduction of an X by 45 degrees, making it appear as a cross. Throughout this test he spontaneously verbalized what he was doing.

Throughout the administration of the Perceptual Survey Rating Scale George engaged the examiner in conversation. George seemed to have below average ability in his control of gross motor movements. He found balancing on the board difficult, particularly when requested to walk backwards. He had equal difficulty in following simple rhythms when jumping, skipping, and hopping. He could not distinguish his left from his right foot and found it necessary to seek clarification from the examiner. He was able to imitate the majority of the examiner's movements, raising and lowering corresponding arms. Only on one occasion did he become confused on this series of tasks. He found it easy to move both arms and legs together, but he had less skill in moving one arm and one leg simultaneously, especially when asked to combine movements of opposite limbs. George also had considerable difficulty in doing such physical exercises as sit-ups and push-ups. He tired quickly on these tasks. On the Ocular Pursuits Test George was able to follow fine movements with both eyes, and with either left or right eye, with comparative ease. (On a previous testing a year and a half ago he had had some difficulty on this test item.) He copied the geometric shapes on the Visual Achievement Form subtests quite hurriedly. When asked if he could do a better job, he was willing to repeat the designs, but did them no better than the first time. He was somewhat critical of his accomplishments on this test, but did not feel that he could do better.

Summary: In this testing situation, George seemed to have slightly better control of his fine than of his gross motor movements. While he was able to perform the majority of the tasks requiring movements of large body parts, he did so somewhat awkwardly. On the more strenuous tasks he tired quickly, not having much physical stamina. When faced with tasks requiring precise movements, George demonstrated greater ability in the manipulation of three-dimensional objects than he did in drawing. On the tasks requiring insight in a problem-solving situation, his accomplishments were considerably above average and he performed efficiently and imaginatively.

We will conclude the case of George with reports from his tutor, from the school principal, and from George's mother.

From Tutor's Report   Age 11 years

George is still a member of the ungraded tutorial group, but is involved increasingly in the activities of the regular fifth-grade classroom. He is able to read some of the fifth-grade material, with help, even though his reading skills are considerably below grade level—about middle second grade. It hasn't been until this year that he has been able to identify all the letters of the alphabet as well as write them. Also, he has finally begun to make the connection between speech sounds and letters. He is much less tense in regard to school work, and is more willing to try to solve problems on his own. His handwriting (manuscript, because attempts to switch him to cursive have been unsuccessful) is neat, legible, and very laborious. Reversals are not as common but still occur occasionally, as do all his language weaknesses, when he is under stress. His motor coordination has been improving constantly. He has made the greatest progress in this area since he has been participating in the strenuous activities of his fifth grade gym class and after-school sports program. He has learned to tell time, but is vague as to days, months, and dates. Arithmetic and science continue to be his strongest areas. He is achieving at grade level here. His wide general knowledge has helped him considerably in social studies. Mastery of language skills will take much more work, but he continues to be highly motivated to overcome his difficulties.

Referring to the tutorial class as a whole, the principal of George's school remarked:

Progress is painfully slow for all children in this special group. Goals set for achievement must be realistic for them. The usual report cards, achievement tests, or teacher evaluations do not encourage the youngsters or do justice to their teachers. The standard report card does not tell their story. Other means of evaluation must be used which will reflect their teacher's optimism and a measure of progress which will be acceptable to the teacher and to the home.

As these children spend part of their days in a regular classroom, it is important that the teachers involved receive information concerning the children's disabilities, understand their problems, and are willing to modify their teaching in order to include these youngsters. Daily communication and joint planning by the principal, the tutorial teacher, and the classroom teachers is essential. Most of all, it is important that a principal be well informed about the specific disabilities of these children, and that he have a sympathetic attitude toward their problems.

In addition to the sharing of information and the ongoing communication among all members of the staff involved, positive relations and frequent interaction between home and school are of the greatest importance for the well-being and achievement of each child.

In a letter to the author written when George was 11 years 3 months old, George's mother vividly described the personality of her son, and also the many ways in which she and her husband attempted to help him to cope with his disabilities. With the parents' permission, we quote here from her letter.

My husband and I feel strongly that we are very fortunate in having a healthy, intelligent son. George has been a joy and a warm, loving companion to both of us. He is left-handed, clumsy, and not well coordinated. He had articulation problems at a younger age and still has difficulty with cluttering or stuttering. His mind works so much more quickly than he can formulate his ideas in words. He is very sensitive and aware of the feelings of others. He often takes an original, creative approach and thinks very clearly and logically. He is also stubborn and determined to do things his way. He makes close and lasting friendships. He has a strong sense of justice and fairness and becomes quite emotional when this is outraged. He is a dreamer and a procrastinator and can be quite frustrating.

George enjoys physical activity, but because of his lack of coordination he is not a truly enthusiastic team player. Last fall he enjoyed participating in soccer and for the past two years he has enjoyed peewee hockey. We have been having family pool games and this winter for the first time, George is able to shoot with a fair amount of accuracy.

George has an eager, curious mind and a good memory for facts of a widely diverse nature. He learns mostly by listening. This weekend I discovered him watching intently a documentary on the life of Gandhi and another TV program of an interview with an artist who was sketching famous men and pointing out personality traits which were evident in their faces. For a child who has such great difficulty in learning to read, TV can be invaluable.

George loves words and has a large vocabulary which he uses to a surprising extent. He has a good sense of humor, too. The other night my husband was complimenting me on our dinner. He asked George: "Where do you suppose I ever found such a mother?" George responded instantly: "I don't know, Daddy. Did you look in the Yellow Pages?"

Not long ago he remarked: "I like school this year, Mother." This is particularly gratifying since he has had so many problems and frustrations in other years. In third grade he had an especially hard year. He didn't complain at all. However, last year when the special tutorial class had been established and he had exceptionally fine and understanding teaching in the fourth grade, he did remark, "This year I really have to work. You know, Mother, last year so much of the time all I could do was dream."

George has always loved to build. He began with the large wooden blocks when he was 2 or 3 years old and has continued building to this day. He still uses those same blocks, Lincoln Logs, straws, paper, building sets, and does so every day or at least several times a week. It is almost a compulsion. He also uses Erector Sets and his train track and trestle and bridge. He also loves soldiers and sets up campaigns and has battles with his friends or even with himself alone. We try to confine this activity to a playroom on the second floor; but on occasion the campaigns range all over the house.

Despite his difficulties in learning to read, George has loved books from the time he was very little. Beginning with nursery rhymes, his father and I have read to him every night and often during automobile trips. Some books had to be read over and over. *Peter Pan* was a great favorite, as were many fairy tales. Animal, adventure, and mystery stories have occupied us often. Recently I have noticed that George anticipates what will happen next in a book—and usually he is right.

George has been in Cub Scouts for the past three years. One of the things I did last year for him was to be a den mother. Since he does not attend his neighborhood school, my having his contemporaries here for Cub Scouts one afternoon a week has helped to keep his friendships alive.

My husband and I feel that physical activity is vitally important for George. Summers we spend many weekends and two or three complete weeks at a fishing camp. For the past three summers we engaged an older boy to be with us at camp. This has worked out well. George and the other boy sleep in a separate building and carry on their own boating, fishing, swimming, snorkling, or hiking pursuits, but they are with us for meals and for family projects.

One thing I should like to point out is the actual physical strain which results from George's work in reading or writing. Learning the alphabet was a real challenge for George. I shall never forget the first time he got through it with flash cards for his tutor and me. He was literally yawning from the effort. The letter *h* was so hard for him that his tutor finally gave him an exercise using his whole body to trace it. Now, even though he can read on his grade level, he can't keep it up for a very long period. To those of us who read as easily as we breathe, this is hard to comprehend or to accept.

Other problems which we have found often are those created by pressure and tension. George, who is an unusually sensitive child, *actually becomes incapable of functioning when under pressure*. It is hard to maintain the delicate balance necessary to keep him operating as effectively as his capabilities will permit.

My husband and I try to help George with homework when necessary and we see to it that he reads some each day. I work in the library at George's school one morning every other week. This enables me to keep in closer touch with George and his work. I also find books which I feel he can cope with and will enjoy reading or which we will enjoy reading to him.

It has been a long struggle since we first had George's problem diagnosed in the spring of his first grade year. We know there will be no easy solution. We are so very grateful to the people who have worked with him in the school system. Our pediatrician also has been a major factor in the total picture giving wise counsel throughout the whole period.

Where we will go with George at the seventh grade level we do not yet know. We do feel that he will still require specialized help, even though he has made great strides.

Not all parents will possess the strength and the resources which would enable them to assist a child with a major learning disability. Garrard and Richmond (1963b) have given a penetrating description of the multidimensional social, psychological, and economic problems which afflict the families of handicapped children. In the group discussed here, the wide variety of possible symptoms and the puzzling combinations of talents and limitations in one and the same child are particularly apt to arouse anxiety in parents. Parents of children with motor-perceptual and language disorders may be exposed to a variety of conflicting diagnoses and recommendations. Even after a competent assessment of a child's difficulties has been made, and an appropriate educational program has been set up, the parents can not be assured that the child's difficulties will disappear rapidly or completely. Frequent informal conferences and communication between principal, teacher, and parents will help the parents to gain a better understanding of the child's approach to learning as well as of the tutor's approach to teaching. In addition, the school psychologist or guidance counselor should meet with the parents from time to time to help them cope with their anxieties and defense mechanisms. The dynamics of this form of parent counseling have been succinctly described by Garrard and Richmond (*op. cit.*).

A final word should be said about a form of group activity for the children in the Wellesley tutorial class, which was initiated, on an experimental basis, by von Sander, one of our school psychologists. The group leader meets with the children once weekly for a period of nonacademic group activities, organized around a building or constructing project, or the learning and playing of various games. The techniques used by the group leader are not those of psychotherapy, but rather of educational therapy or *Heilpaedagogik*. Von Sander observed that the children appeared to gain much from the double track of their educational program: they spend most of the morning in the protective environment of the special classroom, but are exposed during the afternoon to the more complex, multi-stimulating setting of the regular classroom. Coping with this more diversified environment calls for built-in controls against overstimulation, for the maintenance of ego boundaries, and for the ability to shift rapidly from one social grouping to another—ego functions in which these children are notoriously deficient. During the therapeutic play sessions the group leader, in helping the children to work on nonacademic group projects, teaches them not only eye-hand coordination but also methods to anticipate and to cope with change, to shift from one mode of perception to another, to organize various kinds of material and tools, to discover the structure inherent in a situation or even to provide their own structuring if necessary. It is evident that this type of group activity is not set up to induce the children to express their feelings, but rather to help them to contain and organize their feelings and sensations; to anticipate possible frustrations and to develop coping mechanisms; and to gradually shift from a largely concrete experience of their environment to more abstract forms of cognition, thinking, and planning. The therapeutic methods initiated by von Sander, are experimental; the results have been encouraging.

COMMENTARY

The case of George has been presented because we wanted to demonstrate the length of time necessary—with our present methods—to help a perceptually handicapped child learn the basic skills of communication. Longitudinal case studies of perceptually handicapped children have been scarce in the literature. As George is one of the children we have known over an extensive period of time, we chose to describe his development, hoping that it might help the reader to appreciate his complex handicap, as well as his manner of coping with it.

Under the impact of time, maturation, skillful tutoring, and loving guidance at home, George has made slow but continuous progress. While George demonstrates certain difficulties similar to those of other children in this group, we cannot say that his behavior and development are typical of children with motor-perceptual disabilities. As we know, George had severe difficulties in the areas of auditory discrimination and articulation of speech sounds; connected speech; differentiation of and memory for abstract visual shapes; the connection of phonemes with graphemes; hand-eye coordination; gross and fine motor coordination; and drawing and writing. These multiple difficulties were somewhat compensated for by his excellent understanding of the meaning of words; his ability for conceptual thinking and for learning and retaining content through auditory input; and his skill in establishing interpersonal relationships. His continued interest in learning, in spite of all his difficulties, indicates a high degree of ego strength, while his occasional mood swings and his periods of stuttering suggest that below the surface of his friendly and cooperative behavior he may experience much anxiety and anger concerning the adults around him, his peers, and himself. Evidently, beyond the support which George receives from his teachers and parents, he needs more intensive therapeutic help to cope with his accumulated feelings of insecurity, anger, and frustration. Arrangements are being made for George to receive such help from a psychotherapist.

Looking back at the distribution of symptoms presented in Table 11, we realize again that each child in this group is, in some manner, different from every other child. George, for instance, did not show the symptoms of hyperactivity which are found in many of the children and which make their education unusually difficult.

A developmental study of a child with motor-perceptual and language disabilities is bound to have specific limitations. However, following George's development over a five-year period may have helped the reader to perceive the difference between the mentally retarded child and the perceptually impaired child, on the one hand, and between the perceptually impaired and the normal child, on the other.

CHAPTER THIRTEEN

Group C: Children with Multiple Motor-Perceptual and Language Disabilities, II

The program for children with motor-perceptual and language disabilities developed in the Wellesley Schools can best be appreciated if it is viewed against the background of research carried out by other groups. As will be seen, the field is still very much in flux.

TERMINOLOGY AND ETIOLOGY

Interest in the identification, diagnosis, and training of children with multiple motor-perceptual and language disorders has greatly increased in recent years. The literature shows, however, that children with similar multiple symptoms have been described under a confusing variety of headings. We read of children with mild, diffuse, or minimal brain damage; with specific or with general language disability; with alexia, dyslexia, or strephosymbolia; with cerebral or with neurological dysfunction. As Anne E. Bowes pointed out (1966), "perceptual-motor dysfunction" is by itself a broad term which will imply different things to different people and will encompass varied kinds of behavior. In our work we preferred a descriptive terminology, which facilitated communication among members of an interprofessional team.

Different investigators tend to use different levels of abstraction in referring to their observations. Educators might mention a child's short memory span, or his immaturity in figure drawing; research psychologists will talk about "deficits in visual figure-ground perception" (Ayres, 1966). Orthopedists or pediatricians might stress a child's motor difficulties, speech therapists, the speech deficiencies, and reading specialists, the severe reading disorder, while they sometimes may overlook or minimize difficulties in related areas. Understandably, examiners often seem to focus upon specific aspects of behavior which are closest to their respective fields.

Interest in severe learning disabilities goes back to the beginning of the century when J. Hinshelwood, in England, began to describe cases of "Congenital word-blindness" (Hinshelwood, 1900a, b, 1912, 1917), followed in this country by Orton's studies of "Word-blindness in school children" (1925) and of "Specific reading disability—strephosymbolia" (1928a. See also Orton 1928b, 1934, 1937, 1943). Similar studies were carried out, in Germany, by Liebmann (1924), Ranschburg (1916, 1928), and others. Since then, research in the many facets of perceptual-motor and language disorders has greatly increased. Experiments in developing methods of perceptual and language training at present are carried out in this country and abroad, though data concerning treatment results have been scarce.

The following brief excerpts from the literature might help the reader to perceive not only the differences in theory and in categories of classification, but also the similarities in methods of diagnosis and training which are beginning to emerge in this field.

Professor Arthur L. Drew, of the Indiana University Medical Center, includes a discussion of nonretarded children with specific learning disabilities, dysphasias, dyspraxias, and perceptual-motor disabilities in his study, "The clinical neurology of mental retardation" (1966). He reports that the history and neurological examination of these children often reveals delay in motor development; restlessness; poor sleep; frequency of febrile seizures; delayed or incomplete language development; difficulties in learning to dress, to ride a bicycle, to play hand-eye or rhythmic games; hyperactivity; short attention span; and lack of concentration. So-called soft signs, to be considered by pediatric neurologists, include awkward gait, frequent stumbling, slight loss of balance on sudden change of direction. As the child learns to dress himself he has more trouble with buttons, sleeves, and shoe-laces than the majority of children of his age, and he may confuse right and left shoes, raising the suspicion of a dressing dyspraxia. The child also may have difficulty in comprehending and following instructions; he may show awkward control of tongue movements (tongue dyspraxia) and difficulties in spatial orientation, both in intrapersonal and extrapersonal space. Drew also mentions difficulties in the reproduction of geometrical figures and in directionality, and laterality—confusions in paper-and-pencil work. The author considers the diagnosis of children with perceptual-motor learning disabilities as the joint province of the pediatric neurologist and the neuropsychologist. He emphasizes that "probably no other area of neurology, psychiatry, psychology, or education suffers more from lack of basic information, on the one hand, and from hastily evolved, preconceived formulations, on the other" (*ibid.*, p. 42).

As mentioned earlier, children with disordered functioning and with aberrations in development and in the learning of skills have been referred to, at different times, as defective, brain-damaged, or minimally brain-damaged. H. G. Birch (1964) considered these terms "unfortunate diagnostic labels"; he felt that all "designations of nervous system damage, whether they be described as minimal, as diffuse, or as nonfocal, remain presumptive in the absence of well-established data demonstrating the nature of the damage to the underlying structure itself" (*op. cit.*, p. 5). Birch stressed the fact that *for all practical purposes we are not concerned with a neurological designation but with a behavior pattern.* This behavior pattern consists of "varied pictures of developmental lag, of behavioral disturbance, of transient or persistent motor awkwardness, of minor perceptual disturbance, of distractability, of limitation of attention span, of thought disturbance, and of educational and emotional difficulties," suggesting "rather subtle disturbances of the nervous system" (*ibid*). Thus, Birch's concept of the "syndrome of dysfunction" is complex and refers to a wider range of phenomena than those considered in earlier studies.

A report on the motor-perceptual and language disorders of aphasic children by J. Eisenson (1966), also contains much pertinent information. Starting from the steps in the perceptual process known as input, integration, output, and feedback (a check on the appropriateness of the output), Eisenson lists the following functions as basic to language learning (*op. cit.*, p. 23):

1. The capacity to receive stimuli that are produced in sequential order.
2. The capacity to hold the stimuli in mind, to hold the sequential impression, so that its components may be integrated into some pattern.
3. The capacity to scan the pattern from within so that it may be compared with other impressions or other remembered patterns.
4. The capacity to respond differentially, meaningfully, to the perceptual impression.

According to Eisenson there is a "special total population" of children with disturbances in these basic functions. These children differ from others in the delayed development of manual laterality and in the learning of spatial orientation. They manifest awkwardness in gross motor functioning and deficiency in fine motor coordination. They may also show signs of hyperactivity, deficiency in attention span, and considerable variability and lability in their responses to repeated learning situations. The problems in language functioning of these children, while not as severe as those of aphasics, present serious communicative and educational handicaps. A number of these children may have abnormal electro-encephalographic (EEG) findings. Eisenson referred to this special population as "brain-different" rather than "brain-damaged." Similar to Birch, Eisenson doubted the wisdom of referring to these children as having "minimal brain damage," or of using the label "specific language disability" (SLD)—a term which recently has become rather popular. We fully agree with Eisenson that the term *specific language disability* should be changed to *nonspecific language disability*, "because the evidence, if carefully examined strongly suggests that to a lesser or greater degree, a variety of vaguely defined linguistic functions are impaired" (*op. cit.*, p. 26).

In a paper, "Perceptual-motor dysfunction in children: criterion problems," D. A. Leton (1966) suggested a possible framework for a system of classification, based upon observed "syndromes" or "constellations of traits," possible neurological bases, and examination procedures used. A "comprehensive concept of the neurologically handicapped child" was presented by Denhoff, Laufer, and Holden (1959), and comprehensive descriptions of psychoneurological language and learning disorders in children can be found in publications by Myklebust (1956, 1964), Myklebust and Boshes (1960), and Boshes and Myklebust (1964).

Further neurological discussions of the syndrome of cerebral dysfunction or minimal brain damage can be found in the book *Minimal Cerebral Dysfunction*, edited by Bax and Mackeith (1963), and in papers by Bradley (1966), Clements and Peters (1962), Clemmens (1966), Gubbay, Ellis, Walton, and Court (1965), Knobloch and Pasamanick (1959), and Paine (1962).

As severe reading disability must be considered a major social and vocational handicap for all members of literate societies, the syndrome of dyslexia or alexia has attracted particular attention. M. Critchley, a British neurologist, discussed dyslexia in an "aphasiological context" (Critchley, 1964). The author considered the study of dyslexia as a medical province, "invaded" by educational psychologists. Using the terms "specific" or "developmental dyslexia," he defined the disorder as a "specific syndrome wherein the particular difficulty exists in learning the conventional meaning of verbal symbols, and of associating the sound with symbol in appropriate fashion" (*op. cit.*, p. 18). In spite of this initial, somewhat narrow definition, the book ranges widely over the linguistic, motoric, and perceptual difficulties encountered in dyslexic children; the etiology, genetic properties, and clinical manifestations of the disability; and diagnostic testing and training of older dyslexic pupils.

Critchley summarizes the work of many European and American specialists, starting from Hinshelwood's notion of congenital word-blindness, mentioned above, Orton's theory of strephosymbolia, and Bender's concept of maturational lag (Bender, 1957). The discussion of pedagogical issues, however, is perfunctory, and though the author acknowledged the fact that neurological findings differed according to the age of the subject, the early manifestations of motor-perceptual disorders in preschool children are hardly considered.

The phenomenology of dyslexia, as well as its epidemiology, were the topics of The Johns Hopkins Conference on Dyslexia, in Baltimore, Maryland, in 1961. Papers presented dealt with the educational significance of the disorder; its relation to cerebral dominance; form perception and directional sense; language acquisition and concept formation; and problems of visual function (Money, 1962). Benton's paper, in particular, should be read for its discussion of perceptual deficiencies, both visual and auditory, observed in children with developmental dyslexia (*ibid.*, 81–102). He suggested that perceptual deficiencies are found more in younger retarded readers, while conceptual deficiencies prevail in older retarded readers.

Myklebust and Johnson in "Dyslexia in children" (1962), proposed the diagnostic differentiation between two syndromes: (1) a primary deficiency in the ability to visualize, and (2) a primary deficiency in the ability to auditorize. The authors felt that when a precise diagnosis is made which permits differentiation between major and minor learning disorders, language therapy can be planned more adequately, indiscriminate tutoring can be avoided, and the outlook for the dyslexic child is more promising.

Many investigators have agreed that disturbances in intersensory integration are an outstanding characteristic of this special population of children. As Birch and Belmont pointed out, the development of adaptive behavior in children is based upon the gradual elaboration of intersensory relationships (Birch and Belmont, 1964, 1965a, b). Information arriving as inputs from different sensory modalities has to be assimilated and organized to provide multimodal information. In the learning of reading, in particular, visually presented and spatially distributed information must be treated as equivalent to auditorially and temporally distributed stimulus patterns. If intersensory integration is disturbed, the learning of complex skills depending upon multimodal information may become difficult, if not impossible. In experimental studies of retarded readers, Birch and Belmont found that defects in auditory-visual integration contributed significantly to incompetence in reading.

Modifying the experimental technique used by Birch and Belmont, Blank and Bridger (1964, 1966) found that retarded readers differed from successful readers not only in intermodal transfer—the integration of information presented in two different modalities—but also in intramodal transfer. Their subjects were unable to convert temporally distributed stimuli (visual light patterns) into spatially distributed stimuli (visually presented patterns of dots), even though both sets of stimuli had been presented within the same visual modality. On the basis of further experiments, Blank and Bridger considered two possible reasons for this difficulty: (a) a deficiency in general attention affecting a wide range of perceptual and cognitive processes, and (b) the difficulty which the retarded readers had in applying correct verbal labels to the visually presented stimuli. Normal readers, without exception, resorted to some sort of verbal coding to achieve the task of conversion. Retarded readers showed a deficiency in the basic skill of symbolic (verbal) mediation. Blank and Bridger's findings suggest that a deficiency in applying verbal labels to physical stimuli may lead to a relative inefficiency of intermodal and intramodal transfer of stimulus equivalences. We might add that if this hypothesis proves to be correct, the explicit teaching of verbal mediation or labeling may serve as a useful device in improving intermodal and intramodal transfer in children with motor-perceptual and language disorders.

Myklebust (1964) also found that many children with "psychoneurological learning disorders" had serious difficulties in the integration of auditory with visual learning. Borrowing a term from biomedical engineering, Myklebust viewed intersensory function as a "transducing process." The brain, provided with one type of sensory information, works as a transducer, converting for instance, visual into auditory information. Children with neurogenic learning disorders were found to be particularly deficient in the ability to transduce, or to integrate one type of neurosensory information with another.

Of particular interest is Mykelbust's hypothesis that in children with neurological dysfunction, sensations received through one sensory channel might interfere with those received through another channel. This type of disturbance was illustrated in the behavior of children who comprehended another person's speech better when they did not watch the face and lips of the speaker, or who were unable to initiate speech when they watched themselves or their therapist in the mirror.

In our work we made similar observations among children with motor-perceptual and language disorders. As an example we may quote a boy of 7 years who succeeded well in walking backward on a walking board, but had considerable difficulty in walking forward. In walking backward, apparently he relied exclusively on kinesthetic information concerning the position of his body in space, while in walking forward the visual perception of his feet on the board interfered with the motor information he received through the movements of his muscles.

Myklebust proposed the hypothesis that in the case of children with neurological dysfunction *a breakdown in neurological processes occurs when two or more types of information are delivered to the brain simultaneously*. The clinical manifestations of such neurosensory overloading will be confusion, disturbed attention, poor recall, or random movements. The author suggested that a better understanding of such breakdowns would have important implications for the medical treatment, management, and education of such children. Referring back to Blank and Bridger's hypothesis (*ibid.*) the question could be raised whether the teaching of verbal mediation, or labeling of incoming information, derived from varying sources, might possibly serve as a bridge or a connecting link between the different modalities, thus helping to prevent neurosensory overloading.[1]

Other aspects of possible importance have been stressed by European authors. B. Minnigerode (1965), in a study carried out at the ear, nose, and throat clinic of the University of Goettingen, Germany, examined 681 third-grade children, of whom 14.83 per cent demonstrated symptoms of dyslexia and dysgraphia (legasthenia). In a high percentage (43.56) of this legasthenic group, untreated organic ear, nose, or throat diseases were discovered. The examiner concluded that not all children with reading and spelling disorders belonged in the category of *familial legasthenia*, and that poor sound perception, resulting from peripheral hearing or central processing defects, was an important and hitherto unrecognized cause of *acquired legasthenia*. The children in this special group showed a characteristically short attention span, they were easily fatigued, and their ability for auditory discrimination of speech sounds was lower than that of normal readers of the same age. The author felt that the "global" or "look-and-see" method of teaching to read, recently adopted by many German schools, was particularly inadequate for children with a history of hearing difficulty or of respiratory diseases. The relatively high percentage of dyslexic children with ear, nose, or throat pathology revealed the inadequacy of routine school health examinations, particularly with regard to hearing. The author felt that the exclusively psychological and neuropsychiatric

---

1. In this connection see also A. R. Luria (1961).

Johnson and Myklebust systematically present their point of view in *Learning disabilities, educational principles and practices* (1967), unfortunately published too late for discussion in this chapter. The authors have made important contributions through their careful analysis of disorders of auditory language, a topic not touched upon often by other investigators. Of particular importance for teachers will be the chapters on disorders of written language and disorders of arithmetic.

examination of legasthenic children was insufficient for a complete evaluation of their problems. Diagnostic studies, in each case, should be complemented
by a thorough ear, nose, and throat examination, together with audiometric
testing.

Dr. Ánna-Lisa Annell, of Uppsala, Sweden, included a discussion of hyperactive children with severe language and learning disorders in her comprehensive
report, "The psychopathology of the inflammatory diseases in childhood" (1962).
She strongly recommended that all children with multiple disorders be subject to
multidimensional exploration, in which somatic as well as psycho-pedagogical
aspects of their disorders are to be considered.

In addition to the neurological and somatic aspects of the complex syndrome
of multiple learning disabilities, other variables have been subject to investigation.
The clinical aspects of motor disorders in children were discussed by H. Feldmann
(1965), and by Gubbay, et al. (1965), while Rose (1958) investigated the occurrence
of short auditory memory span among dyslexic school children.

Basic research, presently carried out independently by E. J. Gibson at Cornell
University, and P. Meredith at Leeds University, England, promises to enhance
our understanding of the nature of *perceptual learning* in general and of the
learning of reading in particular. Gibson and her collaborators (Gibson, 1963, 1965,
1966; and Gibson, Osser, and Pick, 1963) have carried out a series of ingenious
experiments concerning the development of perceptual differentiation in early
childhood. Gibson assumes that the child's earliest *perceptual learning* is concerned
with objects and space; later with events, related to his locomotor and manipulative
abilities; and finally with pictorial representation and symbols. She considers
filtering a basic principle in perceptual learning: "distinctive features" of the environment have to be extracted or filtered out from "noisy" or irrelevant input.[2]
Gibson stresses that the stimulation which a child receives is not only full of
information, it is actually too full of information; the stimuli the child is exposed
to contain not only invariants but also a lot of "noise," or irrelevant information.
"Reducing this information is the goal and end of perceptual learning" (Gibson,
1966, p. 5). However, in most early life situations there is no teacher at hand to
help the child separate the relevant patterns and structures from the irrelevant
aspects of the environment. The child, actively exploring the environment, develops
"systematic search patterns" which serve him in learning perceptual skills.

Turning to later perceptual learning in school situations, Gibson examined
how teachers can help children to discriminate essential features from noise.
Analyzing the factors which facilitate learning, Gibson concluded that "anything
which enhances distinctive features or impoverishes noisy background in relation
to them should help; exaggeration of contrasts in the case of distinctive features,
and 'showing the bones' in the case of structure" (*ibid.* p. 14). The principles implied
here may remind the reader of our techniques of "lessening the linguistic load"

---

2. Gibson borrowed the term from Jakobson and Halle (1965), who analyzed the "distinctive
features" of phonemes, the smallest units of speech.

and of exaggerating phonemic contrasts in the language training of children with defective articulation.

Gibson has been particularly interested in analyzing how children learn the distinctive features in "printed displays of all kinds," pictures, letters, and numbers (Gibson, 1965). Her studies have ranged from the analysis of the development of depth perception in infants to the learning of grapheme-phoneme correspondence in children in the early grades. Thus, she has investigated various forms of learning in which perceptually handicapped children are notoriously deficient. Gibson's painstaking studies of perceptual learning in normal children should eventually contribute much to our understanding of the idiosyncratic modes of learning characteristic of children with perceptual deficits.

Starting from a different conceptual framework, Patrick Meredith has carried out psychophysical research in reading disabilities at Leeds University, England (1962, 1964), where his laboratory forms part of the Epistemic Communication Research Unit. Meredith, a physicist who moved into psychology, considers the book and the alphabetical shapes on its pages a part of a child's environment and assumes that the child has to master "the geometry of the environment" before he can embark upon the learning of reading. Meredith and his collaborators attempt to analyze the task of reading in its many parts, separately and in combinations. In choosing an "operational approach" to the study of dyslexia, Meredith scrutinizes the operations of literacy, of diagnosis, and of instruction. He suggests that "the teaching of reading has been needlessly complicated by too many ingenious theories. . . . The task should be defined by reference to the structure of language, which is known, rather than by theories of the working of the mind, where we are largely guessing" (Meredith, 1966, p. 14). He also says: "In a literate culture every word is a four-sided structure, having: (a) characteristic phonetic pronunciation, (b) characteristic visual form, (c) analytic alphabetic constitution, and (d) operational mode of graphic production" (ibid., p. 12). The difficulties of the dyslexic child are all operational difficulties and can be identified best in operational terms. At the Leeds reading laboratory a detailed analytical system of specific operational exercises is being developed for the purpose of training the child in spatial orientation, a form of learning which has to precede all instruction in reading and writing. These exercises in "the geometry of vision" are relatively simple, and parents as well as teachers are taught to practice them with the child. Descriptions of these exercises and future reports about the results should be of considerable interest.

Meredith's emphasis upon task analysis as a prerequisite for successful instruction agrees with a similar emphasis expressed by Gibson (1966), who considers it essential for the development of a theory of instruction as well as for a theory of learning.[3] Gibson demonstrated that young children are slow in learning to per-

---

3. Barbara Bateman, in a personal communication, also expressed the opinion that task analysis may hold more promise for the education of perceptually impaired children than continued refinement of diagnostic techniques. A systematic job analysis of the reading process has been used successfully also by Silver and Hagin (1967), in their training of children with "specific reading disability."

ceive regularities and distinctive features which adults may find quite obvious. One could hypothesize that children with a perceptual deficit or with a maturational lag in neurophysiological development may be even slower than other children in developing the systematic search patterns mentioned by Gibson, or that they may be unable to develop them at all without specific teaching. In Meredith's project older dyslexic children receive intensive training in perceptual differentiation of geometrical objects and spatial relationships, aspects of the environment which, according to Gibson, are explored by normal children during the earliest phase of perceptual development.

Meredith also stresses that the teacher's job is to discover and appreciate each child's "personal learning strategies," which help him in circumventing his disabilities. He suggests that teachers using preconceived methods may interfere with a child's personal strategies and thus prevent learning rather than facilitating it. This point of view reminds one of Kurt Goldstein's earlier observations, that each brain-damaged individual develops his own "detours" in learning. Rather than rejecting the patient's idiosyncratic mode of operation, the skillful therapist will assist him in modifying and improving his personal strategies, if at all possible (Goldstein, 1948).

Cluttering

Children with symptoms of cluttering might be considered as a subgroup within the special population of children with multiple motor, perceptual, and language disorders. Cluttering as a specific form of language disability has been mentioned in the European literature since the beginning of the century, but has come to the attention of American investigators only in recent years. Seeman and Novak (1963) compared the motor behavior of 52 clutterers between the ages of 7 and 40 years with that of a control group of normal speakers. The authors were able to demonstrate that cluttering is not a form of "clumsiness in articulation," as was thought previously. The major disturbance in the speech of clutterers was found to be a marked acceleration of speech tempo, the rate of speaking becoming faster within words and within common, everyday phrases (intraverbal acceleration). Cluttering was defined as propulsion of the speech impulse, subcortically located. In contrast to stutterers, clutterers, as a rule, were not aware of their symptom, and their speech improved markedly when they consciously controlled the rate of speech. Other symptoms observed were marked motor restlessness or hyperactivity, and accelerated and often imprecise gestures and movements of locomotion. Motor restlessness during sleep was found also in many cases.

Seeman's and Novak's findings were confirmed by Dumke, Heese, Kroker, and Siems (1963), who analyzed the symptoms and behavior of 8 cluttering children between 8 and 14 years of age. All children were boys of normal intelligence; they were considered to be "extroverts" eager to make contact with others; they showed difficulties in motor rhythm and jerkiness in locomotion and gestures, together with below average musical ability. The tempo of their spontaneous, uninhibited speech differed markedly from "braked" or slowed-down speech, which they used in situations they considered important. Sentence structure and organization of thoughts was poor both in oral and in written language. In speaking the cluttering children frequently used "filler" words and phrases, and repeated syllables and words. Sentences were poorly planned and had to be reconstructed. Similar difficulties have been reported by Liebmann (1900), Froeschels (1925, 1931) Luchsinger (1963), Weiss (1960, 1964), Arnold (undated), and others. In individual cases the coexistence of cluttering with marked difficulty in handwriting or in reading has been observed also (Weiss, 1964; Roman, undated).[4]

A confusing terminology, mentioned earlier, has been evident also in reports on cluttering. Weiss (1964), presented a comprehensive description of symptoms together with a valuable chapter on therapeutic procedures. He theorized that cluttering, a manifestation of pathology in spoken utterance, was part of a more general type of pathology, which he called "central language imbalance." Arnold and his collaborators chose to employ the term "tachyphemia" in referring to cluttering; however, in their joint publication (*Studies in Tachyphemia*, undated), the terms "developmental language disorder," and "congenital" or "general language disability" also were used without further clarification, contributing to the terminological confusion.

Emotional Aspects

It will not be surprising to find that in addition to the clinical pathology described, many children of normal to superior intelligence, handicapped by motor-perceptual and language disabilities, also exhibit symptoms of secondary emotional disturbance. R. D. Rabinovitch, director of the Hawthorne Center, Northville, Michigan, described how bright and sensitive children with marked incompetence in vital areas of school learning react to their inadequacies and frustrations with anger, guilt feelings, depression, and finally with resignation and compromise concerning their hopes and aspirations (Rabinovitch, 1962). E. Z. Rubin,[5] reporting about the Wyandotte Special Class Research Project, strongly suggested that medical and educational personnel should differentiate between children whose learning difficulties are symptomatic of primary emotional disturbance and those who exhibit secondary emotional disorders in reaction to their school failure caused by motor-perceptual dysfunction. Young children who receive an undue amount of negative feedback from the environment because of their inability to comply with the educational expectations of parents and teachers will adopt defensive techniques and will develop behavior patterns which permit discharge of tension. Rubin questioned current diagnostic categories and their

---

4. The combination of cluttering with various other symptoms can be seen on Table 11, cases 2, 8, 9, 10, 11, and 13.
5. Rubin (undated); see also Rubin and Simson, 1960; Rubin, Simson and Betwee, 1966; and Eisenberg, 1957.

pragmatic value for the development of useful methods of intervention, especially in the form of school programs.

ASSESSMENT AND DIAGNOSIS

The refinement of methods for the identification and diagnosis of children in need of modified educational programs obviously is of very great importance. Without proper examination, children with various symptoms of language and learning disability may be labelled prematurely as lazy, mentally retarded, emotionally disturbed, or dyslexic.

A guideline for the diagnostic evaluation of children with minimal brain dysfunction has been released by the National Institute for Neurological Diseases and Blindness, U.S. Department of Health, Education, and Welfare (Clements, 1966). It contains a discussion of symptomatology, followed by recommendations for medical and educational assessement which should precede the development of remedial programs for children in this category. No specific tests or test batteries have been suggested in this guideline, which is supposed to be "phase one of a three-phase project." It is hoped that more specific recommendations for diagnosis and treatment will be presented in future releases.

Generally, it is recommended that the diagnostic evaluation of each case be carried out by a professional team. In a school situation the licensed school psychologist or an experienced guidance counselor most likely will serve as coordinator in collecting the necessary information and in planning curriculum adjustments for children with severe language and learning disabilities. For our own work at the Wellesley Public Schools, we developed the *Clinical Inventory* mentioned earlier. (See Appendix XI). This instrument is being used on an experimental basis and will be modified as soon as further experience and new research findings warrant it.

The information sought for in the *Clinical Inventory* has to be derived from a number of people. The developmental history of each child will have to be procured from the child's parents, the pediatrician, or the family physician. The classroom teacher, together with the principal, and the music, art, and physical education teachers, will be able to contribute valuable observations concerning the child's behavior and skills, his approach to learning and problem solving, his relationships to his peers, and his scores on group tests of ability and achievement. Individual tests of mental ability, perceptual and motor functioning, drawing, writing, reading, speech, and auditory discrimination will be administered by the psychologist, the speech and hearing therapist, and the reading consultant. Finally, the child should be referred to a medical specialist or to a clinic for audiological, neurological, and psychiatric examinations. *Superficial testing by inadequately trained personnel will be detrimental to the child and should be avoided.*

As can be seen from the literature, a large variety of psychological tests have been utilized in diagnostic evaluations of children with multiple learning disabilities. The most widely used are the Wechsler Intelligence Scale for Children, WISC (Wechsler, 1949); the Draw-a-Man Test (Goodenough, 1954); the Bender

Visual-Motor Gestalt Test (Bender, 1938); the Bender Gestalt Test for Young Children (Koppitz, 1964); the Peabody Picture Vocabulary Test (Dunn, 1959); and the Auditory Discrimination Test (Wepman, 1949).

In addition to these, the following tests are being used frequently: the Wide Range Achievement Test (Jastak, 1946); the Lincoln-Oseretsky Motor Development Scale (Sloan, 1948); The Purdue Perceptual-Motor Survey (Roach and Kephart, 1966); the Marianne Frostig Developmental Test of Visual Perception (Maslow, Frostig, Lefever, and Whittlesey, 1964); and the Illinois Test of Psycholinguistic Abilities (McCarthy and Kirk, 1961).[6] A differential diagnosis of *disorders of written language* has been carried out by means of the Picture Story Language Test (Myklebust, 1965).

A number of reading surveys and reading readiness tests also were used in most studies. S. Krippner and others reported about the diagnostic and remedial use of the Minnesota Percepto-Diagnostic Test (Fuller and Laird, 1963; Krippner, 1965). L. L. Lee (1966) developed an interesting method for comparing normal and deviate syntactic development in children's language; the method is time consuming, however, and in its present state may be more fitting for research purposes than for diagnostic testing within a school setting. Valuable information on testing procedures to be used with children suspected of neurological dysfunction will be found in Edith Meyer Taylor's well-known handbook (Taylor, 1959).

Screening and Early Identification of High Risk Children

Many of the tests now in use are more appropriate for older children and young adults than for young children. While the early identification of children with potential language and learning disorders obviously would be highly desirable, so far only a few investigators have developed techniques to predict potential learning difficulties on the preprimary level. Silver, Pfeiffer, and Hagin (1966) made use of a therapeutic nursery school for the identification and differential diagnosis of children with delayed language development.

M. A. White of Teachers College, Columbia University, and M. Phillips, of the Pelham Public Schools, developed a set of group tests for perception and motor coordination, to be administered to kindergarten children (White and Phillips, 1964). The children's scores on these tests appeared to have high predictive value for achievement in later grades. There is a great need for group screening devices which can be used under normal public school conditions.

A predictive index for the identification of high risk children on the kindergarten level was developed by de Hirsch, Jansky, and Langford (1965, 1966; see also de Hirsch, 1957). Starting from a battery of 37 kindergarten tests, the investigators succeeded in arriving at a combination of 10 tests which can be administered individually and scored by trained kindergarten teachers. This index appears to have considerable efficacy in predicting potential reading, writing, and spelling

---

6. See also B. Bateman's summary of studies (1965).

disabilities in children; further validation studies are underway. It is interesting to note that I.Q. ranked only 12th among predictive measures, while 11 other tests proved to be better predictors of subsequent reading performance. The authors also made specific recommendations for the organization of so-called transition classes, grades between kindergarten and first grade, to be used for the motor, perceptual, and social training of children identified by their low scores on the predictive index.

Another test to be given individually and administered and scored by class-room teachers is the Reading Prognosis Test, developed by M. Weiner and S. Feldmann of the Institute for Developmental Studies, New York University (Weiner and Feldmann, 1963; see also S. Feldmann, 1965). The test consists of seven subtests in (a) Beginning Reading (naming alphabet letters and simple sight vocabulary), (b) Language (a vocabulary and a story telling test), and (c) Perceptual Discrimination (two visual and one auditory discrimination test). This prognostic test can be administered in the spring of the kindergarten year or at the beginning of grade one. Validation studies were carried out with children of lower and middle socioeconomic status. The items Beginning Reading and Perceptual Discrimination were found to be the best predictors of future reading achievement. In addition to predictive value, teachers administering the test receive diagnostic information about the level of each child's language and perceptual skills. The authors hope that this information will be useful for the setting up of programs of skill improvement for children with potential learning difficulties.

An excellent summary of diagnostic procedures, together with a "check list of school behavior," can be found in a paper by Connors (1967). The latter should be a valuable instrument in the screening of school populations.

In our work with Wellesley children, our well-trained and highly perceptive kindergarten teachers collaborated with us in identifying children with potential learning difficulties. In repeated conferences, teachers and members of the research staff exchanged observations and ideas concerning the criteria of delayed and irregular maturation in children. In addition, for the last few years, the SRA Primary Mental Abilities Test (Thurstone and Thurstone, 1946) has been administered each spring to all kindergarten children. The children are tested in small groups by their own teachers, and those who score lowest are referred to the school psychologist for diagnostic study. It should be mentioned, however, that many of the high risk children are identified by their teachers and referred for study even before the administration of the SRA Test. Many of the children in this low scoring group repeat kindergarten. While no special transition classes have been set up for them, the children come back in small groups several afternoons a week and receive intensive training in motor, perceptual, and language skills. The training is carried out by their own teachers, with the assistance of speech therapists and psychologists. If at all possible, mothers are included in this training program and are advised how to continue the training activities at home. No objective measurement of the children's progress has been attempted so far, but the children's subsequent school performance is being followed.

EDUCATION AND TRAINING

The theoretical basis of most methods used in the training and education of children with severe learning disabilities can be found in the important research publications by Heinz Werner and his collaborators,[7] and also in the work in psychopathology and education of brain-injured children by Strauss and Lehtinen (1947) and by Strauss and Kephart (1955).

Considerable stimulation in the development of teaching methods also came from an interdisciplinary "demonstration-pilot project" concerning the education of brain-injured and hyperactive children, carried out jointly by Syracuse University and the Board of Education of Montgomery County, New York (Cruickshank, Bentzen, Ratzeburg, and Tannhauser, 1961). Diagnostic techniques, methods of teacher selection, classroom management, and instruction utilized in this study were incorporated in many training programs organized by other groups. In short, though no agreement has yet been reached concerning the cause or causes of multiple learning disabilities, educational practices have been modeled primarily after those found useful in the education of brain-damaged children.[8]

In addition to these influential studies, a number of educators and investigators have contributed valuable methods and material to be used in the education and training of this special population of children.

A developmental program for multi-handicapped preschool children was organized by the Kennedy Child Study Center at Santa Monica, California (Stewart and Coda, undated), where a multidiscipline group provided diagnostic services and training for children under 4 years with deficits in the motor, language, and social areas. Group work with mothers was an essential part of the project. The intelligence level of the children was not reported and no evaluation of training results has been presented so far.

An interesting program for the treatment of "language lags" in young children was carried out at the Child Psychiatry Nursery School of the University of Texas, Medical Branch (Burks, Good, Higginbotham, and Hoffman, 1966). Language training, together with "individualized experiences with color, light, sound, taste, and touch" were provided for young children who varied in socioeconomic background, intellectual functioning, and psychiatric diagnosis. The group included understimulated children, autistic children, and children with a variety of neurological handicaps. Several illustrative case histories were included in this report.

Many educators based their work on the assumptions that cognitive functioning and higher-level learning depend on the acquisition of primary or preacademic

---

7. The late Heinz Werner's many-faceted and seminal contributions to developmental and comparative psychology were the topic of a memorial paper by Witkin (1965). A chronological list of Werner's publications appears at the end of the paper, including his many and varied studies of the mental organization of brain-injured children and adults.

8. In *The brain-injured child in home, school, and community* (1967), W. M. Cruickshank summarized the experiences gained through the "demonstration-pilot project." This book is addressed primarily to parents and teachers of neurologically impaired children.

skills, and that training in these skills will facilitate subsequent learning on a more complex level. Thus, a child's successful learning of reading and writing has been conceived as depending upon satisfactory development in the areas of motor behavior and of visual and auditory perception, discrimination, and memory. Appropriate motor-perceptual and language training during the preschool years, therefore, has been considered as the necessary prerequisite for later satisfactory school learning.

An extensive and systematic motor-perceptual training program was developed by Kephart (1960). He wrote for kindergarten and primary grade teachers who wish to assist the "slow learner" in the acquisition of "basic readiness skills." A Perceptual Survey Rating Scale is provided, which should enable teachers to identify children who are deficient in primary skills in ten different areas of motor and perceptual behavior. Training activities in sensory-motor and ocular control and in form perception are described. Kephart's procedures have been used widely in various educational settings, but so far data concerning the results are lacking.

In addition to Kephart's procedures, the Frostig Program for the Development of Visual Perception has found wide acceptance and application (Frostig and Horne, 1964).[9]

Braun, Rubin, et al. (1965) drew attention to the difficulty of rating the adequacy of perceptual-motor functioning, particularly in the younger age groups, in the absence of reliable age norms for the various functions. At the present time, ratings carried out by teachers of perceptually handicapped children depend on the clinical judgment of the raters. In addition, we do not know yet whether training in specific motor and perceptual functions actually shows generalization to the child's performance in criterion areas, such as reading and writing. In the absence of such data the validity of the widely used motor and perceptual training procedures remains unknown.

Programs for the education of older children focus upon the teaching of reading, writing, spelling and, in some cases, arithmetic. Techniques of teaching these subjects to brain-injured children were outlined in the works of Strauss and Lehtinen, Strauss and Kephart, and Cruickshank et al., already mentioned. A manual, "Diagnosis and Remediation of Psycholinguistic Disabilities", has been presented by S. A. Kirk, of the Institute for Research on Exceptional Children of the University of Illinois (Kirk, 1966).

The literature on the teaching of reading to dyslexic children has been prolific. We can mention here only the publications by Borel-Maisonny (1951), Fernald (1943), Gillingham and Stillman (1966), Hallgren (1950), Money (1962), Silver, Hagin and Hersh (1965), Silver and Hagin (1967), M. F. Stuart (1963), and Zazzo, Ajuriaguerra, et al. (1952). Though authors hold a variety of theoretical positions, the reader will gain from the study of the various teaching techniques described. A

---

9. See also Frostig, 1966, and Frostig and Maslow, 1966. The Frostig Center of Educational Therapy, 7257 Melrose Avenue, Los Angeles, Cal., 90046 will forward, upon request, a list of publications by Dr. M. Frostig and her coworkers concerning the education of children with learning disabilities.

particularly clear and systematic presentation of "some principles of instruction for dyslexia" can be found in a relatively short paper by N. D. Bryant (1965; see also N. D. Bryant, 1962).

The Word Blind Centre of London publishes the *ICAA Word Blind Bulletin* (1966) for the communication of its ongoing research and teaching practices. The Orton Society of Pomfret, Connecticut also disseminates information on teaching techniques through the *Bulletins of the Orton Society*.

The Learning Centre of McGill University and Montreal Children's Hospital, Canada, also has been engaged in the study and training of children from 4 to 17 years of age with severe reading difficulties (M. S. Rabinovitch, 1964). Of particular interest is the carefully planned program of liaison between each child's home, his school, and the Learning Centre. This proved to be a powerful agent in modifying the attitudes of teachers toward children with learning disabilities.

A description of a special program for perceptually handicapped children, together with a list of the materials used, has been published by the New Jersey Association for Brain-Injured Children (R. W. Russell, undated).[10]

Methods of teaching writing to children with severe difficulties in this area were described by Cruickshank *et. al.* (*op. cit.*), by Stuart (*op. cit.*), by Heermann (1965), and by Johnson and Myklebust (1967, Chapter VI).

Extensive recommendations for speech therapy with cluttering children can be found in the publications by Weiss (1960, 1964) and in the *Studies in Tachyphemia* (undated), mentioned earlier. While the authors of both publications consider cluttering as part of the more general disturbance of "central language imbalance" (Weiss), or of "general language disability" (Arnold, *et. al.*), it should be remembered that not all cluttering children will have difficulties in learning visual symbols, reading, and writing. As an example see the clinical profiles of cases 9 and 11, Table 11.

Weiss postulated a close relationship between cluttering and stuttering (Weiss 1950, 1964). As can be seen from cases 2 and 10 on Table 11, some children in this special group showed symptoms of both cluttering and stuttering, while stuttering without cluttering existed in cases 3, 6, 10, and 12. The problems of differential diagnosis regarding these two disabilities are complex and will be discussed further in Chapter 14.

Evaluation of Treatment Results

Stewart and Coda (*op. cit.*) rightly remarked that the examination of children in this special group results in a multiple diagnosis which resembles more a mosaic than a pigeonhole. Because of the wide variability in the characteristics of each child, and the fact that most educational programs are relatively new, it is not sur-

---

10. "Indexed Bibliography on the Educational Management of Children with Learning Disabilities" can be procured from The Argus Press, 3505 N. Ashland Ave., Chicago, Ill., 60657.

prising that reports about treatment results have been scarce. As the diagnostic criteria differ in different studies, and the characteristics of each sample of children studied have not always been spelled out, comparisons between studies have been difficult. Improvement in research methodology will be necessary to facilitate classification and evaluation of the results of educational procedures.

The critical variables were defined clearly in three studies which came to our attention; all of them were concerned with the training of children with severe reading difficulty.

E. G. Roach (1966) evaluated the results of "an experimental program of perceptual-motor training with slow readers." Starting from a study by Rutherford (1965), who had reported positive results following the perceptual-motor training of children between 62 and 80 months, Roach provided similar training for children between 96 and 160 months and measured the gains in reading achievement following this training. Eighty children, participating in an eight-week summer remedial reading program at Indiana University, were divided into two groups, matched according to sex, age, grade placement, reading level, and I.Q. on the Peabody Picture Vocabulary Test (Dunn, 1959). The experimental group was subdivided into small groups of 6-8 children who, for 30 minutes daily, received intensive perceptual motor training, modeled after techniques suggested by Kephart (op. cit.). The control group had a 30-minute period of free play instead, with access to equipment similar to that used by the children in the formal training program. Reading achievement of all children was measured at the end of the summer training period and again six months later. No significant difference in reading achievement was found. Following this experiment in group instruction, the author matched seven of the experimental children with their counterparts in the control group. The seven children in the experimental group received continued individual perceptual-motor training during one semester of the school year. "Dramatic differences" in gained scores were found between the group who received continued perceptual-motor training on an individual basis and the group who did not. The authors concluded that group perceptual-motor training of older children did not seem effective in raising achievement levels in reading; the lower age limit of 95 months, as used in the study, might be too late an age for the modification of perceptual-motor behavior on a group basis.

Abrams and Belmont (1965) assessed the relative value of "different approaches to the remediation of severe reading disability in children." It was the purpose of their study to compare the effects of full-time specialized reading instruction with the effects of the type of remedial instruction given in representative public schools, and also to compare the beneficial effects of individual versus group psychotherapy. Sixteen boys, all severely disabled readers, were matched according to intelligence, age, number of years in school, and socioeconomic status. They were assigned randomly to four types of treatment extending over a two-year period. The forms of treatment were: (1) full-time specialized reading instruction at the Temple University Clinic Laboratory school combined with individual psychotherapy; (2) the same form of instruction and group psychotherapy; (3) no special educational help but individual psychotherapy; and (4) no special instruction but group psychotherapy. It was found that full-time specialized reading instruction proved superior to remedial instruction given in representative public schools. No significant differences were found between the two groups receiving individual therapy and the two groups receiving group therapy. The authors concluded that the most vital step in the remediation of severe reading disability in children was the institution of a full-time specialized instructional program.

Finally, Silver and Hagin (1964) conducted a follow-up study of 41 children who had participated, in 1949–51, in a remedial reading program at Bellevue Hospital Mental Hygiene Clinic in New York City. The children in the original group had fallen into the following three categories. (1) The "developmental" sub-group, who had shown the following symptoms: immaturity in the visual-motor sphere, difficulties in spatial orientation and in visual figure background perception, problems in auditory and tactile perception. This syndrome was present in nine out of ten children. (2) The "organic" sub-group, two of those nine, who in addition to the basic syndrome had shown neurological signs suggestive of structural damage to the central nervous system (abnormalities in the examination of "cranial nerves, muscle tone and synergy, and deep, superficial and pathological reflexes"). (3) A sub-group, approximately one out of ten, that consisted of poor readers who showed no perceptual defects or organic signs.

In 1961–62, information was obtained about 84 per cent of the group, and 24 subjects (59 per cent) were reexamined. It was found that subjects with "organic" reading disability tended to retain their perceptual difficulties in all areas tested, while those with "developmental" reading difficulties had recovered partially or had adopted cues which enabled them to cope successfully with reading. The authors concluded that children with severe reading disability require careful initial evaluation, not only to map out their clinical profiles but also to discover those with organic signs of CNS damage. Conventional teaching methods are insufficient for children with organic involvement and new teaching procedures will have to be devised to assist them.

CONCLUSIONS

From our own work and from a survey of the literature we have come to the following conclusions:

1. Children with multiple motor-perceptual and language disorders constitute a special population, with highly specific problems in development and in school learning. While all of these children show mild to severe deviations or impairments in their motor-perceptual and language behavior, the children differ markedly from each other. Careful assessment of each child's difficulties is necessary. Findings should be expressed in the form of descriptive statements or clinical profiles; labeling or pigeonholing must be avoided.

2. According to American and European literature (Annell, 1962, Clements,

1966), it appears that the number of children with deviations in nervous-symptom function or with delayed and irregular maturation has been on the increase; this increase in dysfunction often is, unfortunately, "the unintentional aftermath of advances in medical knowledge and care" (Clements, *op. cit.*).

3. The causes of this syndrome of motor, perceptual, language, and learning disorders are still largely unknown. More precise classification and terminology are needed for the purpose of reporting to central agencies, program planning, and research. The National Society for Crippled Children and Adults, in cooperation with the National Institute of Neurological Diseases and Blindness, U.S. Public Health Service, have formed a subcommittee on terminology and identification, criteria for diagnosis, a survey of the magnitude of the problem, and a listing of available facilities for diagnosis, therapy, education, and rehabilitation (See Clements, *op. cit.*).

4. In this field—as in the field of mental retardation—the concerns of parents and teachers and their demand for educational services to afflicted children have outdistanced the available scientific knowledge of causation and treatment. Educational administrators and public-school teachers must provide programs for children with multiple learning difficulties, regardless of the exact cause of their disabilities. As Clements pointed out, this demand may lead to "hastily conceived public school programming, involving a considerable expenditure of money, with inadequate provisions and criteria for student selection, teacher training requirements, program supervision, and evaluation" (Clements, *ibid*, p. 1). Imprecise definitions of the problem may contribute further to confusion in this field. However, while social action has preceded the necessary accumulation of scientific knowledge, there is reason to hope that the increased demand for educational services will be reflected in greater awareness of the problems involved, leading to increased research and to subsequent improvement of educational practices.

5. From the present vantage point, the following limited recommendations for the education of children with multiple language and learning disorders seem reasonable and justified.

(A) IDENTIFICATION

Early identification of children with developmental deviations appears to be highly desirable. Screening devices are needed to identify such children during the preschool years or in kindergarten. Among other devices, the Predictive Index, developed by de Hirsch, Jansky, and Langford (*op. cit.*), appears to be a valuable instrument for the identification of high risk children on the kindergarten level. Similar instruments to be used by teachers should be developed for use with preschool children. Children who have been identified with the help of screening procedures, or in the course of mental health check-ups, are likely to fall into several categories: understimulated children; children who generally are immature and slow in developing; emotionally disturbed children; and children with various degrees of nervous system impairment. Individual children may fall into more than one category.

(B) TRANSITIONAL EDUCATION

Children who have been identified as high risk cases should be given the time, the opportunity, and the training necessary for the improvement of their primary sensory-motor and learning skills before they are exposed to the more complex and highly integrated forms of teaching and learning, beginning in grade one. Methods for special training in speech and language have been presented in this book as well as in publications by other authors. Techniques for motor and perceptual training have been developed (see Frostig, *op. cit.*, Kephart, *op. cit.*, and others). Further research is necessary to evaluate the results of such training and to assure the appropriateness of specific training methods for use with specific children. Sensory-motor and language training for high risk children can be provided in so-called transition classes (see de Hirsch, *et al.*, *op. cit.*); or it can be carried out by teachers, speech therapists, and parents working with individual children or with small groups, within the setting of Head Start, preschool, or kindergarten classes. Dissemination of information to professional groups and to parents concerning methods of early identification and training of high risk children is of utmost importance.

(C) ASSESSMENT AND DIAGNOSIS

Assessment and diagnosis of children with severe language and learning disorders or with marked developmental deviations must be carried out by a professional team including educators, psychologists, and physicians. In assessing a child's condition and educational needs it must be kept in mind that the effect of developmental deviation is "markedly influenced by interaction of the child with his physical and social environment" (Clements, 1966, p. iii). Assessment procedures should include the developmental and health history of the child; evaluation and testing of his present behavior, abilities and skills; and evaluation of the emotional climate and the system of language and communication which exists in the child's family and of which he forms a part. If a child is participating in a training program in primary skills, observation and assessement of his rate of progress will contribute to a better understanding of his basic condition and educational needs.

(D) EDUCATION AND TRAINING

Educational planning will have to proceed in a tentative manner, open to later modification, taking into account all available resources in a particular school system, community, and region. Children with mild to moderate handicaps may be able to function successfully in a regular classroom, provided the number of children is not too large and the teacher, the principal, and the parents are being helped to understand and accept the characteristic limitations and modes of learning of the children. Special service personnel, such as school psychologists, counselors, speech and reading therapists, as well as teachers of music, and physical education, should work closely with classroom teachers and parents.

Children with multiple and severe language and learning disorders but with unimpaired intellectual ability will function best in a special class setting, where they can be instructed individually or in small groups by a highly motivated, sympathetic teacher with special interest and training. Part-time participation of such children in regular classrooms seems advisable; it should be arranged carefully with consideration of each child's specific talents and weaknesses.

Teaching methods to be used in tutorial classes have been described in the literature; further research undoubtedly will produce additional and more specific methods and techniques. Instruction in tutorial classes should be matched closely with the actual developmental level on which each individual child can perform comfortably in each area of learning. Lessening of the linguistic load to which each child is exposed, and a type of classroom management which protects children from an overload of stimulation are desirable educational measures. Presenting instruction in small steps and with frequent repetitions will be necessary in most cases. A particularly urgent need exists in the field of curriculum development. The day-by-day work of the tutor would be facilitated considerably by an educational outline to be used for guidance in planning.

The personality of the teacher is of the highest importance. The teacher of children with severe learning disabilities has to be "a flexible person who can tolerate ambiguity well, yet who is able to respond to minimal cues in children" (Burks, et al., 1966). She should be able "to determine quickly what particular techniques and procedures to use at a specific time with a given child with a particular problem" (Cruickshank, et al., 1961, p. 127). She has to be imaginative and creative in adapting known instructional techniques to the needs of individual children and in inventing new techniques as needed, while at the same time she must be able to provide and maintain an orderly and highly structured classroom situation. She must be able to tolerate repetitiveness, but also to modify repetitive instruction sufficiently to make it tolerable for her handicapped but intelligent students.

Beyond all this, programs developed and carried out by talented teachers in the interest of handicapped children will succeed only if they are interpreted to and supported by parents, administrators, professional groups, and the community at large.

CHAPTER FOURTEEN

Differential Diagnosis

In Chapters 6 to 13, three groups of children with disturbances in language development were described. At this point it may be helpful to recall the aims of the research study carried out between 1961 and 1964 and presented in the previous chapters. These aims were: (a) to continue our earlier research in the treatment of stuttering children (Group A) and their parents, using a larger number of cases, more therapists, and improved techniques of diagnosis and treatment; (b) to evaluate the results of treatment; (c) to carry out pilot studies in the diagnosis and treatment of children with severely defective articulation (Group B) and of children with symptoms of multiple motor-perceptual and language disorders (Group C); and (d) to compare the children in these groups with regard to a number of significant variables. We assumed that the results of such a comparison would contribute to a refinement of the procedures to identify children with developmental speech and language disorders.

COMPARISON OF GROUPS

A comparison of the three groups studied was carried out in the following manner.

For the purpose of data analysis, two of the three major groups were divided further into subgroups. The distribution of cases can be seen in Table 12.

As reported in Chapter 7 (Appendix III), an intake interview was conducted with either the mother or both parents of each child in this study. Significant factors concerning the child's history which parents recalled later during their own therapeutic sessions were added to the information recorded on the intake form. Finally, the total information recorded on the 62 intake forms was codified, the significant variables agreed upon were analysed, and the results of this analysis were evaluated statistically.

Possibility of Neurological Dysfunction

As mentioned earlier (Chapter 7), all intake forms were inspected by the pediatric consultant, Dr. J. Brines. If necessary, he attempted to gain further information about the child's developmental history from the family physician or from the hospital where the child had been delivered, or he assisted parents in obtaining a neurological examination for the child. On the basis of all available evidence, Dr. Brines reported five cases as "suspect of neurological dsyfunction." Brief histories of these five cases can be found in Appendix XII.

TABLE 12—DIAGNOSTIC CATEGORIES

A	Stuttering Children	24
B	Children with Severely Defective Articulation	18
B¹	Children with Severely Defective Articulation and Stuttering	11
C	Children with Symptoms of Motor-perceptual and Language Disorders, without Stuttering	7
C¹	Children with Symptoms of Motor-perceptual and Language disorders, Including Stuttering	2
	Total	62

We had hypothesized that Groups C and C¹ (children with motor-perceptual and language disorders) should contain a larger percentage of children suspect of neurological dysfunction than Groups A or B. According to Dr. Brines' findings this was indeed the case; however, the numbers were too small to permit any conclusions concerning organicity as a significant aspect of the syndrome of multiple motor-perceptual and language disorder.

Additional Variables

The remaining information contained in the intake forms was codified and ten variables were identified.

1. Additional problems
2. Child's health history
3. Family health history: parental hearing difficulty
4. Family health history: severe or chronic illness of a member of the family
5. Speech disorders in the family
6. Family mobility (number of dwellings child had lived in)
7. Family size
8. Child's position in the family
9. Other persons living with the family
10. Sibling within two years

The distribution of variables was tabulated and the results were evaluated statistically. A copy of the form used can be found in Appendix XIII.

Hypotheses

We expected the following differences between groups:

1. Group A (stutterers) should show a higher incidence of additional problems than groups B or C.
2. Groups C and C¹ (motor-perceptual and language disorders) should show a higher incidence of children with health problems than groups A or B.
3. Group A (stutterers) should show a higher number of cases with high mobility than groups B or C.
4 and 5. We hypothesized that children with severely defective articulation had not received sufficient auditory stimulation from their mothers. Assuming that a large family, or young children close in age to each other, would occupy a mother's time and prevent her from spending much time with an individual child, we hypothesized that Groups B and B¹ (children with defective articulation) should show more children coming from large families and more children having siblings within two years than either groups A or C.

The following groups were compared with all other groups for each of the ten variables:

1. Group A (stutterers).
2. Group B (defective articulation).
3. Group B¹ (defective articulation plus stuttering).
4. Groups C and C¹ (all motor-perceptual and language disorders).
5. Groups A and B¹ (stutterers with and without defective articulation).
6. Groups A, B¹, and C¹ (all stutterers regardless of additional difficulties).
7. Groups B and B¹ (all with defective articulation).

For all of the above comparisons between groups, χ^2 was calculated on each of the ten variables. (See Appendixes XIV and XV.)

Results

The following results were obtained:

1. Groups A and B¹, stuttering children with or without defective articulation, showed a significantly higher incidence of additional problems than all other groups in the sample (p < .05).
2. Groups C and C¹, containing all children with multiple motor-perceptual and language disorders, showed a significantly higher incidence of health problems in the child's developmental history than all other groups in the sample (p < .05).
3. Groups B and B¹, children with severely defective articulation with or without stuttering symptoms, showed a significantly higher incidence of children coming from large families (four or more children) than all other groups in the sample (p < .05).
4. In Group B (defective articulation), more children were either youngest

or middle children than in either groups A or C ($p < .05$). If groups B and B^1 are pooled, thus containing all children with severely defective articulation regardless of stuttering, this relationship holds at the 1 per cent level of significance.

5. Group B (defective articulation) had a significantly higher incidence of additional adults living with the family than any other group ($p < .05$).

No significant differences were found among the groups with regard to the following variables: Family health history (parental hearing difficulty and severe or chronic illnesses of family members), speech disorders in the family, mobility (number of dwellings lived in), and sibling within two years.

Discussion

Result 1 confirms our hypothesis that stuttering should be considered a psycho-social disorder, occurring frequently in combination with or contributing to various personality difficulties or symptoms of childhood neurosis in the stutterer.

Result 2, together with the medical findings reported above, seems to point in the direction of neurophysiological difficulties related to the syndrome of multiple motor-perceptual and language disorders. Of the 9 children in the sample, 3 had incidents of severe illness, severe accident, or hospitalization under 2 years of age; 6 had such incidents between 2 and 5 years of age, and 1 had repeated incidents from birth to age 5. One might speculate that such incidents may interfere with maturational and learning processes in the areas of speech and language, and perceptual and motor skills.

Results 3 and 4 support our assumption that severely defective articulation occurs in children who have had insufficient auditory stimulation and verbal feedback in the home. It also supports our assumption that such verbal stimulation and feedback has to be provided by an interested adult rather than by other children in the family.

Result 5 is somewhat of a paradox. On first sight it appears to contradict results 3 and 4. One would think that if more adults lived with the family, the child would receive more verbal stimulation. Inspecting the data we find the following conditions:

One mother of 3 children (2 with defective articulation) had a maid living in.

One mother of 2 children (1 defective articulation) had non-American servants while living in Africa.

One mother of 6 children (2 defective articulation), and 1 mother of 4 (1 defective articulation) had to take care of an ailing or invalid grandmother.

One mother of 2 (1 defective articulation) had the help of a grandmother in good health.

It appears, therefore, that in some instances additional adults may have contributed to the child's verbal stimulation, while in others—where there were ailing relatives in the home—the mother's chores may have left her less time to spend with her children. In our long-term work with stuttering children we observed that there was, indeed, a marked difference between additional adults who were helpful to the child in therapy and those who were indifferent or hostile. Evidently, the mere fact of other adults living with the family, without exploration of the adult's role in the family, adds little or nothing to our understanding of children's speech disorders.

The incidence of parental hearing difficulty and of severe or chronic illness of family members was relatively low in all groups. The incidence of speech disorders in the family was unexpectedly high for all groups, amounting to approximately 65 per cent in all groups except group C. (See Appendix XIV.)

It seems of particular interest that in groups C and C^1 (motor-perceptual and language disability) we found, in addition to the highest incidence of health problems in the children, also a particularly high incidence of speech disorders in the family (88 per cent).

Mobility was the highest for group A, lowest for group C, but there was no significant difference between all groups in the sample.

DIAGNOSTIC IMPLICATIONS

A knowledge of the differences found between groups will be useful in attempting a differential diagnosis between conditions which may appear similar. Evidently, no diagnosis should ever be derived from a single symptom, even a prominent one, but should always be based upon a careful analysis of the child's total condition. (See Clinical Inventory, Appendix XI.) In individual cases the differentiation between the following types of disorder may be difficult: (a) primary or developmental stuttering and secondary or reactive stuttering; and (b) cluttering and stuttering.

Primary Versus Secondary Stuttering

A comparison between primary and secondary stuttering is presented in Table 13.

Cluttering Versus Stuttering

H. Freund (1952) and D. Weiss (1950, 1964) expressed the opinion that cluttering was the basis of many or most cases of developmental stuttering. The authors defined cluttering as an inherited speech disorder, forming part of the syndrome of "general language imbalance." Weiss further stated that in many instances successfully treated stutterers may lose their secondary symptoms—blocking or accompanying movements—but may retain a tendency for repeating initial sounds and syllables, a symptom which he considered indicative of cluttering. Thus, these authors hypothesized that an "inherited disposition" underlies the manifestations of both cluttering and stuttering.

Our own research findings do not support this hypothesis. Children in our

TABLE 13—DIFFERENCES BETWEEN PRIMARY AND SECONDARY STUTTERING

	Primary Stuttering	Secondary Stuttering
Beginning of Speech	Usual time (10–20 months)	May be delayed.
Rate of Speech Development	Normal or even rapid.	May be slow.
Articulation	Good to excellent.	May be poor.
Onset of Stuttering	Specific onset, critical period between 2½ and 5 years; onset often related to crisis in mother-child relationship or to family crisis.	No specific onset, parents report: "Speech has always been poor." Stuttering appears as reaction to frustration caused by a primary communication disorder (defective articulation, or motor-perceptual and language disability)
Possible Additional Difficulties: Behavior	Aggressiveness, stubbornness, bedwetting, shyness; later perfectionism, passivity, compulsive tendencies (see Appendix XIII).	Hyperactivity, clumsiness, aggressivesness, stubbornness.
Skills and School Learning	There may be no learning difficulty; stutterers frequently are excellent students. Child may have difficulty in reading *aloud*, but not in the decoding process itself.	There may be difficulties in articulation, in hand-eye coordination, gross or fine motor skills, drawing, writing, reading (see Chapters 11, 12, 13).
Treatment	Communication-and-relationship therapy with child and parents (see Chapters 7–10).	Therapy for the primary communication disorder may be sufficient. In case of severe stuttering, same therapy recommended as for primary stutterer.

sample who had been treated successfully did not, as a rule, show symptoms of cluttering after termination of treatment, or in later years. Also, the behavior characteristics of the stuttering children differed markedly from those of the cluttering children, as described by Seeman and Novak (1963), Dumke, Heese, Kroker, and Siems (1963), Arnold (undated), and by Weiss himself. (See Chapter 13.) We do agree, however, that in individual cases both conditions, cluttering and stuttering, may coexist. Such coincidences have been demonstrated in Table 11.

The characteristic differences between the two conditions have been summarized in Table 14.

TABLE 14*—DIFFERENCES BETWEEN CLUTTERING AND STUTTERING

	Cluttering	Primary or Developmental Stuttering
Definition	A familial, congenital speech and language disability.	An individual, psychosocial disturbance in communication and interpersonal relationships.
Beginning of Speech	May be delayed.	At usual time.
Rate of Speech Development	May be slow.	Normal or even rapid.
Articulation	Poor.	Good to excellent.
Onset	No specific time of onset.	Specific onset.
Course of Difficulty	Continuous; no advanced symptoms develop.	Fluctuating; eventually advanced symptoms appear (see Appendix II).
Combination with Other Communication Disorders	Usually combined with difficulty in articulation, word finding, sentence building, story telling; often also in spelling, writing, reading.	No other speech or language disorder.
Behavior Characteristics	Clutterer tends to be extrovert, gregarious, untidy, hurried, have short attention span, be poor in listening; may retell a story with elaborate detail in some parts and omission of important features in other parts.	Compulsive tendencies, clinging, aggressive, often overly well behaved, tends to deny or repress anger.
Awareness of Speech Difficulty	Clutterer usually is not aware of speech difficulty.	Stutterer is very much aware of difficulty.
Effect of Paying Attention to Speech	Clutterer's speech improves.	Stutterer's speech becomes worse.
Treatment	Consciously focusing attention upon speech; drills and exercises.	Communication-and-relationship therapy, no exercises.

* Compare with table in Arnold, *Studies in Tachyphemia* (undated), 44.

Children with Multiple Symptoms

Finally, the diagnosis of preschool children with combined symptoms of delayed language development, defective articulation, and behavior disorders often is very difficult. It may be difficult for the examiner to determine whether the child's symptomatology is caused by hearing difficulty, by insufficient or inappropriate verbal stimulation, by emotional disorders, by neurological impairment, or by a combination of several of these conditions. Cooperation between a team of professional examiners and an extended period of observation and experimental therapy will be necessary to assess the complex difficulties of such children. Parents, understandably, often dread the length of time and the expense of extensive diagnostic procedures. Additional diagnostic and treatment centers are needed badly in which diagnostic observations and experimental therapy could be carried out by an interprofessional team, at minimum cost to the parents. (See van Thal, 1963; de Hirsch, 1967; Menolascino and Eaton, 1967; also Silverman, Laszlo, and Cramer, 1967).

CHAPTER FIFTEEN

Children in Need of Compensatory Language Training

THE POOR COMMUNICATORS

This book would not be complete without a consideration of the very large group of children with more generalized, all-pervasive deficiencies in verbal communication. The vocabulary of these children is meager in quantity and quality; their articulation of sounds, though not severely defective, may be imprecise and slurred; their spontaneous speech—particularly in school situations—consists of brief utterances, awkwardly formulated and lacking in expressive quality; and they are unable to organize and convey their ideas clearly and precisely. Indeed, some observers have hypothesized that the very paucity of their language may prevent these children from reaching higher levels of concept formation and abstract thinking (Bernstein, 1960, 1964; M. Deutsch, 1963).

The children in this group obviously are poor communicators and within the highly verbal matrix prevalent in our present educational system they are bound to rate low in achievement and status. M. Deutsch and his collaborators at the Institute of Developmental Studies, New York University, found a close relationship between intelligence, as measured by standard I.Q. tests, and language skills (Deutsch, Maliver, Brown, and Cherry, 1964). In the lower-class population studied by these investigators, command of language did not necessarily improve with age and school attendance, but limitations actually were more evident in fifth-grade than in first-grade children (*ibid.*).

Because of the absence of specific speech disorders, poor communicators usually are not referred to speech therapists. In recent years, with the increased interest in children's language and cognitive development and with new trends in the education of disadvantaged children, these poor communicators have finally become "visible," and their need for compensatory language training has been acknowledged. A number of studies of the relationship between social class and language learning have been carried out. As a rule, children of upper socioeconomic status were found to be advanced in the learning of sound patterns, vocabulary, and grammar compared to children of lower socioeconomic status (C. P. Deutsch, 1964; M. Deutsch, 1963; Irwin, 1948a, b; John, 1963; John and Goldstein, 1964; Loban, 1963; Templin, 1957; D. R. Thomas, 1962. See also the review by C. B. Cazden, 1966).

Of particular importance has been the work of the British sociologist Basil Bernstein (Halsey, Floud, and Anderson, 1964). Bernstein started from the assumption that, independent of children's biological make-up and potential intelligence, markedly different environments will affect specific aspects of their language development, in particular their vocabulary and sentence structure. According to Bernstein, the measurable linguistic differences between British lower- and middle-class children indicate important qualitative differences in modes of speech. While middle-class speakers make full use of the structural possibilities of sentence organization, lower-class speech is characterized by rigidity of syntax and by a restricted use of structural possibilities in the construction of sentences. Bernstein thus postulated the existence of two markedly different modes or styles of speech: (a) the formal or elaborate language prevalent among middle-class speakers, and (b) the restricted or public language used by members of the lower class. He further proposed that use of the formal type of language facilitates the verbal elaboration of intent and enhances the possibilities of developing a "complex conceptual hierarchy for the organization of experience" (ibid., p. 292). By contrast, the public language used by lower-class speakers, although adaptable to a wide range of communications, orients the speaker more "towards descriptive rather than analytical concepts" (ibid.).

Of particular interest for us are Bernstein's ideas concerning the linguistic relationship between child and mother. He contends that the middle-class child becomes socialized within a matrix of formally articulated language, in which words become the primary mediators between experiences and feelings. Thus, the middle-class child learns early to pay attention and to respond to shadings in word meanings, or to fine changes in word position and sentence structure, which may signal important changes in states of feeling. Bernstein believes that this early attentiveness to verbal clues leads to an increase in affective and cognitive discrimination in middle-class children. (From the vantage point of our research experience, we would like to add that it also increases the possibility of anxiety becoming attached to specific verbal clues, which we found so characteristic of bright, middle-class, stuttering children.)

Finally, Bernstein asserts that middle-class children learn both the formal or elaborate style of communication, to be used with parents, teachers, and other adults and the restricted style of the public language, to be used in association with peer groups or, later in life, in talking to less educated people. In contrast to this, the lower-class child, who has not gone through a similar advantageous learning process, enters school possessing only the limited communicative tools of a restricted language style. In consequence, the lower-class child "has to translate and thus mediate middle-class language structure"—spoken by the teacher—"through the logically simpler language structure of his own class to make it personally meaningful. When he cannot make this translation he fails to understand and is left puzzled" (*ibid.*, p. 293).

Bernstein's theories have been quoted widely, but there has been little critical discussion or empirical testing of his proposition and, as Cazden pointed out, the danger exists that a stereotype of lower-class children and adults might result, which would be "as unfortunate as the now-discredited stereotype of limited genetic potential" (Cazden, 1966, p. 208). We will return to Bernstein's ideas later in this chapter, after looking at the language deficits observed in various groups of American children of different ages and different social backgrounds.

Preschool Children with Language Deficits

Perhaps the reader will remember Nicky, "the chocolate syrup boy," whom we met in the first chapter of this book. Nicky was 4 years 3 months old at the time of observation, he was the third of five young children, his parents were of lower middle-class origin, and his mother's vocabulary was somewhat limited. In addition to defective articulation, Nicky showed other characteristics of stunted language development: a severely restricted vocabulary and a primitive use of grammar—"I hate you, you dumb!"—of the kind one would commonly expect of a child in the third rather than in the fifth year of life. Through later examinations it was found that Nicky was of average intelligence, his hearing was normal, and there were no signs of emotional disturbance or neurological dysfunction. Because of his poor language development Nicky was kept in kindergarten two years. As his mother had little time or skill to help him in developing his language, Nicky received speech training from his teacher and, once weekly, from a speech therapist. In spite of this compensatory language training, Nicky was slow in learning to read and he remained a below-average student through the elementary grades.

Many children like Nicky, with inadequate or stunted language development, can be found in the Head Start programs, compensatory programs in early childhood education, set up for the purpose of "using pre-school enrichment as an antidote for cultural deprivation" (Hunt, 1964). In evaluating the efficacy of special programs for the fostering of language development in children, it must be noted that there are significant differences between children like Nicky, who come from stable, lower middle- or upper lower-class families, and those growing up in severely disorganized lower-class homes. Pavenstedt, in an important investigation (1965), explored the significant differences between young children from disorganized, "very low-lower class" homes, who showed indications of severe and all-pervasive ego damage, and children from relatively stable, upper lower-class families, who were limited in language development as well as in exploratory behavior, but who were psychologically intact and able to learn when given appropriate training.

Pavenstedt's study suggests that children growing up in disorganized, economically disadvantaged families show many of the characteristics reported in earlier studies of institutionalized children (Bowlby, 1951; Goldfarb, 1945; Provence and Lipton, 1962; Spitz and Wolf, 1946. See also Chapter 2 of this book). In both groups—institutionalized children and those from disorganized homes—similar conditions were found to prevail: The children experienced lack of consistent care from the same person. There was little holding, comforting, and handling involved in child care. The infants were isolated from sensory stimulation during most of the day, they rarely were played with or talked to, and no explanations were given concerning the mother's or another caretaker's behavior or wishes. In short, the varied physical, emotional, and intellectual stimulations of a mutually enjoyable mother-child relationship were minimal (Malone, 1966).

In both groups of children the early deprivation of sensory and intellectual stimulation led to similar consequences: shallow interpersonal relationships; low level of initiative and low interest in exploration of the environment; quiet and docile, or withdrawn, or acting-out behavior; delayed and restricted language and cognitive development; inability to listen to and to comprehend the meaning of verbal messages; and severe difficulties in attention and concentration resembling those found in children with neurological dysfunction (M. Deutsch, 1965; John, 1963; Keller, 1963; Malone, 1963, 1966; Pavenstedt, 1965; Vosk, 1966; Whiteman, Brown, and Deutsch, 1966).

In a review of the literature on cognitive learning in infancy and early childhood Fowler (1962) suggested that concept formation begins early in infancy and that the low level of intelligence found in many disadvantaged children may often be due to the lack of intensive stimulation during the period of early language development. D. McCarthy demonstrated that once children begin to speak, at approximately 1 year of age, they will then steadily multiply the number of discriminations and generalizations of the language system which they are able to grasp (McCarthy, 1954). Hunt, in *Intelligence and experience* (1961), suggested that it might be feasible to discover ways to govern the encounters that children have with their environments, especially during their early years, in order to achieve a substantially faster rate of intellectual development and eventually a substantially higher adult level of intellectual capacity.

Language Tutoring of Infants

Translating Hunt's ideas into action, Earl S. Schaefer, of the National Institute of Mental Health, and Paul H. Furfey, of the Catholic University of America, embarked upon a remarkable project. They attempted to raise the intellectual level of lower-class infants through home tutoring, beginning at 15 months and continuing through 3 years.[1] An experimental group of 30 lower-class Negro infants and a comparable control group was selected on the basis of parental income,

---

[1] I am grateful to Drs. Schaefer and Furfey for permission to refer to their informal progress report.

education, and occupation. The infants were tested at 14 months; tutoring of the experimental group was begun at 15 months. The infants were tested again at 21 and 27 months and will be tested at 36 months. The experimental infants are being tutored in their homes for an hour daily, five days a week, with particular emphasis upon verbal stimulation. The tutors also collect data on the environments and experiences of the children, using rating scales and structured inventories as well as daily narrative reports.

The intimate knowledge of the homes acquired during the tutors' daily visits revealed the severe physical, social, emotional, and intellectual deprivation experienced by these infants. Deprivations included deteriorated housing, insufficient living space, and inadequate quantities and quality of nutrition. Social and emotional conditions included unstable parental relationships and insufficient and inadequate parental care. Intellectual deprivation was attributed to the low educational level of the parents. The parents and other persons in the infants' environments were poor models for language and intellectual development. The investigators assumed that these conditions were directly relevant to the low level of intellectual functioning typically found in children coming from similar environments.

After the 27 months testing, the investigators reported the following preliminary findings:

	14 Months	21 Months	27 Months
Experimental Group	N = 30 Mean IQ = 105	N = 30 Mean IQ = 96	N = 29 Mean IQ = 100
Control Group	N = 32 Mean IQ = 109	N = 31 Mean IQ = 90	N = 29 Mean IQ = 89

These results indicate that the infants were not below the average in infant test scores at the age of 14 months; on the contrary, as the investigators point out, the children appeared to be above the normative group in the sensory-motor skills that were measured at that time. However, by 21 months the scores of these infants had dropped significantly, with a larger decrease for the control group. A six-point difference in mental test scores had widened to 11 points for the partial samples tested at 27 months, with the untutored control cases continuing to drop, but the tutored cases increasing their scores slightly. These trends—together with earlier reports in the literature on cognitive development—suggest that by the age of 3 the control group might reach a relatively stable mean score of approximately 80, while the experimental group may have mean scores of 100. Preliminary analyses of the data showed greater differences between the two groups on verbal than on nonverbal skills.

The results of this pilot project seem to demonstrate the importance of verbal learning during the second and third year of life. It is exciting that approximately four to five hours of verbal tutoring per week—plus the possible effects of the tutor's demonstrations upon maternal practices—could produce sizable differences in test scores between the stimulated and the nonstimulated groups. It suggests that mental growth during the early years is highly related to the amount of intellectual, particularly verbal, stimulation that the child receives.

The investigators plan to continue the tutoring of the children in the experimental group until they are 3 years old, and to follow the future development of both groups through nursery school and later years. Further research is recommended on ways to provide compensatory stimulation for infants whose parents do not have the time, talent, motivation, or resources to provide an adequate educational environment for their children. The amount and type of intellectual stimulation should be varied systematically to determine what would be optimun educational programs for various infants.[2]

OBSERVATIONS OF CHILDREN IN HEAD START PROGRAMS

General Characteristics

In 1966, some of my coworkers and I had the opportunity of observing 55 children attending two Head Start programs in the greater Boston area. The children, who were $4\frac{1}{2}$ to 6 years of age, came from Irish, Italian, and Negro families; most of these families were supported by welfare funds. In 80 per cent of the homes the father was seldom if ever present. The number of children in these families ranged from two to nine, and many siblings had experienced severe problems in school learning. Most of the mothers we met appeared overburdened and depressed, but they expressed a strong interest in the welfare and education of their children. Many of them were eager to visit the nursery school and to attend parent-teacher conferences, which took place in the evenings.

The majority of the children were appealing, attractive, and physically well developed. Several of the children were emotionally disturbed to some degree. Socially, the Head Start children displayed a strong feeling for group cohesion. Early in the program they moved from one activity to the next almost as one; if one child started something, all would follow. Being very accepting of each other generally, they quickly developed friendly relations with one another.

In their relationships with adults, most of the children were friendly, but initially rather cautious. Compliance to the wishes of adults was notable and concern for manners was evident, particularly at mealtime. Minor accidents, such as spilling milk, caused great and contagious anxiety through the group, until it became clear that teachers did not punish for such mishaps. As it became apparent to the children that the teachers tolerated some previously unacceptable behavior—such as saying "no" or spilling milk—the children began acting out of bounds in a provocative manner, testing the teachers' limits of tolerance. This type of group acting-out quite obviously caused the children much anxiety.

---

2. Future detailed reports concerning this project will be most interesting. In particular, one would like to know more about the methods of tutoring employed and the mothers' reactions to the presence of a tutor in their homes.

Consistent, meaningful limitations and standards of behavior had to be established, explained, and enforced. Such limitations were derived from concrete situations and were explained to the children, as for instance: "School is a place where children work and learn and have fun, and teachers are there to help the children do this. If children run all around, shout, and knock things over, teachers cannot help them work."

Emotionally, the Head Start children tended to be more uncertain of the dependability of situations or relationships than middle-class children. This seemed understandable in children coming from homes where fathers, and sometimes mothers, disappeared and where discipline tended to be arbitrary, inconsistent, unexplained, and often brutal. In spite of this background, most of the children were outgoing and easily accessible. They trusted adults to some degree, but they were decidedly anxious when a teacher or helper left the room or was absent. In order to build up trusting relationships between children and adults, it was important to warn the children and to explain in simple words when such a leave-taking or absence was necessary.

Motor Behavior

Most of the children performed very well in the area of gross motor coordination. During the first week they spent a great deal of time outdoors, performing feats of climbing and jumping. It was remarkable to see that up to ten children could be climbing on a single jungle gym at one time and no one was pushed or stepped upon. They attempted to attract the teacher's attention with their physical ability and bravado, upon which their culture placed a premium.

Fine motor coordination was not as well developed in many of the children, although none of them actually was deficient. The girls showed more interest and dexterity in activities dependent upon fine motor skills, such as cutting and drawing, while the boys preferred hammering and building with large blocks. However, many of these girls also enjoyed climbing, wood-working, and building, perhaps to a higher degree than is found usually in non-Head Start groups.

Language Behavior

Intellectually, the majority of the children seemed to be at least of average ability. They appeared to be eager, interested, and desiring to better their own performances. However, there was evidence of a marked lack of experience with many things that most middle-class teachers may take for granted in 4-year-old children. For example, during the second week of school one boy shouted delightedly: "Look! Look! It sticks," when he encountered paste for the first time in his life. Books, as a source of enjoyment, were unknown to most of the children. It was impossible to tell a story to a group, as most children were not yet ready to listen. Some children responded to looking at a book in a small group, probably enjoying the teacher's company as much as the book. Large, bright pictures of familiar objects were received best. The teacher simply named the object, gradually proceeding from single words to short descriptive phrases. Thus, the techniques we had found helpful in working with children with defective articulation (see Chapter 11) proved to be fitting also for these children with language deficits.

The most striking characteristic of their communication was a preponderance of expressive sounds, gestures, or physical demonstrations; the latter sometimes accompanied words but often were used in preference to words. All the children seemed to lack appropriate words and names to express their wishes and needs.

A little girl provided an example of this bodily communication when she backed up to the teacher, holding her bathing suit in one hand and expressing through gestures that she needed help in changing her clothes. In another instance a boy snapped his fingers to get the teacher's attention when he wanted to make a statement. Another girl pointed and grunted to indicate that she wanted food passed along the table.

One little girl was highly verbal, and though her articulation was poor, she and her listeners enjoyed immensely her rich and strongly rhythmical verbalizations. Looking at pictures in a book she would make up a story, which might go something like this: "The sun is up—and it's time to get up—oh yeah. The kids get out—and they look at the sky—oh yeah!" and so forth. The words were simple but expressive and her enticing rhythm and the repetitive "oh yeah" made the whole story move along like a rock-and-roll song. Unfortunately, however, none of these expressive communicative patterns would serve the children well in most of our regular first-grade classrooms!

A dearth of words in certain categories was particularly evident among the Head Start children. Conspicuously lacking were the names of animals, which most middle-class children learn early. The Head Start children had not been exposed to picture books and had not visited zoos or farms, both part of the experience of many middle-class children. However, the same boys who could not identify any animals except cats and dogs knew the words to describe the various parts and functions of trucks and cars.

Nouns and verb forms indicating concepts of time were lacking also or were used erroneously, "yesterday" and "tomorrow" being confused. Terms of spatial relationships such as "middle," "between," or "underneath" were not always understood. However, in contrast to children with neurogenic language disabilities, the Head Start children were able to learn definitions of space and time and to remember new names for activities, if the new words were explained well and used repeatedly in concrete situations. For instance, a teacher's statement: "*Listen* means one person talking and everyone else hearing what he is saying" was immediately successful in gaining the attention of the group.

Before relationships between the children and their teachers were established, verbal communication was at a minimum. Conversation, when it occurred, usually dealt with an immediate experience. Food was the primary topic, until its plentifulness at school was understood. After the children had begun to realize that the adults were always willing to listen to them, they began to trust their teachers, their verbal communication increased, and the topics they touched upon began to broaden, finally including their past experiences and their lives at home.

Changes in the children's faulty syntax and sentence structure were not induced through formal or forceful correction; a good relationship between teacher and pupil, however, opened the doors for mutual imitation and reciprocal identification between them. It seemed wisest for teachers initially to accept the children's own verbalizations, to encourage verbal communication, and to provide corrective feedback in an atmosphere of mutual consideration and delight in each other. "Snobby" speech coming from a teacher was not valued by the children. Standard English was accepted and adopted eventually if it came from a down-to-earth, warm, accepting, and vital person, whom the child could count on to be fair and honest, and with whom he could achieve a straightforward relationship.

Examples of Teaching and Learning

Teachers who previously had worked primarily with children with normal or advanced language development had to discover new modes of communicating with the Head Start children. At the beginning of the program the children were interested primarily in motor activities but hardly at all in the verbal mediation of experience, as the following example illustrates.

A teacher and a group of five children were observed sitting around a tub filled with earth, getting ready to plant petunias. The teacher gave each child a plant. Speaking very carefully in short sentences she described what they were going to do, why they would plant the flowers, where the earth came from, how they all would water the flowers, and what colors the flowers would be. After each statement the teacher tried in vain to elicit some reactions or questions from the group. The children showed no interest in the name of the flowers nor were they curious as to their colors; all they wanted to do was have a turn in planting them. The teacher seemed surprised and discouraged about the children's lack of response to her explanations. While she carefully had used simple words and short sentences in talking to the children, she had not been aware of the fact that her own communications did not refer to events which were "here and now"; talking about the future colors of the flowers, the distant place where the plants and the earth came from, she had lost track of the children's desire to do something actively and immediately, namely planting.

At noon the children were sitting in small groups around a table, eating lunch with their teacher or a helper. The teachers sent some of the children to a serving table to bring food back to their group. At the serving table the head teacher sliced bread and vegetables and passed out the food.

During the second week of the program, a 5-year-old boy was observed coming to the serving table with his empty bowl. He just stood there, not saying a word. The teacher asked in a friendly voice: "What do you want, Jimmy?" Jimmy said nothing. The teacher asked: "Do you want carrots or do you want cucumbers?" He still said nothing. The teacher then realized that Jimmy did not know the names of the different kinds of vegetables at the serving table. She pointed to each one in turn, saying: "These are the cucumbers and these are the carrots. Do you want cucumbers or do you want carrots?" Jimmy now pointed to the carrots. "Oh, you want carrots! Here are the carrots," said the teacher, filling Jimmy's bowl. She added: "I think you did not know the names for these." Jimmy replied: "I know them now!" He picked up his bowl and walked back to his table. It would be fine if the story ended there. The adults were much impressed with Jimmy's sturdy and positive statement: "I know them now!" However, when Jimmy got to his table, ten seconds later, he put his bowl down and announced happily: "Here are the cucumbers!"

The teaching he had received was specific and appropriate, indeed, but it had not been frequent enough. Also, Jimmy had listened passively to the teacher, but had not had an opportunity to use the words himself. If we look back at the example of the 2-year-old boy in the London taxicab (p. 7), we realize that what 4-year-old Jimmy needed was verbal stimulation and frequent reinforcement of a new word coming from an interested adult, combined with his own frequent repetition of the word. Only in this manner would he succeed in associating the word with the specific image and, eventually, in storing the combined image-symbol in his memory.

In the seventh week of the program three boys were observed sitting around an adolescent male teacher who was reading to them. The teacher came to the word "ten" in the story: "There were ten trucks." A little boy interrupted him to ask: "What is ten?" The teacher said: "Oh, Tom, you know what ten is!" "No, I don't," said Tom. The teacher asked: "How many fingers do you have?" Tom replied: "I don't know." The teacher proposed: "Let's count your fingers!" Tom, who already had spent a year in kindergarten, then counted his fingers with the teacher's help. When they had finished counting, the teacher said: "Now you know what ten is." After finishing the story, the teacher spent the next half hour counting other items in the room, until finally the nature of "ten-ness" was understood by Tom.

This example is of particular importance. It was highly unusual for any child in this group to ask an adult a question when a subject was not understood. It was even more unusual for a child to pursue the subject and force the teacher to explain a puzzling problem in great detail. It seems likely that Tom never would have asked his question earlier in the program, nor would he have pursued his questioning unless he was sure of being accepted by the teacher. Undoubtedly, in our crowded classrooms there must be innumerable occasions in which communication between teacher and child breaks down because the teacher does not remember or does not have time to find out whether the incoming information matches the information the child already has stored, and whether new information can be handled comfortably and effectively by the child.[3]

---

3. Concerning the match between incoming information and that already stored by the listener, see Hunt (1964); also Chapter 1 of this book.

A word should be said here about the use of picture books and of story telling in working with young children with insufficient language training. In Chapter 11 we mentioned the kind of simple, uncluttered pictures which we found helpful in training preschool and kindergarten children with severely defective articulation. Such pictures, however, might be inappropriate at the beginning of a program for disadvantaged children. The children we observed were not interested in pictures or stories and would leave in the middle of a story if anything happened at the other end of the room. Language training might profitably begin with some of the motor activities the children enjoy so much. The boys, for instance, were engrossed in building with blocks intricate roadways, bridges, and tunnels, and quite obviously they wanted to talk about their constructions. Not knowing the words to refer to them they enjoyed learning these words, rather than learning about trees, zoo animals or other one-dimensional items contained in picture books. The girls—like most little girls anywhere—enjoyed playing mother, working in the doll kitchen, and ironing clothes for their doll children. A little girl who had refused to speak at the beginning of the program communicated in a nonverbal manner with the other children playing in the housekeeping corner, pointing out through gestures when she wanted to use the ironing board. One of the helpers, a teen-age girl, spent much time in the doll corner with the nonspeaking child. As the summer went on, the little girl began to speak with increasing frequency to this helper, whom she learned to trust and to whom she was able to relate in a very personal manner.

Observing a story hour, we once experienced an example of language training which was quite inappropriate for the children concerned. The teacher, experienced in kindergarten work, had chosen to read a book with advanced vocabulary, *Little Toot*, the story of a tugboat.[4] The teacher read rapidly, and from time to time she turned the book around to let the children see the pictures. Only one child paid attention to the story and seemed capable of grasping at least part of its meaning. The other five children in the room were restless and uninterested, as well they might have been in view of their utter lack of familiarity with the objects in the story and the advanced vocabulary and sentence structure used by the teacher. Three student teachers were standing by, trying to calm down the children, whispering to them: "Now, be quiet and listen to the story." It was unfortunate that this teacher had chosen such a story to read to a group of deprived children, functioning linguistically on a 3-year-old level.

A very different type of story hour was presented by another teacher, who had taught in the neighborhood from which the Head Start children came and who knew and understood their circumstances and deprivations. Her stories were simple in style, dealing with the immediate environment and with concrete events in the lives of the children, and full of descriptive words and repetitive sounds and noises. When the ball in the story bounced, the teacher said: "Bumpity, bumpity, bump!"; she made hissing noises and other funny sounds related to the stories. The

---

4. Hardie Gramatky, *Little Toot* (New York: G. P. Putnam's Sons, 1939).

children listened to her with obvious pleasure, paying attention to her words, occasionally asking questions, or joining her in making noises. Whenever a child responded to the teacher, she in turn reacted to the child's communication and repeated what the child had said, thus bringing it to the attention of all the children. For instance, in telling a story about a cat, the teacher asked the children whether they knew what the cat would say. "Meow," answered one of the children. "Yes, meow, meow," responded the teacher, and she continued to repeat the word until all the children in the group joined in, saying "meow." When the milk was passed out, the teacher said: "The milk is white. Can you find anything else that is white?" Speaking the word "white" repeatedly, she had the children find white pieces of paper or straw, and induced them to repeat the word in finding the objects. One of the children needed a straw at juice time. Not knowing the word for it, he asked to be given "one of them." The teacher immediately said: "Charley needs a straw. Eric, please pass the straw, he needs a straw." In spite of the fact that some of these children had already spent a year in kindergarten, their language development was so stunted that they needed and enjoyed the mutual exchange of repetitive sounds and words, much in the manner of 2- to 3-year-old children.

Such repetition of familiar words gave the children a sense of reassurance, of feeling at home with the person sharing words with them. In contrast to this, new words used by a relatively strange person, or a new way of saying things, might arouse mistrust, anger and even anxiety in the children, leading them to withdraw, stare at the adult speaker, and break off communication. A visiting student was looking at a picture book with a little girl, who seemed to enjoy the activity. At one point a child in the story was putting something on a windowsill. The little girl stopped listening and looked perplexed. The student tapped the windowsill nearby explaining: "This is a windowsill!" The little girl turned her head away from the adult and did not want to continue with the story. By introducing a new and unknown word, the adult had "switched the code," both linguistically and psychologically, and the child had lost contact with the adult. If we remember Heinz Werner's observations (Chapter 3) that words in early life have a concrete and physiognomic quality and are perceived as a part of the person who speaks them, we will understand why children with a minimum of experience in the use of language will react strongly, both positively and negatively, to strange adults approaching them with verbal stimulation.

Dr. Vera P. John, of Yeshiva University and the Institute of Developmental Studies, reminded Head Start teachers of the crucial importance of listening in the language training of young children (John, 1965). In many homes—and not only in those of low-income families—there is little if any ongoing communication between an interested adult and a young child. In families with many children, and particularly under crowded urban conditions, a great deal of "parallel talking" occurs rather than true communication between speech partners. Adults talk about their problems and express their moods in the presence of young children, and the noise of simultaneous talking by several family members is exacerbated by the almost continuous flood of words spilling from radio and television. The effect of such auditory flooding and the continued impact of diffuse verbalizations upon young children may be two fold: (1) The children learn early to tune out; "Instead of listening, they learn not to listen" (*ibid.*, p. 10). (2) The children predominately have a passive experience of language. They hear but they are not being heard, nor do they receive corrective feedback. However, "It is only when there is the opportunity to hear and be heard that language acquisition is implemented and facilitated" (*ibid.*, p. 9).

Listening to the children's language and finding ways to make the children interested in listening to the teacher should be among the first goals of Head Start teachers. Dr. John suggested that in the first few days teachers should talk as little as possible, introducing the children in a practical concrete manner to the new rooms and to the current routine. By helping the children go through various familiar experiences, such as dressing, washing, sharing a meal, and similar activities, and by using a minimum of language initially, the teacher at first will establish a preverbal bond with the children. Bit by bit the teacher then will attach verbal symbols to familiar experiences. Mrs. John remarked: "We tend to talk too much and want to achieve too much by means of language with children who we feel have been very limited in their previous lives. We tend to shower the children with what we have ready to give. *And at times a very active showering just continues the history of tuning out on the part of the children.*" (*Ibid.*, p. 11. author's italics). If the teacher uses language sparingly she inspires a kind of suspense and the children will want to hear what she has to say. Dr. John feels strongly that orienting children to listen in a classroom situation would be one of the most important achievements of a Head Start program, difficult though it may be for research workers to measure the listening capacity of young children.

The tuning out and the unwillingness to listen which result from overloading children with diffuse verbal stimulation will interfere with the children's learning of discrimination between speech sounds. In several research studies, in which the Wepman Auditory Discrimination Test was administered to large groups of young children, it was found that first-grade children of low socioeconomic status made significantly more mistakes than middle-class children (John, 1964; Katz and Deutsch, 1963; Templin, 1957). Similarly, Clark and Richards found that economically disadvantaged preschool children exhibited significant deficiencies in the ability for auditory discrimination, compared to a nondisadvantaged preschool group (Clark and Richards, 1966).

It is interesting to see that Mrs. John's recommendations for the training of children with general language deficits have much in common with the techniques we found helpful in working with children with severely defective articulation. In both instances, cutting down the linguistic load has been considered basic for successful speech training. The adult listens to the young child, he takes his cues from the child, he speaks sparingly, using simple words and short phrases together with clear articulation and a pleasant tone. Thus, the adult acts as a good listener, a good speech model, a source of corrective feedback, and as participant in delightful verbal games, played with the child. The child is not urged to repeat words or sounds right after the teacher. Repetitive practice is provided through the use of simple songs, nursery rhymes, or rhythmic repetition of words and phrases the children find enjoyable.

For very shy and noncommunicative children, individual help from an interested and skillful adult will be necessary. A child who may be too timid to speak in a group should spend some time every day alone with "his own" helper. Developing at first a preverbal relationship with a trusted adult, the child gradually enters into verbal communication with his helper. The same provision which we found of primary importance in working with young, stuttering children and children with severely defective articulation appears to be valid also in compensatory language training of deprived and intimidated young children.

Technological devices also have been used successfully in language training by the staff of the Institute for Developmental Studies. The ingeneous technique of the Telephone Interview was developed to record children's spontaneous speech in natural play-settings (Gotkin, Caudle, Kuppersmith, and Wich, 1964). A similar technique should prove useful in involving shy children in verbal communication with an adult. The Listening Center, consisting of a tape recorder and sets of earphones for six to eight children, also was used and described by members of the Institute (Gotkin and Fondiller, undated). Listening Centers since have become available commercially, and teachers of all age groups are beginning to experiment with their use in compensatory language training.

Work with Mothers and Other Adult Caretakers

In view of the mother's pivotal role in the speech training of young children, attempts must be made to involve mothers of Head Start children in the training program. In our contacts with Head Start, we found that the methods we had previously used in working with middle-class mothers had to be modified. Some mothers could be reached through evening group meetings, and many mothers made a considerable effort to attend such meetings. We soon learned that the consultant in language development—similar to the speech therapist working with the mothers of stuttering children—must show great tact and understanding in working with mothers from low-income groups. Many have become "tired of the kids being miseducated," and "tired of being called disadvantaged and culturally deprived," as David Spencer stated forcefully at a meeting of the Parent and Community Coordinating Committee in East Harlem.[5] The teacher or speech consultant will be perceived easily as being critical of the mother, as a person who tells her how to be a "better parent." Working with the so-called helpers as intermediaries proved to be a successful way of reaching parents. The services of a consultant in language development might best be employed in the following manner: She would assist Head Start teachers in identifying children with speech and hearing disorders and with general language deficits; she would contribute to the diagnostic

---

5. L. Buder, "Ford Fund Helps a School Project," *New York Times*, July 7, 1967, p. 38.

evaluation of children with speech and language disabilities in cooperation with the medical and psychological consultants; she would instruct Head Start personnel in language development and language training; she would be available for demonstration of procedures and supervision of teachers and their helpers. The helpers, as a rule, are of the same ethnic background and come from the same neighborhood as the children's parents. It has been found that these helpers have easy access to the children's homes and during their visits are in a good position to transmit to the mothers information concerning improvement of educational practices, nutrition, and language training.

It would seem highly desirable if teachers and helpers would meet regularly with consultants to discuss the best ways of working with parents. Sarason, Davidson, and Blatt (1962) pointed out that teachers do not receive "the slightest bit of training" in the difficult skill of talking with parents, though this is considered one of their regular functions. Professional people and lay helpers will have to learn from each other how to be most helpful, not only to children but also to parents of diverse social, educational, and ethnic backgrounds.

PROGRAMS OF COMPENSATORY EDUCATION FOR YOUNG CHILDREN

Within the last few years, compensatory programs for disadvantaged young children have been organized in large numbers, many of them supported by grants from the U.S. Office of Education. In the following section we will discuss briefly five programs illustrating varied assumptions concerning the nature of preschool enrichment.

1. An Enriched Nursery Program

Undertaken by the Institute for Developmental Studies, this three-year demonstration and research program for 4-year-old children was sponsored by the Ford Foundation and was carried out in cooperation with the Board of Education and the Department of Welfare of New York City (Feldman, 1964). While the curriculum was based on common nursery-school practice, three features were of particular importance: (1) The curriculum emphasized training in language, concept formation, and perceptual discrimination; (2) Teachers were the central figures in the program; they received intensive theoretical training before and during the program and they helped to prepare the curriculum; (3) Parent participation was considered of vital importance. Teachers made home visits to gain first-hand knowledge about the children's backgrounds, and discussed with parents specific ways in which they could supplement the school program—for instance, through reading stories to the children at home.

The methods used were derived from research studies mentioned earlier, carried out by members of the Institute. It appears that some of the principles developed early in the century by Maria Montessori for the teaching of Italian slum children (Montessori, 1959) and techniques used by Cruickshank in the education of children with neurogenic learning disabilities also were utilized. Room arrangements and routines were specified clearly, providing a setting for the teaching of concepts of order, space, and direction. Perceptual stimuli, such as toys, simple furniture, and uncluttered equipment were so organized and presented as to make singular properties more observable, one at a time, without the distraction of competing and more complex elements. As concepts of routine and order were poorly developed in the children, classroom routines were introduced slowly and explicitly through repeated motor demonstrations, and verbal directions alone were given only after the routines had been fully understood. Language training began with the labeling of objects and people. Among other items, snapshots of the children themselves were used for language activities. Eventually all equipment and activities were referred to by name, and in choosing a piece of equipment or an activity, children were induced to verbalize their choices instead of simply pointing. Expressive language was stimulated through individual contacts between teacher and child; in time, common class experiences led to group language activities. Conversations over toy telephones, dramatization of rhythms, action songs with repeated sequences all served to improve listening skills and led to improved articulation and increased vocabulary. Books containing large and uncluttered pictures, and the telling of simple stories, served to develop language and concepts. The children's favorite stories were tape-recorded so that a child might listen to a story repeatedly and on his own initiative, at the same time watching the pictures connected with it. (See Gotkin and Fondiller, undated). Specific equipment was used to teach discrimination of sizes, shapes, colors, and numbers.

A teacher, an assistant, and 15 children met for a two-hour session four days a week during one school year. No formal evaluation of results was reported in Feldman's paper. The teachers observed, however, that by the end of the year the children were using short sentences instead of one-word utterances. Also, they were able to listen and respond to verbal directions, and their attention span appeared greatly increased. In particular, both children and parents showed increased interest and even enthusiasm toward school-oriented activities. Children enjoyed looking at books and taking part in group experiences, while parents became more aware of their potential roles in stimulating their children's speech and in preparing them for school.

In the light of our present knowledge on language and cognitive development, the methods used in this program appear highly appropriate. However, in the absence of a control group it is impossible to assess whether the improvement in the children's language behavior was caused by the methods employed or simply was a result of time and maturation.

2. The Early Training Project

An experimental preschool program for culturally deprived children, referred to as the Early Training Project, was carried out by Susan W. Gray and Rupert

Klaus of George Peabody College, Nashville, Tennessee (Gray and Klaus, 1965). It was the purpose of this project to explore whether it might be possible, by specially planned techniques, to offset the progressive retardation in cognitive development and school achievement which has been found characteristically in culturally deprived children.

The subjects studied were 60 Negro children in a Southern city, plus an additional group of 27 children in a nearby town, who served as a distal control group. All parents' incomes were below the "poverty level," the level of parental education was eighth grade or below; the median number of children in the families was five; the father was absent in almost half of the homes.

The theoretical assumptions of the study were formulated in terms of stimulus-potential and reinforcement dimensions, which appeared applicable to the observation of young children. It was assumed that the children in the project, at age 3 or 4, would have their behavior "not too well under the control of adult verbal directions"; that they would be "highly responsive to adult reinforcement of a non-verbal sort (hugs, pats, being carried, and the like)"; and that because of their upbringing the children would tend to approach new experiences by inhibiting behavior rather than by exploring the situation. The study was centered around changing the attitudes toward achievement in the children as well as in the parents. Perceptual and cognitive development and language learning were stressed in the daily activities of the program. The work with parents was carried out through weekly home visits by a specially trained preschool teacher.

The general design of the study provided for four treatment groups. At the time of publication of the report, the first group had had three special summer-school experiences of ten weeks each, plus weekly contacts between the parents and the home visitor over the remainder of the year. These contacts continued during the children's year in the first grade. The second group had had a similar program, which began a year later. The third group, called the local control group, had received the same tests as the children in the two experimental groups, but except for a two-hour play period once weekly during the third summer, the group had had no contact with the project. The fourth, or distal control group had pre- and post-tests, but no further contact with the project.

The teaching personnel of the two experimental groups consisted of a specially trained head teacher and teaching assistants who were either college students or doctoral students in school psychology. The assistant staff was divided equally as to race and sex, and each assistant was in charge of four to six children. Because of the low adult-child ratio it was possible to reinforce children immediately for any desired behavior, to individualize scheduling and types of reinforcement, and to provide a large amount of verbal interaction between child and adult.

Apparently, books were of particular importance in this program. Picture books relating to subjects familiar to the children were used several times a day, though the workers recognized that during the first summer the children "could not pick up the meaning of a picture as adequately as middle-class children." Many books were available in several copies so that children could follow the pictures as a story was read to them. Also, children were given small books as rewards for performance.

Between May 1962 and August 1964, tests were administered at the beginning and the end of each summer session. On the Stanford Binet Test (Terman and Merrill, 1960) as well as on the Peabody Picture Vocabulary Test (Dunn, 1959), the differences between the experimental and the control groups were significant at the .05 level and beyond. The Illinois Test of Psycholinguistic Abilities (McCarthy and Kirk, 1961) was administered twice during the study and, again, the children in the experimental groups proved to be "significantly (at the .05 level) superior to the control children on all subtests except that of motor encoding." On entering first grade, all children were given a battery of preschool screening tests. The experimental children did conspicuously better than the controls, tending to approximate the nondeprived children in the school; they were superior also on reading readiness tests.

The authors are planning to follow all groups through several years of their school performance; they feel that only after the children have been in school for some years will it be possible to know whether or not the effects of a deprived home environment have been overcome through intensive, early compensatory training.

In addition to its encouraging results, this study presents several important features: a careful research design, skillful translation of theoretical variables into relevant operational processes, intensive training and involvement of teachers, and well planned and prolonged work with parents. Finally, one must admire the extensive and skillful work carried out with the children, characterized by appropriate and continued verbal stimulation and by frequent, immediate corrective feedback or reinforcement.

3. *A Program of "Pattern Drills"*

An experimental preschool program which differed markedly from the two programs described was carried out by Carl Bereiter and his collaborators at the Institute for Research on Exceptional Children at the University of Illinois (Bereiter, Engelmann, Osborn, and Reidford, 1966; Bereiter and Engelmann, 1966). The project was "academically oriented" with emphasis on giving 4-year-old children highly structured training in language, arithmetic, and reading. The authors were convinced that the usual enriched nursery-school program was insufficient to help the culturally deprived child overcome his extensive deficits in the primary skills. The program was highly task-oriented; its aim was not to increase generally the children's intellectual abilities, but rather to concentrate the teaching efforts "on what seems most significant for academic success."

In the programs described earlier, attempts were made to establish a trusting relationship between adult and child, prior to getting the children to talk. The methods used in these developmental programs were modeled after the processes of verbal interaction between parent and child, observed in cases of successful language development. Bereiter, *et al.* departed from the developmental model and disregarded the children's already established, primitive language patterns. It was their conviction, derived from Bernstein's theories (*op. cit.*, p. 255), that the language of culturally deprived children represents not merely an incorrect version of standard English "but is a basically non-logical mode of expressive behavior which lacks the formal properties necessary for the organization of thought" (Bereiter, *et al.*, 1966, p. 113).

The subjects of Bereiter's study were 15 4-year-old Negro children coming from "the lower stratum of the culturally deprived ghetto." At the beginning of the program these children showed severe and general language deficits, such as severely defective articulation, extremely limited vocabulary, inability to make statements or ask questions in connected sentences—in short, the stunted language commonly observed in preschool children from the lowest income group.

The teaching model adopted by Bereiter and his collaborators was that of foreign-language teaching; an attempt was made to teach the children a "different language," which should eventually replace their own impoverished form of communication, at least in school settings. So-called pattern drills, commonly used in foreign-language teaching, were the basis of this form of compensatory language training.

In teaching the children "statement patterns," emphasis was given to "achieving clear pronunciation of the particles which distinguish one statement from others that may involve the same lexical elements." The authors rightly pointed out that many logical distinctions in English are conveyed by small words or particles which are slurred over easily or misperceived, such as *and* versus *or*, *than* versus *and*, *is* versus *isn't*.

Bereiter's report has to be studied in the original in order to appreciate fully the logical approach which the authors used in the teaching of language, arithmetic, and rudimentary reading. As an illustration of their teaching methods, we quote a paragraph describing the teaching of prepositions.

The children were not able to pronounce, use, or understand the functions of prepositions and conjunctions in a sentence. Prepositions selected to be learned were *in, on, above, under, beside, between, in front of, in back of.* A child was instructed to sit on a table; if he didn't do this correctly, the teacher helped him and said, "You are sitting on the table." The child and teacher repeated the statement. The teacher asked the child "Where are you sitting?" The child would say, "On the table." T—"Now say the whole thing." C—"I am sitting on the table." Eventually, one child was able to give another child the orders to sit under the table, stand beside the table, hold a hand above the table, etc. In translating words into actions the underlying logic of grammatical forms becomes apparent to the child so long as the specified or implied operation is physically possible. In correctly following an instruction to sit under the table, the child demonstrates to himself the connection between word and action. The next and more difficult step is to have the child describe the relationship between action and word. The teacher puts a pencil between a red block and a green block; the child must describe the action. Tasks of this type give children practice in manipulating the verbal machinery necessary to transfer words into action, action into words. (*op. cit.*, pp. 116–17).

Most readers probably will be reminded immediately of their school days, which may have included such lessons as: *"Le chapeau est sur la table. Où est le chapeau? Il est sur la table."* Such rigidly structured methods and drills have been found useful in teaching foreign languages to adults, and also in the training of aphasic adults and children. Furthermore, Bereiter's approach to the teaching of basic arithmetic and reading may well contain elements which might prove helpful in the teaching of children with severe perceptual-motor language disabilities. However, the question must be asked: is this highly structured method, used exclusively, the best way or even a desirable way of teaching a primary language to young children?

Bereiter's program for 4-year-olds ran for two hours a day, five days a week. The school day consisted of three 20-minute sessions devoted to the teaching of language, arithmetic, and reading, separated by a period for refreshments and singing, and one session for free-play activities. Instruction in each subject was given by a different teacher, who worked with groups of four or five children. The effectiveness of the program was measured through scores on three subtests of the Illinois Test of Psycholinguistic Abilities: the Auditory-Vocal Automatic, the Auditory-Vocal Association, and the Vocal Encoding subtests. The children gained "approximately 20 points in three months" in the three language areas tested, and the authors felt that "their progress in three months' time seems to compare rather favorably with that of culturally deprived children in the first grade, and these children are two years younger." They added, however, that judged by absolute standards, the children were still a long way from mastery of language, arithmetic, and reading.

A final evaluation of the methods employed, of course, will be possible only after the children and their school achievements have been followed over several years. The program has been much discussed and criticized. Many observers objected to the rigidity of the instruction, the extensive use of rewards and punishments, the lack of interest in diagnosis, and the apparent disregard for the values of inter-personal relationships. One might wonder also what effects the discouragement and even inhibition of spontaneous verbalizations may have had upon the children's initiative, personality development, and interest in further learning.

4. A "Learning to Learn" Program

A study concerning curriculum development and learning materials for early childhood has been conducted at the Learning to Learn School, Inc., in Jacksonville, Florida, under the direction of Dr. Herbert A. Sprigle (Sprigle, 1967).

It was the purpose of the project to develop a sequential curriculum for early childhood education and to innovate materials specifically designed to be used with the curriculum. Sprigle feels that deprived children, like all other children, must learn how to learn; thus, the focus is not on the deficiencies frequently found in educationally deprived children. In his opinion, many children in all classes of society do not know how to learn because educators fail "to reduce the complexities of the adult world to the child's level of understa ndingand interest." In addition, most of the commercial materials now available do not motivate and challenge children "to find ways to go beyond what is obvious and on the surface."

The experimental curriculum is based upon Piaget's theory "that mental development proceeds along an orderly sequence of motor-perceptual-symbolic phases, with periods of transition." According to Piaget, repeated encounters with objects which the child can move and explore lead to the development of images which, in turn, lead to the acquisition of symbolic language. In the process of establishing some kind of relationship between sense impressions, actions, and words, eventually the child reaches the stage of symbol formation, which enables him to talk about things and events even in their absence.

The curriculum is organized around developmental tasks which the author designed and for which he provided real and miniature objects and raw materials. The educational processes of this program require two classroom areas: a work-play area, which is large enough to accommodate all children for a variety of activities; and a smaller room used for work with four children in learning tasks. The small room is nearly bare, except for the learning materials, and most work is done on the floor rather than on tables.

Orientation programs were conducted for teachers and students to give them a good working knowledge of the curriculum and its objectives. The aims of the program and problems of children's home management are discussed with parents in discussion groups, and parents are encouraged also to observe the classes frequently.

In his paper of March, 1967, Dr. Sprigle discussed the educational procedures he developed, but research findings have not been published yet.[6] The study is of great interest because of the translation of Piaget's developmental theories into educational practices. Sprigle's curriculum, in which the child, as an active participator moves from stage to stage in a planned yet individualized manner, appears to be in marked contrast to Bereiter's, in which the child appears in the role of a passive recipient of standardized inputs. To learn more about both studies and to follow the children in both projects over several years will be most enlightening.[7]

5. An Unsuccessful Enrichment Program

Gerald D. Alpern, of the Indiana University Medical Center, reported "The failure of a nursery enrichment program with culturally disadvantaged children" (1966). A group of 42 4-year-old Negro children, living in a federal housing

---

6. A further and more comprehensive report of the Learning to Learn Program has since appeared (Sprigle and Sprigle, undated). Both groups of lower-middle class children participating in the study made large gains in verbal skills and in creativity. Follow-up data also indicate "superior abilities in using mathematical concepts." The area least affected by the program was that of activities involving motor coordination. Children who were behind in their intellectual development initially received most benefit from the experimental program.

7. Piaget's concepts were applied also in another preschool intervention program; the Ypsilanti (Perry) Preschool Project (see D. P. Weikart, Ed., undated).

project in a slum area of Indianapolis, was divided into two groups matched for sex, age, intelligence, and reading readiness. Before treatment all children were tested at the Indiana University Riley Child Guidance Clinic, where the Stanford Binet Intelligence Scale (Form L–M) and the first three subtests of the Metropolitan Readiness Test (Form R)[8] were administered. One group of children was selected randomly to attend a nursery-school program, while the control group received no nursery school education. All children were retested again at the end of the program and a follow-up study of all children was accomplished 17 months later, when they were in first grade.

The nursery group, which eventually consisted of 15 children, met three times each week for a two-hour session over a seven-month period. One teacher and two "trained volunteers" were in charge of the children. All mothers attended at least one of the 13 teacher-parent meetings, and eight of the mothers "participated in the preschool sessions." Approximately 50 per cent of the class time was devoted to free play, 25 per cent was spent in outdoor activities, and 25 per cent was given to "specific enrichment training." The program suffered from "spatial and financial limitations." The teachers and assistants were "creatively involved in the project" and conducted weekly staff meetings "for the purpose of consistently upgrading all aspects of the curriculum."

The hypothesis underlying the study was that a group of preschool, disadvantaged children who attended an enrichment nursery school would be better prepared for public school and would function better there than would a matched group who had not attended nursery school. However, no significant differences were found between the two groups in intelligence or reading readiness following the seven-months' preschool experience, nor were there any differences between the groups in their academic achievement when they were tested again in the first grade.

On the basis of these negative results Dr. Alpern questioned certain assumptions concerning the benefits of preschool enrichment programs for poverty stricken children, and emphasized the essential value of the use of control groups in assessing the effects of preschool programs. He further suggested that "perhaps ultimately the most fruitful approach will involve not a changing of the child during his preschool years but an altering of the elementary school systems" (*ibid.*, p. 16).

A few remarks concerning this study might be justified. In his paper the author presented a precise and detailed report of the statistical aspects of the study, but there is little information provided about the educational process. We learn practically nothing about the specific training of the teacher and the trained volunteers. We do not know in what particular manner parents were approached, nor to what extent and in what roles the eight mothers mentioned participated in the project. We do not really know what methods were employed in the so-called enrichment training. We do know, however, that the time spent with the children

---

8. The first three subtests are Word Meaning, Sentences, and Information.

was rather limited: "The average attendance of the 15 children was 72 sessions" (*ibid.*, p. 9). We also know that the program extended over seven months, consisting of three two-hour sessions per week, and that only 25 per cent of each session was given to "enrichment training." This means, in fact, that 15 children in the care of three adults were given approximately three and a half hours of language training per month. Even if we assume for the moment that the methods of language training used were appropriate, we can hardly assume that the training was frequent enough. One only has to observe the interaction process going on between a young child with satisfactory language development and his parents to realize that successful language training consists of a total immersion of the child in verbally stimulating and rewarding experiences. The failure of this particular program may be due to inherent shortcomings and may not justify abandonment of preschool training programs for educationally deprived children. *It may well be that we need both well-designed and well-staffed preschool programs and radical changes in elementary education, if we wish to compensate children successfully for the lack of adequate training and stimulation at home.*

PRINCIPLES OF COMPENSATORY LANGUAGE TRAINING FOR YOUNG CHILDREN

Comparing our own observations, reported earlier, with the reports of these five preschool programs, we found more similarities than differences. We found similarities in the language deficits observed in deprived children and in the teaching methods used in the majority of projects, and differences in the theoretical frameworks chosen by the investigators. On the basis of our present information it seems feasible to formulate some preliminary principles, which should be helpful in planning and setting up programs in compensatory language training.

1. Language training alone almost never is, and should not be, the sole purpose of a compensatory preschool or kindergarten program for deprived children. The training in the correct use of symbolic language in all its facets has to be an integral part of an overall developmental program—a program of guided learning in all areas of motor, perceptual, symbolic, and social development, organized, in Fowler's words, as "a sequence of encounters between a child and the environmental stimulation he cumulatively experiences" (Fowler, 1967).

2. Time should be allotted for the careful and systematic planning of compensatory programs. All staff members—administrators, teachers, helpers, and consultants—should meet for intensive exchange of ideas prior to the beginning of the program and should continue to meet in regular workshops during the period in which the program is in operation.

3. Provisions should be made for diagnostic and consulting services from professionals in the fields of health, psychology, speech therapy, language development, and reading instruction. Children with physical or mental health problems, sensory impairment, speech or hearing disorders, or mental retardation should be

identified and referred for medical treatment or remedial education where necessary. Children who are advanced in development should also be identified. Consultants should be available to assist the teaching staff in working with children with developmental deviations.

4. In language training proper, the principles stated frequently in this volume should be applied: New information should be presented to the child in a manner which he can handle comfortably, carefully matched with information he already has received and has organized cognitively. The adult should provide the child with appropriate and frequent verbal stimulation and corrective feedback without "overloading the system." The teaching should occur in a setting of mutual delight, enabling the child to feel accepted and adequate, and encouraging him to develop initiative and enjoyment of learning.

5. In all compensatory training programs for young children, a small teacher-child ratio is of vital importance; an adult should not be responsible for more than four or five children. Semiprofessional helpers, mothers, and volunteers should be trained and employed in order to guarantee this ratio. In the case of severely deprived, traumatized, or extremely shy children, a one-to-one adult-child relationship should be provided, at least in the early phases of the program.

6. If possible, parents should become involved in their children's training programs, contacts with parents should be planned carefully, and the procedures used should be flexible and adapted to different situations and social and ethnic groups. The work with parents has two important aims: to enlist the parents' help and enhance their skill in stimulating the child's language development; and to assure the parents of their parental adequacy and worth, thus enhancing their self-respect which is crucial for their own learning and personality development.

7. If possible, pre- and post-tests should be administered in order to evaluate the results of training and to improve future programs.[9]

Unfortunately, except for programs connected with research projects or university training centers, few preschool programs for disadvantaged children have had well-designed and systematic approaches to language training. Often there has been little time for planning, staffs have been poorly prepared, and consultants have been hired midway through a program to impart urgently needed technical information in a condensed and abbreviated form. Although teachers and helpers invariably have been hard-working, dedicated, and enthusiastic, many so-called compensatory projects in actuality have amounted to nothing more than non-specific nursery school programs. In addition, even when programs were well designed and executed and the progress reported was encouraging, initial gains

---

9. The reader will be aware of the fact that many of the methods described in this chapter, and the principles stated above, will be applicable, though with some modifications, to the early education of children with perceptual-motor and language disabilities. These methods will be useful also in so-called transition classes for high-risk children, as described by de Hirsch, Jansky, and Langford (1966, Chapter 9). In the case of brain damaged children and those with severe perceptual-motor handicaps, emphasis will have to be placed on a simplified environment, a highly structured program, and much repetitive practice of skills.

often were wiped out later when the children involved had to attend overcrowded and poorly conducted elementary-school classes. We are reminded of Alpern's recommendation (*op. cit.*), that "an altering of the elementary school systems" will be needed in order to improve the language and cognitive development of approximately one third of the school population.

Professor William Fowler, of the Ferkauf Graduate School of Humanities and Social Sciences, Yeshiva University, New York City, expressed himself forcefully on this matter:

The concept of social disadvantage has served a useful purpose in capturing the popular imagination and energy in remedying social injustices to the poor. However, this concept can be used as no more than a crude guide in designing educational programs for the children of the poor. While there are a number of personality and intellectual problems that appear more frequently in children of the lower working class than in children of the more socially and economically advantaged classes, the problems appear in different combinations in different children. They are, moreover, not limited to this group of children. Personality traits such as apathy, withdrawal, hyperactivity and low impulse-control; and intellectual difficulties, including general and specific cognitive and language deficiencies; and perceptuo-cognitive diffuseness are to be found in nearly all populations of children (Fowler, 1967).

DIAGNOSTIC FINDINGS IN KINDERGARTEN AND FIRST GRADE CHILDREN

Some statistics from the Wellesley Elementary Schools seem to bear out Dr. Fowler's statements. These statistics were collected in the school year 1965–66, when 903 children attended kindergarten and grade one. The social class of the parents ranged from lower-middle to upper-middle class. Of the 903 children, 326 (36 per cent), were referred by teachers because of some form of speech difficulty. All children were examined by speech therapists; 178 (19.5 per cent) were found in need of speech therapy, while the speech of the remaining 148 was judged to be well within developmental norms. Of the children assigned to therapists, 103 had moderate difficulties in articulation, 12 spoke with severely defective articulation in the absence of hearing loss, 7 showed symptoms of perceptual-motor and language disabilities of various degrees of severity, and 4 were stutterers. Speech therapy was carried out with the cooperation of mothers and teachers in the manner described earlier in this book.

In addition, kindergarten and first grade teachers referred 50 children (5.5 per cent) to the office of the school psychologist for diagnosis. Teachers were asked to describe their concerns in terms of observed behavior rather than by using diagnostic labels. Almost all of the children were referred because of multiple difficulties, and teachers reported altogether 153 observations concerning these 50 children. All children received diagnostic examinations by licensed school psychologists. It was found that the intelligence of this group ranged from borderline to highly superior. Later, all written referrals made by teachers and all reports written by psychologists were analyzed and categorized, to assess the problems presented

TABLE 15—ANALYSIS OF PROBLEMS PRESENTED BY CHILDREN RE-FERRED TO SCHOOL PSYCHOLOGISTS FROM KINDERGARTEN AND FIRST GRADE, 1965–66

Problems		Identified by	
		Teachers	Psychologists
A. Attention			
1. Short attention span		12	21
2. Inadequate attention to environment		4	2
3. Daydreaming		2	1
	Total	18	24
B. Speech and Language			
1. Poor articulation		10	14
2. Substandard grammar		1	1
3. Poor language comprehension		1	5
4. Rate—too fast or unusually slow		2	5
5. Delayed development		4	3
6. Does not follow verbal directions		4	2
7. Volume of voice inappropriate		0	2
	Total	22	32
C. Motor			
1. Overactive, restless		6	8
2. Clumsy gait		6	5
3. Inferior small muscle coordination		14	23
4. Very slow movements		1	2
5. Marked motor-perceptual difficulties (Bender Test)		0	14
6. Handedness not established		0	1
	Total	27	53
D. Emotional			
1. Aggressiveness		6	5
2. Withdrawal		3	0
3. Marked, sudden mood shifts		2	0
4. Passivity		3	8
5. Immaturity		14	12
6. Lack of self confidence		2	7
7. Impulsiveness		4	7
8. Overdependence		5	6
9. Bed-wetting		1	2
10. Timidity, shyness		6	10
11. Temper tantrums		1	0
12. Anxiety		3	4
13. Thumbsucking		0	2
14. Nightmares		1	0
15. Vomiting		1	0
16. Low frustration level		0	3
	Total	52	66

E. Learning
    1. Does not remember routines   2   3
    2. Cannot learn content (numbers, letters, etc.)   6   6
    3. Overall accomplishment poor   8   2
    4. Has reading difficulty   4   2
    5. Does not finish work   1   0

                           Total   21   13

F. Physical (Medical)
    1. Hearing difficulty   1   0
    2. Visual difficulty   2   3
    3. Generally immature   4   2
    4. Health problems   1   2
    5. Neurological impairment   0   5
    6. Fatigue   1   3
    7. More than one month premature   1   1
    8. Cerebral palsy   2   2
    9. Drooling   1   0

                           Total   13   18

G. Promotion
    1. Transfer from other school system   2
    2. Transfer to another grade   1

Total number referred   50
    Observations noted by teachers   153
    Observations noted by psychologists   206

Rank Order of Problems Identified

Teachers		Psychologists	
Emotional	52	Emotional	66
Motor	29	Motor	53
Attention	28	Speech and language	32
Speech and language	22	Attention	24
Learning	21	Physical (medical)	18
Physical (medical)	14	Learning	14

by this group of children and to compare the observations made by teachers with those made by psychologists. The findings of this analysis are presented in Table 15.

These findings most likely could be matched in similar suburban schoool systems. The percentage of children in the early grades in need of speech therapy (19.5 per cent), or of compensatory language training (3.1 per cent), probably will be very much larger in school systems with a majority of children from disadvantaged homes. Therefore it is urgently necessary to explore whether compensatory programs in language training could be built successfully into the curricula of elementary schools and whether such programs might promise results if carried out later than the preschool years. A look at some groups of older children with language deficits may shed some light on these questions.

OLDER CHILDREN WITH LANGUAGE DEFICITS

A Group of Fifth Graders

In the fall of 1966, a Wellesley fifth-grade teacher found herself with a group of 23 children, 9 boys and 14 girls, most of whom proved to be highly deficient in verbal communication. Twelve of the children had repeated grades. The class met in a new elementary school, to which the majority of the children had been transferred from two other schools in the community, while a small number of pupils had come from other states. Thus, the children did not share a common educational background. The ages of the children ranged from 10 years 2 months to 12 years, and their I.Q. scores on the California Short Form Test of Mental Maturity (Sullivan, Clark, and Tiegs, 1957) ranged from 97 to 127, with a median of 100. Most of the children were poor spellers. Their reading skills, according to their scores on the reading section of the S.R.A. Achievement Series (Thorpe, Lefever, and Naslund, 1964) ranged from the 3.2 level to the 10.3 level. Two of the children had been referred for speech therapy because of marked articulation difficulties. The socioeconomic status of the parents ranged from upper-lower class to upper-middle class. In spite of these marked intragroup differences, all children, except one, were strikingly poor communicators. The one pupil who expressed himself well was a boy with an I.Q. of 125, the son of a business manager, and the youngest of three children.

The teacher, a very experienced and highly skillful person, tried hard to improve the verbal skills of the children in her class. She insisted that they answer questions in complete sentences, she called upon them to read aloud in class, and she requested that they give oral reports about books read or about personal experiences. The children responded with sulkiness, resistance, and avoidance of the assignments. One of them remarked "Do we *have* to do all that talking in class?" It was evident that these children, who communicated freely with each other in the playground, had developed inhibitions and feelings of incompetence concerning the more formal communication manner required in a school setting. The teacher then turned to the speech therapy services, requesting assistance in her efforts to improve the linguistic performance of her pupils.

The children's difficulties were discussed in a staff conference and a speech therapist, formerly a member of our research staff, was assigned as consultant to the fifth grade. As this was an ad hoc experiment and not a research project, no formal evaluations were carried out. We did hope, however, that our research experience might provide us with guidelines for compensatory language training fitting for this group.

Having observed teacher-pupil communication in the classroom, the consultant concluded that the teacher's demands—though appropriate for fifth graders with more advanced language development—were too complex for this particular group of children. Following our basic principle of matching verbal instruction with the level on which a child can function comfortably, the consultant considered the possibility that these children might respond positively to a simple language task, but be unable and unwilling to respond to a highly complex one.

The Wepman Test of Auditory Discrimination (Wepman, 1958) was administered to each child individually and it was found that all but one child missed between two to six word comparisons presented in the test; thus, these pupils functioned in auditory discrimination on the development level of 5- to 6-year-old children. Consequently, the consultant began her work by teaching the children auditory discrimination between speech sounds. Simple sound and word games were demonstrated to the class once weekly by the consultant, while the teacher continued working with the children along the same lines during the week. To the teacher's surprise, the children reacted pleasantly to this type of auditory stimulation. Focusing upon a part-aspect of language behavior—listening to likenesses and differences between speech sounds—was not an easy task. But after three weeks of practice, they finally had a successful language experience. Their tension and resistance disappeared and their obvious delight in succeeding was evident in their frequent laughter and in the expressive quality of their voices.

As the students' auditory discrimination improved, the therapist demonstrated other and increasingly more complex verbal games. Naturally, it would have been offensive to these older children to be asked simply to label pictures. Instead they were challenged to find the most appropriate and most colorful word to describe a picture or an object; later they were encouraged to describe pictures, objects, and events in simple connected statements, and eventually to make up brief stories about them. Intragroup communication in the classroom was stimulated through question-and-answer games played among the children and through the sending of verbal messages in the manner of Simon Says. Finally the children engaged in spontaneous telling of imaginative stories, which they recorded on tapes. The children also evaluated their own and their classmates' communications with increasing interest and understanding.

Choral speaking of simple poetry also became a part of the project, and selections of spoken poetry were presented successfully by the group at a school festival. Principal and teacher felt very satisfied with the success of this training program. The children no longer avoided verbal communication in the classroom and they expressed themselves freely and easily. Continuation of the program is planned for the sixth grade.[10]

A word should be said about the incidence of poor auditory discrimination in this group. Wepman and his collaborators (Wepman, 1960, 1964; Morency, Wepman, and Weiner, 1967) found that approximately 20 per cent of normal

---

10. As this book goes to press, we have begun a pilot project in compensatory language training for disadvantaged children with language deficits, to be carried out at two Wellesley elementary schools from kindergarten through grade six. The program is supported by a Title I grant from the U.S. Office of Education. Reports will be available in 1969.

speaking populations may have poor auditory discrimination. Many children with poor auditory discrimination have difficulty in reading, spelling, or both. The authors suggested that children who are poor in auditory discrimination should be considered as being "at the lower end of the developmental scale rather than as defective" (Morency, et al., 1967, p. 336). These children should be grouped separately for the teaching of fundamental reading skills and should receive special training in their area of weakness. Interestingly enough, the same investigators found that only one third of the children with articulatory errors had poor auditory discrimination. So far we do not really understand how children with poor auditory perceptual ability succeed in learning to produce correct sound patterns. In the experiment with our fifth graders we discovered that some children continue to go through school with poorly developed auditory discrimination, and also that specific auditory training may contribute to overall improvement in communication skills.

The reader will have realized that a basic element of this program can be found in the temporary regression to earlier forms of language behavior, a regression to a style of communication which might be employed successfully even with preschool and kindergarten children. Psychologically, it was important that the consultant encouraged the teacher to permit herself and her children to regress temporarily to this more primitive level of verbal behavior and enjoyment of words. Evidently, a great deal of flexibility is necessary for a teacher to tolerate temporary regression in one area of instruction while insisting on more advanced forms of behavior and control in other areas!

In addition to temporary regression, a second principle proved of fundamental importance in the language training of this fifth-grade group. The teacher was urged to *increase the frequency of verbal interaction between herself and each child in the room*. Carrying out this procedure is not as easy for a teacher as it might seem at first.

In general, one would assume that children who express themselves poorly are likely to be less frequently included in teacher-child interaction than those who express themselves well. This assumption was tested by Ursula Wiesenhuetter, who studied the frequency with which teachers call upon children during school hours (Wiesenhuetter, 1961). The author was aware of the fact that many children today are in particular need of increased stimulation from teachers to compensate for the deficit in verbal and intellectual training caused by working parents' extended absences from the home. In her study she explored whether or not teachers provided such compensatory stimulation.

During 170 teaching hours, Wiesenhuetter observed teacher-pupil interaction in grades three to eight of a coeducational public school in a medium-sized German town. As one might expect, she found that frequency of teacher-pupil contact depended upon a number of interrelated variables; teacher's personality and teaching style; child's personality and behavior; sex of the teacher and sex of the students; subject matter; lesson plan; and such field factors as time of day, size of room, and the place of pupils in the classroom.

A more extensive distribution of teacher-student contacts occurred at the beginning and at the end of most teaching hours, while a distinct tendency toward diminishing contacts was evident at the time when teachers presented new material. All teachers showed tendencies toward "perseveration" during periods of intense concentration on their topic and during periods of marked fatigue. Perseveration was manifest in a teacher's successively calling upon one and the same student— usually a high achiever—without being aware of this repetitive contact; simultaneously, perseveration also was apparent in the teacher's repetitive use of phrases, examples, or figures of speech.

The author analyzed statistically the frequency of teachers' calling upon children and identified the characteristic differences between children who ranked high in frequency of teacher contact and those who ranked low. Children with high ability or high achievement, as well as children with disturbing behavior, were called upon during warming-up or practice periods or at times when homework was assigned or checked, while children with high ability or achievement were most frequently called upon when teachers presented new material. *Quiet and inhibited children, without exception, were lowest in teacher contact in all types of teaching situations.* Within the framework of this study, the author had no way of finding out whether the inhibitions and verbal paucity of these children had existed prior to school entrance, and whether they were caused by unfavorable home conditions, innate personality factors, or negative school experiences.

It seems worth reporting also that in this particular sample, children with sensory deficiencies (vision or hearing), physical defects, or chronic illness frequently were called upon by some teachers but were neglected by others. This was in spite of the fact that they occupied at all times seats in the front row, to which they had been assigned, presumably, to receive the teacher's attention.

The findings of this study appear to have relevance for the problems of poor communicators. Apparently there is a high probability that children who enter school with well-developed language skills, acquired within the matrix of favorable interaction patterns in the home, will receive frequent verbal stimulation and feedback from their teachers. However, children with language deficits or deficiencies in communication (indicative of disability, or insufficient parental stimulation, or both) are apt to receive infrequent verbal stimulation at school. This deplorable state of affairs will contribute to the "cumulative language deficit" observed by M. Deutsch and his collaborators (1964) in older disadvantaged children.

The experiences with our fifth-grade students, together with the findings of U. Wiesenhuetter, suggest that in our search for successful strategies to enhance language development in children, we should consider not only diagnostic findings related to a child's past history, but also "the social and cultural contextual patterns of learning in the classroom" (Fowler, 1967).

The fifth-grade teacher who participated in our training program succeeded in distributing her attention and verbal interactions evenly among her students because she was intensely aware of their deficiencies and anxious to help them improve their communication skills. As practically all the children in her room were poor communicators, the teacher was not tempted to call upon highly verbal children more frequently and neglect the children with underdeveloped language skills. Her task would have been more complicated, and the program would have had to be designed differently, had only a few children been in need of compensatory training.

Evidently, flexibility and consideration of given populations will be important in the design of language training programs. Each program should start from an assessment of the level of language skills represented in a particular group—an assessment for which, as yet, no tests or guidelines have been developed.[11] Depending upon the number of poor communicators in a given classroom, a program should be carried out either with the whole group or with a smaller subgroup working independently. Care must be taken, however, not to antagonize the children in the subgroup by labeling them "the poor communicators."

In whatever manner such a training program might be organized, however, involvement of the classroom teacher will be essential. Participating actively in training procedures, the teacher encounters the students in a situation in which she does not teach content but rather teaches communication. As the teacher has the opportunity of evaluating each child's style and level of communication, "meta-communication" becomes the subject matter of her encounters with the students. In communicating with the teacher about the means and effects of communication, the children become aware of hitherto unknown aspects of language and its use: auditory discrimination between sounds; listening to others and comprehending the meaning of their messages; appropriate choice of words, development and enrichment of vocabulary; ordering and conceptualizing experiences through the use of words; and finally, extensive and meaningful verbal expression together with the enjoyment of precision, beauty, and originality in the use of language.

Language Training of Older Disturbed Children

An experimental program not unlike the one described here was carried out with a smaller group of children in a different type of setting (Minuchin, Chamberlain, and Graubard, 1967). The subjects were six 10- to 12-year-old, emotionally disturbed, delinquent children from disorganized, lower-class families, who were in residential treatment at the Floyd Patterson House, Wiltwyck School, New York, N.Y. Communication patterns in the boys' homes had been erratic and unpredictable, characterized by a "deficit of information through words" and a lack of "the attendant rules which regulate the communication flow" (ibid., p. 559). The children had grown up suspiciously watching the persons they were dealing with, rather than paying attention to the verbal content of messages. This type of experience had interfered with their learning of verbal symbols to the degree that they functioned approximately on a 5-year-old level in communication, even though

---

11. A teachers' rating scale for children's communicative skills is being developed through the Wellesley Title I Project, mentioned earlier.

their mental ages were only slightly lower than their chronological ages. This deficit made it difficult if not impossible for the children to succeed in school learning. An "intervention curriculum" was designed, therefore, to instruct the children in the communication system used in public schools and also to train them in observation of themselves and others.

During a five-week period a remedial educator, assisted by a therapist, conducted ten class sessions during which the children assumed alternate roles, either participating in the curriculum or observing their classmates through a one-way mirror. The following skills were taught: listening, understanding the implications of noise, staying on a topic, taking turns and sharing in communication, telling a simple story, building up a longer story, asking cogent questions, categorizing and classifying information, and finally, role playing. The lessons were sequentially organized and were presented in the form of ingeniously devised games.

After the first few lessons, the children began to hear themselves, to judge themselves and others in positive terms, and to become aware of some formal aspects of language. The teacher was, at all times, explicit in her definitions and expectations and new topics were geared to the children's level of readiness. Role playing eventually brought the children to a level of awareness where they could label their own actions accurately. While the children had been noisy and disruptive at the beginning of the project, their ability to maintain focal attention improved markedly within a few hours and from the fifth session on, disruptive behavior and noise were diminished and concentration upon process and achievement became general. At all times the teacher de-emphasized her role as a controller or rewarder of behavior and the children were reminded that the "judges" were their peers and thus, by implication, themselves.

It is interesting to note that when the teacher moved too quickly for the children or was not explicit enough in her definition of goals, the children were unable to maintain structure and control, and hyperactive and disorganized behavior reappeared.

The experimenters were surprised to observe that within the short time of five weeks the children were able to progress from simple skills to complex and formal operations, such as categorizing and role playing. Obviously, the time was too short to permit internalization of newly learned patterns, and most of the children still regressed to previous patterns of communication outside of the therapeutic setting. The overall results of the experiment, however, confirmed the authors' belief that educational intervention could be carried out successfully with children much older than 4 years of age, and that a positive change in the communicative and cognitive style of 10- to 12-year-old children could be initiated.

If we compare these two studies carried out with such widely divergent populations, we discover certain similarities. In both projects the curriculum was sequentially organized, leading from discrete and simple skills to complex and formal uses of language; and in both the basic principle observed was that of matching the incoming information to a level on which the children could operate comfortably and successfully (Hunt, 1964)

CONCLUSIONS: ENVIRONMENTAL FACTORS RELATED TO LANGUAGE DEVELOPMENT AND LANGUAGE DEFICITS

Looking back over the observations and studies reported in this chapter, we come to the conclusion that—notwithstanding Bernstein's theories—social class, though important, should not be considered the most important environmental variable affecting the rate and quality of language development in children. Obviously, significant intragroup differences exist in all classes, or as C. B. Cazden of Harvard University expressed it, "the contrast is between what parents are and what they do" (Cazden, 1966). Looking over the results of various training programs, we concluded also that age of the child is not the most decisive variable determining the outcome of developmental or remedial language-training programs.

In an excellent critical review of interdisciplinary studies, "Subcultural differences in child language," Cazden discussed a number of mediating variables, or critical features of the environment, which are related significantly to language development in children (*ibid.*). We will comment briefly upon some of the significant variables mentioned in her review. The reader will recognize that several of them already have been topics of discussion in various sections of this book.

Affective Quality

The quality of the mother–child relationship is of primary importance for language development. This has been demonstrated particularly through comparisons of the effects of home versus institutional care of infants. (See Chapter 2 of this book.)

Adults Versus Children

Cazden reports that it is still an unresolved question whether conversation with adults or with other young children is more important for language development. Our own findings (Chapter 14) agree with those of Koch (1954) and Nisbet (1961), that only children, or children in small families, who have more opportunity for verbal interaction with parents, show superior speech development and that speech disorders are more frequent among children in large families than in small.[12]

---

12. W. A. Stewart (1964) observed children of second generation Negro families in Washington, D.C., whose parents spoke standard English, while the children's speech was much closer to that of their playmates who had recently immigrated from the rural South. I wonder whether Stewart is talking about the children's accent, rather than their vocabulary and language patterns. I grew up as an only child in a family of adults, my language development was excellent, and I spoke Viennese German, but during our long summer vacations I regularly adopted a rural accent from the children I played with. Nana (Chapters 3 to 5) learned most of her vocabulary and sentence structure from her mother, but did not adopt her mother's foreign accent. Nana's marked Cantabridgian accent frequently caused observers to ask questions about her upbringing. As Cazden suggested: "The opportunity to talk with adults may determine largely the complexity of the 'programs' for constructing and understanding utterances

Contextual Variety

Varied surroundings and experiences, combined with verbal interpretations from a more mature individual, will lead to more advanced language development in a child. Children who live in narrow and unstimulating environments, having only a limited number of close personal contacts, will show a more limited language development than children who are exposed to varied and stimulating experiences (see Pavenstedt, 1965). It should be remembered that young children growing up in affluent American suburbs often live in narrow and unstimulating environments.

Signal-to-Noise Ratio

A high noise level, as found in overcrowded and disorganized homes, induces "habitual inattention" in children, thus interfering with language learning (M. Deutsch, 1963). Television may add to the amount of noise in the home, without having a positive effect on language development in young children.

Quality and Quantity of Stimulation Received

Fiske and Maddi (1961), found that increased variety in language stimulation may increase attention in the child. Differences in the quantity or frequency of verbal stimulation received appear to affect language development, "although frequency of exposure may matter only up to some threshold, beyond which no additional benefits may accure" (Cazden, *op. cit.*, p. 198). Reinforcement or corrective feedback appears to be necessary, or at least very helpful, for language development, particularly during the first three or four years of life. So-called "expansions" are examples of corrective feedback and are important particularly for the child's learning of grammar and syntax. (For further details consult the review by Cazden, and also Chapters 1 and 3 of this book).[13]

---

which a child can handle, while conversation with peers has more effect on specific details of those 'programs,' such as features of phonology and morphology" (*op. cit.*, p. 195). This is a thought-provoking hypothesis worth following up; at present the mediating variables are not understood fully.

13. Readers who are organizing compensatory language training programs for poor communicators, from kindergarten through the ninth grade, will find many stimulating ideas and useful material in the following publications of the National Council of Teachers of English: Corbin and Crosby, 1965; Loban, 1963, 1966.

CHAPTER SIXTEEN

Summary: A Comprehensive Approach to Communication Disorders in Children

At the beginning of this book we proposed that the "medical model," which considers the child outside of his social context, is insufficient for an understanding of normal as well as of deviating language development. This statement did not imply an underestimation of the important contributions of the medical sciences to speech pathology and therapy. The so-called organic speech disorders—deficiencies in the biological equipment of the speaking and listening person—would never have been understood or ameliorated without the pioneering work of audiologists, otolaryngologists, neurologists, dentists, surgeons, and speech pathologists. However, a child's acquisition of language and the posible deviations in his language development cannot be understood through a merely biological approach.

Let us go back to Edward Sapir and remember his statement that language cannot be defined "as an entity in psychophysical terms alone, however much the psycho-physical basis is essential to its functioning in the individual" (Sapir, 1921). Once we have accepted Sapir's thesis that speech is a noninstinctual, cultural function, a purely human method of communicating ideas, emotions, and desires by means of voluntarily produced symbols, we can no longer treat the social and cultural aspects of language behavior as mere epiphenomena, as is done so often in medically oriented textbooks. On the contrary, these environmental aspects must be perceived as variables of primary importance. If we think of a child's acquisition of language as a process occurring within a given communication system, of which the child is learning to become a part, it becomes mandatory for research workers as well as for teachers and therapists to pay as much attention to the kind of input the child is receiving as to the biological equipment which enables him to receive, analyze, store, and transform this input.

Focusing upon the interpersonal network of which the growing child is a part, we began our investigations with an analysis of the effect of mother-child interaction upon language learning in children. The process of this interaction was conceptualized through the diagram of the speech chain (p. 18). Through the analysis of examples and case studies we demonstrated that certain types of adult-child interaction appear to facilitate language development, while others tend to inhibit or disrupt the learning process.

Looking over Debby's history (Chapter 2), we noticed the negative effect of parental deprivation upon her language learning and the shortcomings of an institutional environment, in which verbal stimulation and corrective feedback were accidental, diffuse, and insufficient. The effects of a disrupted mother-child relationship and of the unmeshing of well-established interaction patterns were demonstrated in the case of Nana (Chapters 3–5). They were elucidated further in the reports of our work with stuttering children and their parents (Chapters 6–8). The negative effects of insufficient or inappropriate verbal stimulation upon the learning of the phonological features of language (articulation) was discussed in Chapter 11. Chapter 15 was devoted to the whole spectrum of deficient communication observed in children who were educationally deprived or who grew up in disorganized homes with a high signal-to-noise ratio.

In the course of our investigations we extended our interest from the role of the mother as the primary speech model to that of other adults acting as verbal stimulators: fathers, teachers, and other helping adults. We also touched upon the possible influence of brothers, sisters, and playmates upon a child's language learning—an area in which further research is needed.

As far as we know, all children in the above groups were free of constitutional or acquired deficiencies, and their communication disorders could be understood only through an analysis of the verbal input they had received and the human relationships they had experienced. In the case of children with multiple motor-perceptual and language disabilities (Chapters 12 and 13) we were dealing with highly complex syndromes: children with malfunctioning neurophysiological equipment responded to often inappropriate inputs, provided by baffled and anxious adults, who themselves responded to the children's idiosyncrasies in ways which interfered with their own ability to function as successful speech models.

In talking about "communication disorders" rather than "speech disorders," we considered language in all its manifestations: listening, speaking, reading, and writing, all of which children in our culture are supposed to learn within the first eight to ten years of their lives. Keeping all these forms of language in mind, we must remember also that, on the one hand, communication is more than language, including preverbal and nonverbal modes of interaction; and, on the other hand, that spoken words have a primacy over all other forms of communication. W. J. Ong, in his brilliant essay, "Breakthrough in Communication," stressed the paramount importance of sound in establishing meaning. He stated:

> The development of communication is one of the central activities of man—indeed, in one sense, it is his central activity. . . . Human thought as we know it . . . cannot come into existence outside a communications system. A child does not learn to think first and to talk

afterward. He learns both together and the two processes of communication and thinking remain correlatives throughout life.

Communication strikes deep into the consciousness ... [It] brings the human person himself not only to knowledge of things and other persons, but also to his own self-awareness. ... I become aware of myself as myself only through communication with others.

Man communicates through all his senses, and in ways so complicated that even at this late date many, and perhaps most of them never have been adequately described. But in some mysterious fashion, among all forms of communication—through touch, taste, smell, sight— ... communication through sound is paramount. Words have a primacy over all other forms of communication. No matter how familiar we are with an object or a process, we do not feel that we have full mastery of it until we can verbalize it to others. And we do not enter into full communication with another person without speech. Verbalization, speech, is at root an oral and aural phenomenon, a matter of voice and ear, an event in the world of sound. Written words are substitutes for sound and are only marks on a surface until they are converted to sound again, either in the imagination or by actual vocalization. ... Meaning thus focuses in a peculiar way in sound itself.

The curious primacy of sound in establishing meaning ... is obvious enough but very difficult for us today to grasp. The original ... spoken word has become all but inextricably entwined with writing and print. ... When we talk about words, we are seldom sure whether we mean spoken words or printed words or all these simultaneously. ... We have to make a supreme effort to establish a sense of vocalization as such. And yet, if we lack this sense, we cannot understand the development of communications systems in any real depth.[1]

It is of the utmost importance that teachers, tutors, and therapists assisting children with various kinds of communication disorders make this "supreme effort" and broaden their understanding of the nature of language and of communication systems. What is needed most is not just more research; research in children's language behavior has been more extensive since the middle of this century than in any previous period in the history of psychology. What is needed, however, is the distribution of available findings and their interpretation for the many professional and semiprofessional groups working with children. It is hoped that this book will serve as one avenue leading from research findings to educational practice.

Some procedures for *primary and secondary prevention* of communication disorders can be deduced reasonably from the material presented in this book.

Pediatricians, psychologists, and other medical and paramedical specialists should be cognizant of the interpersonal aspects as well as of the time scale of language development in children. For example, physicians who are familiar with the timetable of children's learning of speech sounds (see page 200) will notice at what point a child's articulation should be considered deficient or developmentally delayed. The physician then can instruct a mother in how to become a more effective speech model, thus helping to eliminate most of the child's difficulty before he enters school. In other instances, the physician's evaluation of the child's speech patterns, together with observations of his motor skills and general behavior, may lead to early identification of multiple motor-perceptual and language disabilities.

---

1. Walter J. Ong, *In the human grain: further explorations of contemporary culture*, New York, The Macmillan Company, 1967. Copyright © Walter J. Ong, S.J., 1967.

Furthermore, as I mentioned in an earlier publication (Wyatt, 1965), physicians, social workers, and teachers of preschool children should alert mothers and other caretakers of young children about the child's vital need for appropriate verbal stimulation and corrective feedback; such enlightenment would be the first step toward primary prevention of developmental speech disorders. Caretakers of young children should be made aware of the possibility that prolonged separation of mother and child or unavailability of the mother during the critical period of language learning—age 2 to 5 years—may lead to disorganization in the child's language behavior, unless a familiar mother substitute (father, relative) is available, who enjoys the child and is willing to provide corrective feedback and verbal stimulation. Finally, once a child has developed symptoms of stuttering or speaks with severely defective articulation, early intervention is desirable as a form of secondary prevention. As described, the emphasis in such early forms of therapy should be on the parents, in particular on the mother. She should be strengthened in her role as the child's primary speech model, provider of corrective feedback, and loving partner in the speech and language games so thoroughly enjoyed by the young child.

Speech therapists also need a more comprehensive understanding of the role of language in child development. European speech pathologists often are constricted in their perception of language behavior by their predominantly physiological orientation. The perception of American speech therapists frequently has been narrowed because of their preoccupation with teaching methods and their insufficient familiarity with theories of human development. Rather than using the medical model, many American speech therapists seem to apply a "machine model" to language behavior. "Incorrect" sounds or "nonfluencies" in a child's speech are treated as isolated deficiencies to be repaired by mechanical means: replacement of parts (teaching new sounds for old ones) or repetitive exercises and drills. The bio-socio-cultural totality of the child-within-the-family-system is often disregarded by speech technicians attempting to correct the faulty performance of a child.

Speech therapists need more comprehensive training in child development, which would lead to a wider and more refined definition of their role as mediators in the interpersonal systems of family and school, within which the growing child acquires his command of language. Thus, speech therapists gradually might turn into child-development consultants. Working with a team of clinical and counseling services provided in school systems, speech therapists would be cognizant not only of the child's speech and hearing but also of his social and emotional status and his sensory-motor and intellectual capacities. Those therapists, in particular, who wish to assist stuttering children and their parents must transcend the machine model in order to function successfully as specialists in crisis intervention, in the manner described in Chapters 7–10.

Finally, going beyond specialists, research findings must be distributed to and interpreted for all the primary caretakers of children: parents, teachers, and volunteer workers. In recent years a variety of channels have been developed to facilitate the distribution of information within professional groups; distribution of information between groups and to so-called lay people has remained woefully slow and inadequate. Hunt's principle of matching the incoming information with the information the recipient already has and can use comfortably is as sound with regard to interprofessional as to interpersonal communication. This, of course, implies that research findings have to be translated into diverse conceptual languages and reformulated on various levels of abstraction, in order to be meaningful for varying groups of adults taking care of children. Such dissemination of useful information should be carried out not only by means of the spoken word (lectures) and the printed work (publications). Other media, such as audio tape, film, and television also must be utilized. Communication with varied audiences must occur by means of demonstration as well as of explanation.

Integrated multilevel programs of child care, education, remediation, and therapy are needed urgently and are emerging in many places and in a variety of patterns. (One possible design for such an integrated multilevel program is presented in Appendix XVII.) At some point in their professional lives specialists working with children must transcend their specialities and become generalists. Only then will a meaningful interprofessional communication be possible, and only then will children be served well.

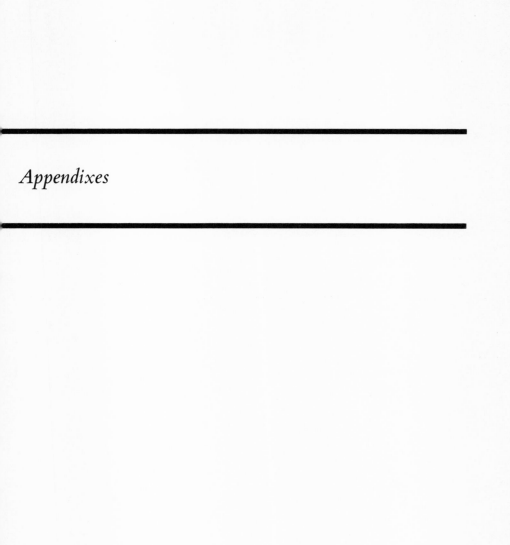

Appendixes

Description of the Mother-Child Relationship (MCR) Test

The MCR Test consists of the following:

Five pictures of the Children's Apperception Test (CAT).[1]

Card 1. Hen and chickens, feeding situation.
     4. Mother kangaroo, child kangaroo on bicycle behind her, baby in her pouch holding a balloon.
     6. Mother, father, and baby bear lying in a dark cave.
     9. Rabbit in a crib in a dark room, open door.
   10. Big dog and small dog together in a bathroom.

Three pictures of the Thematic Apperception Test (TAT).[2]

Card 1. Boy with violin and a sheet of paper on the table before him.
     5. Woman looking through open door into a room.
   13b. (For boys) Little boy sitting on the threshold of a cabin.
   13g. (For girls) Girl walking up a stairway.

The picture tests are administered in the customary manner (see original manuals).

Seven story stems, called Story Completion Test "Episodes."
Story stems 2, 3, 4, and 5 were taken in modified form from the Duess Fables.[3]
Story stems X, Y, 1, 6, and 7 were developed for the purpose of the MCT Test.

---

1. L. Bellak and S. S. Bellak, Children's Apperception Test (1949).
2. H. A. Murray, Thematic Apperception Test (1943).
3. Louise Duess, Fabeltest (1946).

Note: The two introductory stories, X and Y, are not scored but serve only as transition from the picture to the story part of the MCR Test.

ADMINISTRATION OF THE STORY COMPLETION TEST

The experimenter introduces the test, saying: "I will now read you some stories. I will read the beginning of each story and you help me find an ending for it. All right?" Experimenter then reads each story-stem aloud, ending with a question. The child's answer is recorded verbatim. The experimenter reads the next question and records the answer, and so on. The headings of the stories are not read to the child.

If the subject is a boy the story is read in the following form: "Tommy was a little boy. He lived with his father and mother. . . ." If the subject is a girl the story reads: "Susy was a little girl. She lived with her father and mother. . . ."

Introduction

Tommy was a little boy. (Susy was a little girl.)
He (she) lived with his (her) father and mother and some brothers and sisters in a nice house with a backyard.

X. *Turning for help to X* (not scored)

One Sunday afternoon all the children were playing in the yard making toy houses with pieces of wood and clay. Tommy had a hard time building his toy house. He needed some help. Whom did he call to help him?
Did X help him?

Y. *Aggression expected from X and reaction to it* (not scored)

The next day Tommy came home from school. He went into the yard to play with his new toy house. Somebody had broken the little house all to pieces. Who had done it?
What did Tommy do when he found out who did it?

1. *Expectation of anger on the part of X and reaction to it*

One day Tommy was playing in the yard. All of a sudden he heard a loud angry voice from his house. Somebody was very angry. Who was so angry?
Why was X so angry?
What did Tommy do when he found that X was so angry?

2. *Expectation of damage to child's property or body, caused by X*

Tommy had a little elephant which he loved very much and which was very pretty, with its long trunk. One day when Tommy came back from school he found that his elephant had changed. How do you think it had changed? What had happened to it?

What did Tommy do when he found out about it?

3. *Something is of value to the child. What does the mother do with it?*

Tommy had made a tower with clay which he thought was very, very pretty. His mummy asked him to give it to her. Do you think Tommy gave it to her?

What was she going to do with it?

4. *Anxiety fable*

One day Tommy said to himself: "Oh, I am so afraid!" What do you think he was afraid of?

5. *Bad dream fable*

One morning Tommy woke up all tired and said: "Oh, what a bad dream I had." What do you suppose he had dreamed?

6. *Story to investigate anxiety about loss of the mother*

One day Tommy came home from school and his mother was not in the house. He looked for her all over the house and in the yard but she was not anywhere. What do you think had happened to her?

What did Tommy do?

7. *Fairy tale about the lost child and a woman in maternal role*

One day Tommy was walking through a deep, dark wood and he could not find his way out of the wood. After a while he saw a little house. He knocked at the door. "Come in," said a voice from inside. Tommy opened the door and looked into the house. There he found a woman all alone in the house. What do you think the woman was doing?

Tommy was very hungry. He asked the woman for something to eat or to drink. What did the woman do when Tommy asked her for food?

What happened afterwards?

Definition of Terms[1]

STUTTERING

(or Stammering. The two expressions are considered to be synonymous.)

Stage I

(Initial) Child speaks with frequent, compulsive repetition of initial sounds or syllables.

Stage II

(Transitional) Child's speech shows compulsive repetitions as in Stage I, also occasional prolongation of vowel sounds and blocking of speech. Child is beginning to show overt signs of frustration and anger in connection with his difficulties in communicating.

Stage III

(Advanced) Child exhibits symptoms listed above. In addition, such symptoms may be observed as compulsive movements of some parts of the body, avoidance of specific sounds or words, stilted sentence structure, long pauses, withholding of speech, labored breathing, vibration of the nostrils, tendency to avoid looking at the speech partner, tendency to avoid certain topics or speech situations.

---

1. It is expected that no child will show all symptoms described here, but that certain children will show several symptoms. The term difficulty should always be defined as relative to the child's age and social background and to the average performance expected of his age group.

RATING SCALE

Severity of Stuttering

7. Frequent severe stuttering
6. Infrequent severe
5. Frequent moderate
4. Infrequent moderate
3. Frequent mild
2. Infrequent mild
1. Normal speech, appropriate for child's age

CLUTTERING

Propulsive impulse to speak expressed in increasing acceleration of speech, leading to irregular, nonpredictable distortion and omission of consonant sounds, occasionally to rapid repetition of syllables. The clutterer is usually not aware of his symptoms; speech improves markedly when the clutterer consciously controls his speech tempo, that is, when he slows down.[2] (In contrast, the stutterer is usually painfully aware of his symptoms and his speech becomes worse when he is asked to slow down and to control his speech consciously.)

SEVERELY DEFECTIVE ARTICULATION

The child's speech is largely incomprehensible to a listener who is not familiar with the context of the child's utterances. The child speaks with frequent omissions or substitutions of speech sounds. Substitutions usually occur within specific *clusters* of consonants. These clusters are:

Plosives: p, b, t, d, k, g (in go)
Fricatives: f, v, th (in think), th (in there), s, z, sh, zh (in Asia).
Liquids: l, r

The child also has difficulty in articulating double and triple consonants. The substitutions and omissions occur in a regular and predictable manner.

DIFFICULTIES IN SPEECH RHYTHM

Speech rhythm is uneven, speech melody often becomes distorted as the various phrases within a sentence are produced with different speed. Simple rhythm tests (clapping hands, marching) often show that the child cannot repeat correctly a simple rhythmic pattern or change correctly from one type of beat to another. Usually there is, however, no flattening of the dynamic accents of speech, as often can be found in the speech of advanced stutterers.

---

2. After M. Seeman and A. Novak (1963).

DIFFICULTIES IN WORD FINDING

These can be observed when the child tells a story or describes a picture, or in response to certain items on the WISC. For instance, on the item Picture Completion, an 8-year-old child pointed correctly to the missing parts, but had difficulty in naming them. Examples: teeth of the comb were called "needles"; leg of the table, "one wood"; cat's whiskers, "that thing"; spade on the playing card, "one things"; and a rooster's spur, "a hand." Perseverations also occurred. The child used the same word several times in succession even if it was inappropriate.

DIFFICULTIES IN SENTENCE BUILDING

Child makes more grammatical errors than are expected at his age. Child also shows a tendency to leave out parts of speech. Examples are word definitions by the same child on the WISC. A sword defined as "for fight in the war"; brave, "you brave for fight." Describing pictures he said: "The man and the lady be walking down—the man be running home."

DIFFICULTIES IN GROSS MOTOR COORDINATION

Awkward in walking, climbing stairs, skipping, running, playing ball, riding bicycle, and so on.

DIFFICULTIES IN FINE MOTOR COORDINATION

Difficulties in writing, drawing, making a circle, a zero, a figure 3; difficulty in specific control of tongue and other speech muscles. In some cases trembling; unsteady hands in drawing, writing, cutting out paper.

SEVERE DIFFICULTY IN READING AND SPELLING

Difficulty in perceiving and remembering printed and written symbols (letters, figures) in spite of normal or superior intelligence. Child shows a persistent tendency to confuse letters which are alike in form but different in orientation such as b and d, p and q (Orton). Extreme difficulty in associating auditory perceptions of sounds (phonemes) with visual images of letters (graphemes).

APPENDIX III

Information Sought During Intake Interview

Name of Child   Sex
Date of Birth   School
Grade   Teacher
Diagnosis
Parents' Address

                                               Telephone

Father   Age
Education
Occupational History
Family History: (Grandparents, Position in Family, etc.)

Mother
Education
Occupational History
Family History: (Grandparents, Position in Family, etc.)

Have Parents or Near Relatives Had a Speech or Hearing Deficiency?

Who Else Lives with the Family?
Family's Mobility
Vacations
Name and Address of Family Physician

                                               Telephone

Who Referred the Case?
Report to Be Sent to Dr.

List of All Children, Beginning with the Oldest Child

Name   Sex   Date of Birth   Speech (Hearing)[1]

Other Pertinent Information

Developmental History

Mother's Pregnancy

Birth of Child

Infancy

Preschool

Kindergarten and Elementary

Later

Language Development

First Words Spoken

Articulation of Speech Sounds

Onset of Speech Difficulty (Details)

Previous Treatment

Present Condition of Child: Home and School Situation

---

1. Categories: normal speech, delayed speech development, defective articulation (how severe), stuttering, cleft palate, other speech disorders. Hearing loss, deafness.

Rating Scales

I. Severity of Stuttering

7	6	5	4	3	2	1

7. Frequent Severe
6. Infrequent Severe
5. Frequent Moderate
4. Infrequent Moderate
3. Frequent Mild
2. Infrequent Mild
1. Normal Speech, Appropriate for Child's Age

II. Social Effectiveness of Child's Family

5	4	3	2	1
Severely disturbed family situation.	Outwardly functioning, but contains source of chronic disturbance.	Functioning, but with frequent disruptions; ineffectual.	Well functioning, in spite of difficulties or disruptions.	Well functioning.

III. Mother's Cooperation and Therapeutic Readiness

4	3	2	1
Uncooperative.	Cooperates superficially, but avoids involvement.	Willing to cooperate but not always able to utilize counsel constructively.	High therapeutic readiness, fully cooperating, imaginative use of counseling.

Ratings Before and After Therapy

Name of Child: ————————————————————————

A. *Rating at Beginning of Treatment*

I. Stuttering

$$\cdot \quad \cdot \quad \cdot \quad \cdot \quad \cdot \quad \cdot \quad \cdot$$

7	6	5	4	3	2	I

II. Social Effectiveness

$$\cdot \quad \cdot \quad \cdot \quad \cdot \quad \cdot$$

5	4	3	2	I

III. Mother's Therapeutic Readiness

$$\cdot \quad \cdot \quad \cdot \quad \cdot$$

4	3	2	I

B. *Rating at Time of Evaluation*

I. Stuttering

$$\cdot \quad \cdot \quad \cdot \quad \cdot \quad \cdot \quad \cdot \quad \cdot$$

7	6	5	4	3	2	I

II. Social Effectiveness

$$\cdot \quad \cdot \quad \cdot \quad \cdot \quad \cdot$$

5	4	3	2	I

III. Mother's Therapeutic Readiness

$$\cdot \quad \cdot \quad \cdot \quad \cdot$$

4	3	2	I

Ratings at Beginning and End of Treatment

Case No.	No. of Sessions	Age at Start of Treatment (Years)	Change in Severity of Stuttering (Ratings)	Improve- ment	Change in Family's Social Effective- ness (Ratings)	Change in Mother's Therapeutic Readiness (Ratings)
1	91	13	7—4	—	4—4	3—3
2	88	6	7—2	+	3—3	2—2
3	82	8	5—4	—	4—4	4—2
4	79	8	7—3	+	2—1	2—1
5	78	9	3—2	+	3—2	3—1
6	72	10	3—2	+	4—4	3—2
7	71	7	5—3	—	5—4	4—2
8	64	11	7—1	+	2—2	3—2
9	62	9	7—2	+	4—4	3—2
10	59	9	5—2	+	4—3	2—2
11	56	11	7—2	+	1—1	2—1
12	55	6	7—2	+	3—3	3—2
13	49	11	5—6	—	4—4	2—2
14	46	6	5—3	—	4—3	4—2
15	36	6	3—1	+	1—1	3—2
16	29	7	3—2	+	2—2	2—2
17	27	3	5—2	+	1—1	3—2
18	26	6	5—4	—	2—2	3—3
19	25	7	3—1	+	2—1	3—2
20	23	6	5—1	+	1—1	1—1
21	12	5	3—2	+	1—1	1—1
22	10	7	3—1	+	1—1	1—1
23	9	3	5—1	+	3—2	2—1
24	5	6	3—1	+	2—2	2—2
25	5	3	3—1	+	3—3	1—1
26	3	4	3—1	+	3—3	1—1
27	3	2	3—2	+	2—2	3—2
28	3	2	3—1	+	1—1	1—1

Treatment Sessions

For All Cases: Range 3—91

$N = 28$

Median $= 41$

For Improved Cases Only: Range 3—88

$N = 22$

Median $= 28$

HYPOTHESIS I: SEVERITY OF STUTTERING VERSUS LENGTH OF TREATMENT

Ratings in Severity: 5, 6, 7 $=$ high

3, 4 $=$ low

For All Cases: $N = 28$

	High	Low
No. sessions > median	12	2
No. sessions < median	4	10

χ^2, Yates Correction $= 7.15$

$p < .01$

For Improved Cases Only: $N = 22$

	High	Low
No. sessions > median	7	4
No. sessions < median	3	8

χ^2, Yates Correction $= 1.19$

Not Significant

HYPOTHESIS II: FAMILY'S SOCIAL EFFECTIVENESS VERSUS LENGTH OF TREATMENT

Ratings in Family's Social Effectiveness: 5, 4, 3 = low

2, 1 = high

For All Cases: $N = 28$

	High	Low
No. sessions > median	3	11
No. sessions < median	11	3

χ^2, Yates Correction = 7.00

$p < .01$

For Improved Cases Only: $N = 22$

	High	Low
No. sessions > median	5	6
No. sessions < median	8	3

χ^2, Yates Correction = .7

Not Significant

HYPOTHESIS III: MOTHER'S THERAPEUTIC READINESS VERSUS LENGTH OF TREATMENT

Ratings in Mother's Therapeutic Readiness: 4, 3 = low

2, 1 = high

For All Cases: $N = 28$

	High	Low
No. sessions > median	5	9
No. sessions < median	9	5

χ^2, Yates Correction = 1.2

Not Significant

For Improved Cases Only: $N = 22$

	High	Low
No. sessions > median	5	6
No. sessions < median	8	3

χ^2, Yates Correction = .7

Not Significant

Additional Variables: Individual Differences

CHARACTERISTICS OF THE CHILD WHICH CONTRIBUTED TO PROGRESS IN THERAPY

Impressed therapist as highly intelligent	18
Related easily and well to therapist	13
Was popular with peers	8
Understood the meaning of therapy	5
Took the initiative in establishing communication with parents ("He pushed for time with his mother.")	5
Had a particular talent (science, music, art, sports)	5
Had great ego strength, was a "fighter," had an intense desire to cope with his difficulties	2
Mastered reading in the course of therapy	2
(Young child) responded well to mother's attention and word games	2

CHARACTERISTICS OF THE CHILD WHICH WORKED AGAINST PROGRESS IN THERAPY

Abilities

Limited in verbal expression	3
Great difficulty in expressing feelings	3
Great difficulty in communicating with parents	2
Great difficulty in learning to read	1

Relationships

Superficial, shallow relations with others	2
(Young child) unresponsive to mother's stimulation	1
Extreme shyness	1

Physical Characteristics and Behavior

Unattractive appearance	3
Extremely stubborn, dominating	2
Hyperactive behavior	1

Psychosexual Characteristics and Defense Mechanisms

Inability to cope with aggressive feelings; either had rages or repressed his feelings	5
Perfectionism, unrealistic goals	3
Confusion of sex role, boy's identification with mother rather than father	3
Passivity	3
Excessive worrying	2
Intensive denial as primary defense	2
Intense resistance to therapy	1
Masochistic tendencies	1
Compulsive tendencies	1
Delayed adolescence	1

APPENDIX IX

Additional Variables: Life Situation

FACTORS IN CHILD'S LIFE SITUATION WHICH CONTRIBUTED TO PROGRESS IN THERAPY

Helpful Adults

Stable home situation, friendly, helpful parents	10
Stable home situation though parents were weak and inept	7
Other helpful, interested adults (teachers, relatives, neighbors)	10
Good camp; happy camping experience with parents	2
Good nursery school	2

Other Factors

Child relieved from pressures by siblings or grandparents	4
Child relieved from school pressures	2
Success at school	3
Mother gets paid help and spends more time with child	2
Father's promotion	1
Older boy's success with girl friend	1
Older girl's success as public speaker	1

FACTORS IN CHILD'S LIFE SITUATION WHICH WORKED AGAINST PROGRESS IN THERAPY

Mother found little time for child because of family pressures	7
Severe illnesses in the family	6
Defective or disturbed sibling	4
Moving, general confusion	4
Intense marital discord	4
Parents' financial difficulties or preoccupations	3
Numerous and continuing moves	3
Strong pressures from achievement-oriented parents	3
Pressures on family by ailing grandmother	3
Death in the family	2
Father frequently absent because of work	2
Alcoholism in the family	1
Both parents frequently absent, traveling	1
Mentally retarded family helper	1
Mother's limited education, poor social skill, and timidity	1

APPENDIX X

Follow-up Study

CHILDREN UNDER 7 YEARS AT TIME OF ORIGINAL REFERRAL

No.	Sex	Treatment Result	Time Elapsed in Years	No Stuttering	Mild-Moderate Stuttering	Severe Stuttering	No Further Treatment	Further Treatment
O1	m	+	5	x			x	
O2	m	+	5	x			x	
R3	m	+++	5	x			x	
S4	m	+++	5	x			x	
T5	f	+++	11	x				Psychoanalysis
A6	m	−	5		x		x	
B7	m	+++	10		x			Individual counseling, public school
Bo.8	f	+++	10		x			Individual counseling, public school
D9	m	+++	5	x			x	
G10	m	+++	7	x			x	
M11	m	+++	6	x			x	
Ga.12	m	−	6			x		Psychotherapy and parent counseling
Ge.13	f	+	6	x			x	
Br.14	m	Moved before termination	3	x			x	
W.15	f	? ?	5	x		x		Conventional speech therapy. Public school and rehabilitation clinic
Ro.16	m		5	x			x	

CHILDREN OVER 7 YEARS AT TIME OF ORIGINAL REFERRAL

No.	Sex	Treatment Result	Time Elapsed in Years	No Stuttering	Mild-Moderate Stuttering	Severe Stuttering	No Further Treatment	Further Treatment
K1	m	+	6	x			x	
BA.2	f	++	5		x			Psychiatric therapy
Jo.3	m	++	5	x			x	
Lo.4	m	−	5			x	x	Individual counseling, public school
P5	m	+	5		x			Psychotherapy and parent counseling
F6	m	−	5		x			Psychotherapy and parent counseling

Evaluation of Children with Communication Disorders

Clinical Inventory

A. *Child's History*
  1. Identifying Information
  2. Medical History
  3. Developmental History

B. *Observations of Child's Behavior and Skills*
  1. Spontaneous Speech: articulation of speech sounds; word finding; grammar, syntax, sentence building; cluttering; stuttering
  2. Speech Tests Administered
      Story Telling
      Peabody Picture Vocabulary Test (Dunn)
      Wepman Auditory Discrimination Test
      Hejna Developmental Articulation Test
  3. Motor Behavior
      Gross: clumsiness, awkwardness; poor rhythm; hyperactivity; handedness
      Fine: pencil use
          Drawing Tests:
              Goodenough Draw-a-Man Test
              Bender Motor Gestalt Test (Koppitz scoring)
  4. Handwriting: directional difficulties, reversals, other findings
  5. Reading: names, dates, and results of reading tests administered; specific difficulties
  6. Spelling
  7. Other Difficulties
  8. Intelligence Tests Administered
      Wechsler Intelligence Scale for Children
      Stanford-Binet Intelligence Scale
      Group Tests

9. Child's Personality and Behavior
   a. Behavior observations at home, at school, in the neighborhood, camp, peer relations, etc.
   b. Projective Tests Administered
      Children's Apperception Test
      Thematic Apperception Test
      Story Completion Test
      Mother-Child Relationship Test

C. *Family, Home*
   1. General condition of home
   2. Number of adults in home and relationships among them
   3. Education of parents and other adults
   4. Number and ages of siblings
   5. Intrafamily communication
   6. History of communication difficulties in family (speech, hearing, reading)

D. *Diagnostic Summary and Treatment Plan*

Test References

BELLAK, L. and BELLAK, S. S. (1949) Children's Apperception Test. New York: C.P.S. Co., P.O. Box 42, Gracie Station.

BENDER, L. (1938) A Visual-Motor Gestalt Test and Its Clinical Use. *Res. Monogr. No. 3.* New York: Am. Orthopsychiatric Assoc.

DUNN, L. M. (1959) Peabody Picture Vocabulary Test. Nashville, Tenn.: Am. Guidance Service, Inc.

GOODENOUGH, F. L. (1954) Measurement of Intelligence by Drawings. New York: Harcourt, Brace and World.

HEJNA, F. (1955) Developmental Articulation Test. Storrs, Conn: University of Connecticut.

KOPPITZ, F. M. (1964) The Bender Gestalt Test for Young Children. New York: Grune and Stratton.

MURRAY, H. A. (1953) Thematic Apperception Test. Cambridge, Mass.: Harvard University Press.

TERMAN, L. M. and MERRILL, M. A. (1960) Stanford-Binet Intelligence Scale (3rd Revision) Form L-M, Cambridge, Mass.: Houghton-Mifflin Co.

WECHSLER, D. (1940) Wechsler Intelligence Scale for Children. New York: The Psychological Corporation.

WEPMAN, J. (1958) Auditory Discrimination Test. Chicago, Ill.: Language Research Associates.

WYATT, G. L. Mother-Child Relationship Test (See this book, Chapter 6, Appendix I.)

Brief Histories of Five Cases Suspect of Neurological Dysfunction

1. CASE B, MALE, AGE 7 YEARS 6 MONTHS. MULTIPLE MOTOR-PERCEPTUAL AND LANGUAGE DISORDER

B. was the product of a full-term, normal pregnancy. However, labor was less than 45 minutes and he was born on arrival at the hospital. The umbilical cord was wrapped tightly around his neck at birth, he was rather cyanotic, and was kept on oxygen for 24 hours because of "too much mucus." Early infancy was normal except that he never cried, he choked easily, and had a very weak voice. His coughing and sneezing also were described as weak. At the age of 3 months he was seen at a children's hospital and it was noted that his vocal cords contracted rather weakly. He turned over at 5 months, sat at 8 months, and walked at 14 months. Although these gross milestones of motor development seemed normal, his parents felt that he was rather awkward in the use of his hands and feet (unable to go quickly up and down stairs without a rail until age 5, very slow dresser with particular difficulty in buttoning, still unable to tie shoes). Although fine movements with his hands remained awkward, he learned to draw well and apparently is a very fast runner at school. However, he has never been able to learn how to either throw or kick a ball. In most activities he has been right-handed but frequently, when learning new tasks, has used both hands alternately. He first began using "funny words" whose meanings his parents understood at age 3½. He began using single words at age 4. By age 5, he was using sentences but still had difficulty pronouncing many consonants correctly.

On examination, he is rather shy and withdrawn. He answers questions with single words or a nod. He cooperates quickly and follows commands readily. On cranial nerve examination, his visual fields are full and his acuity is normal. Optic fundi are normal. His pupils are equal, react symmetrically, and his ocular movements are full. Facial sensation and strength are normal. Gag, swallow, and tongue movements are normal. His gait is normal and limb strength, tone and coordination all appear intact with the exception of very slight spacticity of the left arm and leg which seemed to vary on repeated testing. Reflexes were symmetrical and somewhat brisk; planter responses were flexor. There was no clonus. Sensation was intact. B's present neurological status probably is related to anoxia during labor and delivery which resulted in cerebral damage.

2. CASE G, MALE, AGE 10 YEARS. MULTIPLE MOTOR-PERCEPTUAL AND LANGUAGE DISORDER

In the first month of life, the family physician felt that this infant's anterior fontanelle was closing prematurely. Examination and follow-up visit at a children's hospital indicated that the infant was showing normal growth and development. However, he was noted to have a bilateral sixth nerve palsy.

He was seen at 8 years of age at the medical outpatient department at the same children's hospital, with the complaint that his development seemed delayed. He had not walked until approximately 18 months. Onset of speech was delayed, articulation defective. His behavior at home consisted of a great deal of loud, seemingly purposeless activity and screaming.

On physical examination, he was found to be between the fiftieth and twenty-fifth percentile for height and weight; head size in the tenth percentile. There was persistence of bilateral sixth nerve palsy, fundi negative. General physical examination was in normal limits. On neurological evaluation, the child was cooperative only for short periods of time. There was evidence of short attention span, inability to do any tasks requiring concentration or significant coordination. Gait was somewhat floppy and shuffling and feet poorly coordinated. Impression was that there was an evident amount of psychomotor retardation present with probable subnormal intelligence. Psychometric testing and possible speech therapy with school placement, in accordance with findings of these tests, was recommended. (Note: On the Stanford-Binet, Form L, given at the age of 10 years, G. had an I.Q. of 100.)

3. CASE H, MALE, AGE 12 YEARS. MULTIPLE MOTOR-PERCEPTUAL AND LANGUAGE DISORDER

H's mother had some bleeding off and on during pregnancy, at times requiring bed rest. Labor began approximately two months before the expected date. Delivery was of short duration and without anesthesia. Baby's birth weight was 3 pounds 14 ounces. There was no resuscitation. The infant had no unusual difficulty postpartum. Neonatal course was uneventful. He was discharged at the age of 8 weeks, weighing 5 pounds 6 ounces.

In October, 1956, at the age of 3 years 9 months 12 days, he became drowsy, vomited a few times, and complained of headache. There was question of some blurring of vision. He was known to have fallen, striking the back of his head, two days prior to the onset of these symptoms. He was hospitalized for observation and study. Neurological examination, lumbar puncture, electroencephalography, and skull x-rays were negative for intracranial injury. He seemed to have recovered completely at the end of five days, without any residual neurological findings.

4. CASE M, MALE, AGE 14 YEARS. STUTTERING

Moderate respiratory distress was present shortly after birth and during the first 24 hours of life. The baby seemed jittery and exhibited brief seizure activity. Subdural taps were negative. Lumbar puncture yielded a moderate number of red blood cells. Neonatal tetany was considered and infant was given calcium therapy by mouth. No further treatment was believed to be indicated. Recovery seemed prompt and his subsequent course uneventful. Mother has continued to show anxiety and overreaction to this newborn episode and seems to see this boy as having suffered some permanent damage during that period.

5. CASE L, MALE, AGE 6 YEARS 6 MONTHS. SEVERELY DEFECTIVE ARTICULATION

Delivery was one month prior to the expected date. Birth weight 4 pounds 9 ounces. Newborn period was uneventful; the baby went home from the hospital at age 2 weeks. When seen for the first time by his present pediatrician, he was 3 months old and said to be progressing very well. He weighed 13 pounds 4 ounces, was sleeping well and taking his feedings well. He was responsive and healthy with negative physical examination. He was seen again at age 5 months, at which time the parents showed concern over his seemingly slow motor development. In the pediatrician's opinion, the baby's development and neurological status was normal, but there was poor muscular and ligamentous tone present. Subsequent history has shown no evidence of any nervous system disorder or injury. His parents continued to show anxiety about his development and what they considered to be inadequate food intake throughout his infancy.

APPENDIX XIII

Analysis of Intake, Differences Between Groups

Name: ————————————————————————Sex: ————————
Diagnosis: A. Stuttering
　　　　　B. Severely Defective Articulation
　　　　　　　B-1. Severely Defective Articulation + Stuttering
　　　　　C. Motor-perceptual and Language Disorder
　　　　　　　C-1. Motor-perceptual and Language Disorder + Stuttering

Additional Problems: ———None   ———Discipline problems
                        ———Bedwetting   ———Passivity, shyness
                        ———Nailbiting   ———Stubborn, temper
                        ———Hyperactivity   tantrums
                        ———Learning Difficulty   ———Other

	Under 2 years	2–5 years	Over 5 years
Child's Health History·			
None			
Chronic Illness			
Severe Illness			
Hospital			
Temporary Hearing Difficulties			
Ear Infection			

Family Health History:		Yes	No
Parental Hearing Difficulties	Mother		
	Father		
	Other		
Severe or Chronic Illness	Mother		
	Father		
	Other		

Speech Disorders in Family:	M	F	B	S	A	U	C	G[1]
Stuttering								
Articulation								
Slow Development								
Undefined								
None								

Family History:
     Number of dwellings child had lived in: ————
     Family size: Large (4 or more children) ———— Small (1–3 children)
————
     Position in family: Only —— Oldest ——Youngest ——Middle———
     Other persons living with family: ————————————
     Sibling within 2 years ———————————————

---

1. M = Mother, F = Father, B = Brother, S = Sister, A = Aunt, U = Uncle, C = Cousin, G = Grandparent

Analysis of Intake

	Additional Problems		Health Problems		Family Hearing		Family Illness		Family Speech Disorders		Dwellings Lived In		Family Size		Position In Family				Others Living In		Siblings Within 2 Years	
	Yes	No	Yes	No	Yes	No	Yes	No	Yes	No	1	1+	L	S	Only	Old.	Yng.	Md.	Yes	No	Yes	No
A	14	10	12	12	5	19	7	17	14	10	6	18	10	14	1	8	5	10	3	21	11	13
B	5	13	8	10	1	17	3	15	10	8	5	13	13	5	1	0	11	6	7	11	6	12
B¹	8	3	3	4	0	11	2	9	7	4	5	6	7	4	0	1	6	4	2	9	6	5
C	4	3	6	1	3	4	3	4	7	0	4	3	2	5	0	3	1	3	0	7	6	1
C¹	0	2	2	0	0	2	1	1	1	1	1	1	0	2	0	1	1	0	0	2	1	1

Groups: A Stuttering
B Severely Defective Articulation
B¹ Severely Defective Articulation and Stuttering
C Motor-perceptual and Language Disorder
C¹ Motor-perceptual and Language Disorder and Stuttering

Analysis of Variables

Groups	Additional Problems (Child)	Health Problems (Child)	Family Hearing	Family Illness	Family Speech Disorders	Dwellings Lived In	Family Size	Position In Family	Others Living In	Siblings Within 2 Years
A										
B								9.14	4.56[1]	
B[1]										
C & C[1]		4.24[1]								
A & B[1]	4.20[1]									
A & B[1] & C[1]										
B & B[1]							6.57	13.37[2]		

Only χ^2 significant at the 5 per cent level are recorded.
1. Yates Correction for Continuity.
2. Significant at the 1 per cent level.

Verbatim Transcript of a Tape-Recorded Interview Between a Therapist and the Mother of a Stuttering Child

CHILD'S HISTORY

At the time of the interview Dick was 6 years 4 months old and attended the first grade. His father was a professional man, his mother a former school teacher. His brother Jim was 8 years old. Dick was born in a Western state; the family had moved East when Dick was 3. The pregnancy of Dick's mother had been uneventful, Dick's birth had been "easy and fast," and except for the usual childhood diseases, Dick's health had always been excellent. The mother reported that she had not been overly concerned about Dick's toilet training. Urinary and bowel control had been accomplished by the time he was 3 years old. Dick began to speak when he was 20 months old, his articulation had always been "normal," and he began to speak in short sentences at the age of 3. Stuttering had been observed first at age 3, when the family planned to move. His stuttering had fluctuated and had become more severe during the six months preceding the recorded interview. At the Intake Interview, Dick's mother complained particularly about his frequent severe temper tantrums; trivial incidents, often connected with his brother, would lead to wild outbursts of temper. Dick's mother felt helpless; she had tried reasoning, spanking Dick, isolating him, but to no avail. She mentioned that Jim often teased Dick quite badly. Both parents were concerned about Dick's stuttering as well as about his behavior.

THE RECORDED INTERVIEW

With the mother's permission, the recording was made during the third interview. Abbreviations used in the transcript are: M. = Mother, Th. = Therapist.

The Transcript

Th. How are things going on with Dick?

M. Very well, I think. Good.

Th. In what way?

M. Well, I think we can see some improvement.

Th. You mean in his speech?

M. Yes (Th. uh-huh) I think so, although at times, still, particularly around the table (Th. uh-huh)—and—ah,—you know—he will repeat sometimes as much as six or eight times (Th. uh-huh). It seems to be mostly when all four of us are together—(Th. uh-huh)—and while we do everything we can to not let this be a competitive speech situation—particularly if it's telling about something that his older brother, for instance, knows about—(Th. uh-huh)—and maybe there's a little bit of a—you know I have to hurry to tell this—(Th. uh-huh)—although now always it is only a natural situation. And I remember the last time you asked me if he did much repeating—ah—during—when he and I were sitting down alone together and so I made a mental note of it this time, and I found that he does do it some, even when no one pressured him to—ah—

Th. When you say he does some—how much repeating does he do? Just occasionally he has trouble on a word, or in every sentence? Or how is this?

M. It seems to be more when he is trying to tell a complex idea—or a rather detailed happening.

Th. A harder thing for him to organize?

M. Yes, then he will repeat, not only on the first word of a sentence, but sometimes on the first two or three words within the sentence.

Th. Are there any times when his speech is fluent?

M. Oh yes. Oh yes.

Th. When are these times?

M. They are completely mixed. (Th. uh-huh)

Th. Sometimes he does have difficulty and at other times he doesn't.

M. I do think this feedback technique helps. Because I find when I slow down and repeat back—match his words—that he is more likely to come back with a fluent sentence.

Th. Uh-huh. Very good.

M. I guess what I'm pointing out here is perhaps not when we're using the feedback technique but more a regular spontaneous conversation—

Th. Then, it is a more difficult language task, really, isn't it?

M. Yes, That's right.

Th. Does he enjoy sitting down with you? Is he having fun doing it?

M. Oh yes (laughs)—I think so, because he—ah—you know, this means he really has mummy all to himself, for quite a while, as much as anything.

Th. Right, right. And who wouldn't like that? What kinds of things do you do? Do you usually use books?

M. Ah—I'd say half and half—maybe half the time with books—or his school papers that he brings home—(Th. uh-huh) or sometimes we just talk—(Th. uh-huh) about things, you know.

Th. And he likes to do that?

M. Oh yes—and I tried to follow up on this idea we talked about last time—(Th. uh-huh). At the time one feels sort of almost ah—ah—hostile—ah—hostile is too strong a word here—but ah—ah—sort of like punishing him for something he's done—antagonistic, I guess, is the word I'm trying to think of—(Th. uh-huh) ah—to realize that this may be the time when he needs the most reassurance (Th. uh-huh) and I think this has helped because—instead of—perhaps before I had a little bit ah—the attitude that—well, I mustn't be *too* overtly affectionate with him because ah—you know, this might seem to make a distinction between his older brother and himself.

Th. Yes, you mentioned that.

M. His older brother doesn't need it.

Th. Because Dick does like this, hugging and sitting on your lap kind of thing?

M. Yes—ah—but I have made less effort to—ah—sort of this—ah—you know, "Grow up Dick !" (laughs). I have had that attitude, not that I've ever said it.

Th. This is your feeling.

M. In other words, if he seems to indicate *any* wanting to sit on my lap then I just, you know, welcome him. So I think there's really been more of this and a little more freely given and done on my part—(Th. uh-huh) and he seems to—to—

Th. Respond?

M. Yes, uh-huh.

Th. In what way can you—ah—evaluate his responses as being acceptable?

M. Well he has taken the initiative, for instance, in coming and crawling on my lap (Th. uh-huh) and whereas before I might have said "Oh Dick, I'm busy now, I'll hold you later" or ah—

Th. Well, it's a little distasteful for you to do—for a boy this age—isn't that about what you're saying—you thought it was not grown-up—as much as a boy his age might be?

M. I don't know that I really felt that way so much—it was more a case of—ah—perhaps feeling that this sort of—taking him on my lap, sort of thing was—well, maybe I'm just saying what you are saying in a different way, but thinking that maybe that was more what you would do with a 3-year-old, you know, or a 2-year old or a baby, but if I—well, I guess what I was afraid of perhaps was—perhaps—you know, sort of smothering with motherly affection (Th. uh-huh) ah—at a time when maybe he really needed to divorce himself from this—(Th. uh-huh). This was my thought and I really sort of—although I'm not sure that I have verbalized this before, but I think that I was—you know—sort of at the point of thinking that he probably would like to get out from under it a little bit, you know, (Th. uh-huh) because I know my natural inclination has been to show more affection toward Dick because he's been a cuddly child. I think I've said this before—

Th. Right—

M. —whereas the 8-year-old has been easy to—you know—I can sit down and talk with him almost as with an adult.

Th. In a way you're saying that you can easily understand Dick's dislike of a change, maybe, going to a new school or to first grade for the first time, because he is the kind of child who likes to feel close to you and closeness is important to him.

M. Uh-huh.

Th. Even at this age when he is in school a good part of the day he still wants the extra kind of closeness to you.

M. Uh-huh. Well, yes, and I think I was—in the fear of being overly motherly, you know, I sort of (Th. uh-huh) shunned it a little bit. Now, after our talk two weeks ago I felt well, maybe he needs this (Th. uh-huh) maybe he really isn't ready to be shut off quite yet as much as I am doing it, even though I wasn't doing it a great deal, I didn't think.

Th. I assume you might assume this, especially since his teacher gives such good reports about how he manages in school. Didn't you say she mentioned he does very well—does a good job in first grade? Maybe he's just relaxing a little bit when he's at home and can act a little bit younger than he needs to act in school.

M. Yes. And I found too that—ah—the times when I need to scold him for something—if I then—as soon as possible—clear the air, you know, by reassuring him (Th. uh-huh) you know, take him on my lap and—

Th. You give him immediate feedback letting him know that you still like him.

M. Yes.

Th. Even though he has—

M. Yes, I think that that has helped, rather than to ah—it's helped not to prolong the feeling of alienation that he probably felt from my affection, when I scold.

Th. Very good. How has he been with his tempers?

M. That is another thing I wanted to tell you. He hasn't had any storms—

Th. That must be easier for you—

M. (laughs)—really full blown ones since the last time I saw you.

Th. What have you done to prevent these?

M. Well, the one I really felt I did prevent—I asked him one day to go upstairs and get something for me from my desk and he suddenly—you know, it is the sort of thing you can never anticipate—whether it is going to be—suddenly it just goes from nowhere—and he said "No, I don't want to!" you know—and—ah—so then having made the request and very kindly—I said "Oh, please"—you know—"please, Dicky—mummy's legs"—you know—"get tireder than yours and you can help mummy by doing this," and he said "Why don't you ask Jimmy to do it—you always ask me to do things" he said. And (laughs) of course the truth of it is, his older brother does about ten jobs, you know, to his one, but anyway—so I said "Well, I ask Jimmy to do some things that I think he can do, and I ask you to do some things that I think you can do." (Th. uh-huh). "And, this is a job that I know you can do for mother, so would you please go upstairs and get"—whatever it was, I can't remember what it was, but anyway—so he said—ah—he just got—you know—real angry and he said "Well, you're just an awful mummy" and, you know, I don't remember exactly the words he used but he said "You always make me do things and you never do anything for yourself, you never do anything for me, you always make me work," you know—

Th. He's carrying quite a load, isn't he?

M. (laughs)

Th. What was your reaction when he said this?—

M. Well—excuse me—go ahead.

Th. No, go on.

M. So then I did—you know—what you had suggested before to say right then, because he was really in a—you know—just almost to the point of tears, he was worked up about this, which—you know—seems—probably sounds ridiculous to you, because it does sound like such a silly thing—you know—for him to feel so strongly about—really—but anyway—

Th. It isn't silly if he feels that strongly about it.

M. Well, I guess that's right. So, anyway, I looked at him and I said—you know—real calmly—"Well, Dick, you really do feel angry, don't you, toward mummy," and I said "Well, that's all right, lots of times children do feel angry toward their mothers, and sometimes mother feels angry with you. I know how you feel, I know you feel angry. All right, if you don't want to do it right now, why, that's all right. You can do it later or I'll do it this time, and some other time you can help mother." And—you know—it was just like magic (Th. uh-huh). It really was gone just as fast as it came—and—

Th. What was his reaction to that? Did he say anything—did he make any comments to you about that?

M. Uhhh—no, I don't think so, other than that he may have acknowledged when I said "You do feel angry."

Th. It must have hit the spot—because his behavior changed so dramatically.

M. Uh-huh. This—you know—just—the verbal recognition right in the middle of it, that he felt angry, I think helped.

Th. Actually you showed a high level of control with him without really controlling him in a way that would aggravate him. Right?

M. Well, I suppose—

Th. You intervened, in a—ah—very positive way, with him having a real outburst of temper, and what he probably was objecting to was what we've talked about before—his wanting to control and set rules and laws for himself.

M. Well, I felt this was good—ah—in two ways. One, in that it did have the dramatic effect right then (laughs)—and—you can't argue with that! You know, by the time he'd sat on my lap for five minutes—and—ah—you know—we talked about something else then—

Th. Oh, you stayed with it? You stayed with him and—?

M. Oh, yes—(laughs)

Th.—and he sat on your lap and you talked?

M. Yah. I don't know what we talked about—I guess about something else and (Th. uh-huh)—you know the air was clear, and then, of course he was ready to go and do it then, you know—

Th. He did it for you?

M. (laughs) Oh yes.

Th. Was it his suggestion to go back?

M. No, he just went up and did it without saying anything about it—you know—

Th. So what he was arguing about no longer existed?

M. That's right—and you know—and—so I thought that was good, in that respect and also that we had been able to do this on something that didn't have to be drawn to the extreme (Th. uh-huh). Because there are situations when if it would have been something that I would have to force through (Th. Right) you know, obviously—(Th. Right)—but this was a case where—you know—it didn't matter this much, really whether he did it or whether I did it (Th. uh-huh)—and to me it didn't seem essential that I insist he do it, simply because I had made just an off-hand request "Would you run upstairs and get something?"—you know, so I was able to give in and I felt that it was good because there were—you know— there are and will be and have been instances where it wouldn't be a situation—that would be right for as much give and take, I mean, for instance—if it was "Come on, now, go to bed", well—you know!

Th. Right. And I think it's best for him that you are firm in those situations, don't you?

M. Yes, I do.

Th. It interests me that you didn't seem at all upset—ah—with the fact that he was saying, if not in specific words, in some way, "You're an awful mother." You used the word awful, when you told me about it—this was the impression he gave you. Isn't that what you meant?

M. Oh, well, he's done this before.

Th. It didn't aggravate you in any way? It didn't get you mad or upset you to think that he—?

M. I don't think it usually has—at other times. He has—you know—(Th. uh-huh) at other times, in a burst of anger said "You're an awful mother" before ah—he's never come out and said—you know—"I hate you" (Th. uh-huh) or anything this strong—but—ah—I think words either "You're an awful mother" or "You're a bad mummy," or something like that—(Th. uh-huh). I think I have recognized these for what they were (Th. uh-huh) and I don't think that I have entered emotionally into that. This is things children say.

Th. How has he been getting along with Jimmy—he hasn't had any outbursts against Jimmy recently?

M. Ah—well (laughs)—just the usual brother-brother teasing that sometimes gets to be almost too much—

Th. Anything like the door-slamming episode that you mentioned before?

M. No, oh no. Nothing that Jimmy didn't start. I really, sometimes, you know, I suppose any mother does get at her wits' end at the sort of teasing—

Th. It's more tiring for the listener than it is for the ones who are doing it.

M. That's right, I'm sure, and having heard other mothers say that this is normal with brothers, I don't know (Th. uh-huh) why—I don't think its indicative of anything, particularly— (laughs) it hasn't —in at least these two weeks—gotten to be something that Dick emotionally couldn't seem to handle.

Th. You mentioned the last time I saw you that a neighbor's baby would come to visit once in a while, and that Dick would react so strongly while the baby was there. Has the baby seen visiting lately?

M. Uh—I don't think—she's been there since I saw you last. I can't remember whether I told you about this or not, but the last time she was there—ah—I had him come sit in the chair beside me.

Th. Uh-huh?

M. And—ah—ah—so this helped. I can't remember much else about it, however. We have seen them—ah—for instance, out on the sidewalk, and Dick's been very interested— she's just learning to talk—she's not 2 yet—and—so—ah—she's been able to say Tim—you know—for Jim. (Th. uh-huh) but she didn't say Dick's name for quite a while, so he's been very interested in her learning to say his name. So—(laughs) when he sees her, he'll say "Dick—say Dick"—(laughs) and then Sunday they had us over for dinner and he was very good with her.

Th. He didn't take her teddy bear away or her toys?

M. No. He didn't seem to try to aggravate her.

Th. Then, there are some changes in the last few weeks that you've noticed.

M. Yes.

Th. His tolerance for her seems to be better.

M. Yes, I think so. Now, it could be—if the situation involved just the baby—and me— and him together. But the three children played well together—you know—and there seemed to be tolerance on his part for her antics. And—ah—I noticed that she had her doll and—ah—he was interested and sat by me and he was folding the cover over it and so on, but Patty's attention was, happily, taken up with something else—so—you know—she didn't mind him having her doll and (Th. uh-huh) she came and took it once and when she laid it down he went and got it again (laughs) and brought it back to *my* lap.

Th. But that's different than his taking away the teddy bear. He really wanted the doll for a minute but—he didn't want to get in her way by taking it. That was different, really, wasn't it?

M. Yes, it was.

Th. Would you say—when you look at his papers from school—how is he doing in school? I haven't talked to his teacher at all.

M. I have talked with her since I saw you last and—ah—she says he's doing very well at his own rate—ah—I think that his reading group is the slowest of the three reading groups but they have graduated to the hard-back books, at last, and he's very thrilled about it, because they started in them yesterday.

Th. They are in the hard-back books already in the slowest reading group?

M. Yes.

Th. Well, that school—you know—is —has a group of children who are very bright.

M. Really?

Th. So when you speak of the "slow" reading group in *that* first grade, it could be the adavnced reading group in another school and in another first grade.

M. Oh, really? I didn't realize that.

Th. They have—ah—a very advanced group of children in that school.

M. I didn't realize that.

Th. So, if he's in the hard-cover book by now it doesn't sound like he's having any particular difficulty with reading. Right?

M. Well—I don't think so—I am not really concerned about this.

Th. Does the teacher mention that she hears Dick stuttering in school?

M. No, she said she doesn't. And I really think she does not realize how severe it can be at home.

Th. Uh-huh?

M. And I think it would be—you know—she really—ah—well (laughs) thinks I exaggerate. I think she thinks I worry a little bit needlessly about it, because she doesn't— you know—hear it in school. She mentioned that the other day was the first time that she had been aware of it.

Th. Isn't that nice that he has a lot of times in school when he is speaking very fluently. One possibility is that he has much less difficulty in school than he does have at home; but the other is that his teacher may be very insensitive to repetition of sounds, and this would be a nice thing for Dick, wouldn't it? If it doesn't bother her at all, if she doesn't pay any attention to it and only notices it once in a great while, I think he's in a good spot.

M. Yes, I do too.

Th. This might be part of her assessment of his problem. She may just not pay much attention to it when he does do it—since he does it so very seldom in school.

M. Yes, and she said something else that I thought was good. We were talking about library books and—his interest in reading is beginning to expand—and you know, things— beyond his reader, I mean he's realizing that he can read some words in the newspaper.

Th. Very good!

M. Or also in books we have, and so, and—ah—so he's taking an interest in that and figuring out things on his own, which I think is good, and when they get to that point, you know, they really begin to get over the hump!

Th. As a former schoolteacher—you must find that—fun to see it happen?

M. Uh-huh. Yes, and he's figuring out some words on his own. He had brought home a library book—ah—oh, a couple of weeks ago, one that was easy to read—you know what I mean.

Th. Pre-primer?

M. Well, the kind with a controlled vocabulary. I think it's sort of nice to be able to go to the library and pick out a story book that has a vocabulary that he can read.

Th. Right.

M. So, anyhow, ah—he brought one of these home and—ah—I was amazed to find that he could read—really—all the way through the book. I had to help him, of course (Th. uh-huh) with some of the words he hadn't had, but there were enough words he had had that he could feel he was really reading (Th. uh-huh) the book, and I was really quite amazed that he got through it, you know, so I was saying this, how surprised I was, that he could read most of his library book. And the teacher said that Dick had a very good sense of what he was able to do and what he wasn't able to do. She thought he had been choosing books wisely.

Th. In other words, he seems to really like to do it—to find things he can do and can read. Things seem to be going pretty well with Dick, don't they?

M. Yes, I think so as far as his school work is concerned. He's happy. Now, one thing that he's hardly ever participated in in school is Show and Tell. (Th. uh-huh). And—ah—his teacher said that of course some children would—you know—do it all the time (Th. uh-huh) every day they have it. So she had tried to encourage the children who weren't quite as actually aggressive to—ah—participate, and so one day she—it must have been a month ago—she apparently specifically asked Dick that morning if he could bring something that afternoon for Show and Tell. So he came home at noon that day and said "I have to take something for Show and Tell"—you know. So we found something and he took it back and she said he did such a fine job, and she suggested that I encourage him to bring things. And she said that he did such a good job in explaining this before the class—oh, I know what it was, it was a shell—ah—a thing made of shells we got last summer in California. And so I tried several times, you know. I said "Oh, Dick, today is Show and Tell, let's see, what could you take," and several things I've suggested have been things that other children have brought, and he's said "Oh, no, they've seen that." So apparently he wants something really distinctly different. And he's never, never wanted to do it, since. And —ah—both the teacher and I had praised him, you know, the one time he did it. So anyway, Sunday at church he made—at Sunday School he made a little pine cone figure—an elf—and it really is just as clever as can be. So he took it yesterday afternoon to show his reading group when he went back.

Th. Was that his idea?

M. Yes, his idea. He wanted to take it, and—ah—I said "Oh, I bet they'd just *love* to see that, Dick" you know (Th. uh-huh) "because this is something so different, no other child has it" (laughs) and—ah—so anyway, he said they really liked it and when he came home he said "You know why I didn't bring my elf home with me?" and I said "No, why." "My teacher wanted it to save it to show to the *whole* class today.

Th. She's very clever in picking things up, isn't she?

M. Yes. And so, sure enough this afternoon they were to have it. He mentioned that he was going to show his elf. He seemed to be very pleased to do this.

Th. It looks like things are going well in every way for him, doesn't it?

M. I think so, yes. I guess I would be happier if there was more marked improvement—(Th. uh-huh) but—ah—but

Th. In his speech, you mean?

M. Ah—uh-huh.

Th. But actually, his symptom is a very mild one, when he only repeats initial sounds. And he has such little difficulty in school that we can just wait and see what happens. It's really been a very short time, to see improvement.

M. I suppose. And then, too, it may be that it will be a by-product—you know—improvement will be a by-product of little more improvement—ah—in his relationship at home, too, you know, it may be that—ah—more assurance—

Th. I'm sure you are a help to him. He has shown you, in many ways, that you are a help to him by responding to his kind of approach. I'm sure that it's good for him that you can operate the way you do with him. The only difficulty is that we cannot predict when children might give up the symptom of stuttering. Actually it's been a very short time that you've been sitting with him and working with him that closely—and—ah—"feeding back words" to him. So I think that the best thing to do might be just to wait and continue going along the way you are going. I'm wondering about Christmas. It's usually a very difficult time for stuttering children. Is Dick really excited about Christmas yet?

M. Ah—yes, I think he is. Ah—

Th. Have you decided to stay at home or to go away?

M. We'll be home, yes—uh-huh. I think Dick's excited but I don't think overly excited. (Th. uh-huh). He hasn't been in the stores much. I hate taking him to the stores at Christmas anyway, because it's so terrible—I hate to go myself.

Th. Right, right.

M. And so—ah—I don't think he has sensed as much the extra excitement of the season as maybe I have, you know—

Th. You keep the stimulation down a little bit?

M. Yes, I think so. Now, we—you know, started putting up decorations (Th. uh-huh) and Christmas cards and we're going this afternoon to get our tree—we don't have it yet—we talk about it, but you know—as far as being excited about it, I don't think so.

Th. Have you been excessively busy during the season, shopping and—has it made a difference how much he had of your time?

M. I don't think it has. Ordinarily I—ah—most years I know that I am busier (laughs).

Th. *D*h-huh.

M. But then I've had a part-time job—as—the last two years (Th. uh-huh) which ended in October this year, so that I think that's made this period seem a little easier to me than it has for the last couple of years. I really do have more time—we're still working on cards but I haven't let it—you know—consume me (laughs). I've worked at it but I really don't think that I have—ah—been—you know—more nervous and too overly busy yet, so I don't think that I have had less time for him.

Th. Uh-huh. That's very nice. You're really organized getting things done so that there isn't a real rush.

M. Uh-huh. Right.

Th. And it's not a week where you're not available.

M. That's right. Yah.

Th. Very nice. You have a lot of insight into what happens with your children.

M. Well—ah—(laughs)—Thank you. You know what Dr. Spock always says—he says that people who have been to college and studied a little spychology are the worst parents.

Th. (laughs) I hate to think of that as being true. It doesn't seem to me today that you have any questions or anything that is really bothering you—

M. I really don't—

Th.—in connection with Dick.

M. I don't have anything particular, you know. Last night when I was sitting down with Dick and we were reading the titles in Jimmy's book, and we were doing this while Jimmy was practicing—Jimmy suddenly said—burst out with—"You always do things with Dick but not with me" (laughs).

Th. Here it comes! This is what you were waiting for!

M. So I thought he was beginning to notice. So I said "Well, you come here, Jimmy, and sit down with me," so I sat down beside him for a little bit, you know (Th. uh-huh) but Dick came, and I said "Dick, you can go and sit on the stairs or go on up and get on your pajamas, I'm going to talk with Jimmy a minute," but Dick didn't leave and I didn't persist. I let him stay, but I did talk quietly with Jimmy a little bit.

Th. Could you explain to Jim that—you think that Dick needs a little extra amount of your time right now for whatever reason, that Jim might understand?

M. Yes, I could, and I do intend to—I didn't want to say it right then (Th. right) in front of Dick.

Th. It's not easy to deal with two children, is it?

M. I will—I've been thinking that I'm—you know—when I have a few moments when I can really talk to Jim alone (Th. uh-huh)—tell him that I have been doing this intentionally with Dick—and—ah—so I don't think it was really so much jealousy for spending more time with Dick than with him, as it was more just disappointment—I feel good that Dick hasn't had a real blown-up temper tantrum. I'm not sure that I'd know how to handle it any better the next time. But maybe—

Th. That was the thing that made you feel most uncomfortable about Dick, these kinds of outbursts?

M. Yes.

Th. Now it seems possible to avoid them, at times.

M. Right.

Th. Very good. Well, let's make an appointment for our next meeting. It will be after Christmas.

COMMENTARY

This transcript has been reproduced because it illustrates *four important factors* which must be considered in working with mothers of stuttering children.

1. The Child's Need for Closeness and the Mother's Difficulties in Responding to It

These were evident in the mother's discussion of Dick's sitting on her lap; also in the scene when Dick brought the baby's doll to his mother to put it on her lap. The therapist suggested to the mother keeping the Christmas holiday quiet and relaxed and avoid a hectic family situation, which might make the mother inaccessible to Dick.

2. The Mother's Fears of the Child's Aggressiveness and of Her Own Counteraggression

The mother could not find the "right words" to describe her feelings about Dick; she felt "hostile" or "antagonistic" toward him; she needed the therapist's permission to permit Dick to regress to more infantile behavior, to treat him at times as if he were "a younger child." She recognized that in the past she tended to "shut him off," urging him to "grow up" and not bother her. The therapist helped the mother understand her own anger against Dick and to react more constructively to Dick's outbursts of anger.

3. School Problems

The mother was very anxious to have her child succeed in school; she pushed him to participate in Show and Tell time. The therapist pointed out in a tactful manner that Dick's teacher was more tolerant of Dick's symptoms; the teacher made Dick feel more comfortable and less ambivalent than he felt in the presence of his mother; consequently his speech at school was much better than at home.

4. The Atmosphere of the Counseling Session as an Important Factor in Therapy

The therapist closely followed the mother's words and responded to her feelings with interest and sympathy. The therapist constantly stayed in contact with the mother, using eye contact as well as voice contact, hence her frequent utterances "uh-huh," of which she was unaware until she heard them on the recording. The therapist reassured the mother that in spite of her ambivalent feelings toward Dick she was not a destructive person but a competent adult, able to guide her children wisely.

Design for a Comprehensive, School-Centered Program of Teaching and Therapy for Children with Communication Disorders

Type of Difficulty*	Adults Involved in Diagnostic Procedures	Adults Involved in Teaching, Remediation, or Therapy
1. Defective articulation, mild to moderate, in young children (preschool, kindergarten, grade 1).	Teacher, speech therapist.	Speech therapist instructs teachers and parents in such techniques as providing corrective feedback, lessening the linguistic load, etc. (see Chapter 11). Also specific teaching of auditory discrimination between speech sounds, if necessary. This blends eventually into the teaching of phonics for beginning reading.
2. Severely defective articulation in young children (preschool, kindergarten, grade 1).	Teacher, speech therapist, audiologist, pediatrician.	
3. Primary or developmental stuttering in young children.	Psychologist, speech therapist.	Crisis intervention, communication therapy, carried out by professional persons trained in psychotherapy and parent counseling, or by a lay therapist assisted by a mental health consultant. For details see Chapters 7–10; also Table 5, p. 130.
4. Advanced stuttering in older children.	Psychologist, speech therapist, psychiatrist, social worker.	
5. Cluttering.	Speech therapist, neurologist.	Speech therapist works with child; training should be reinforced by parents and teachers. See Table 14, p. 252.

* Individual children may have two or more of the listed communication disorders simultaneously, presenting complex syndromes which require various patterns of comprehensive services.

6. Brain damage, cerebral palsy. Child may be of normal intelligence or mentally retarded.	Medical and psychological examiners, speech therapist.	Special class or regular classroom teacher, assisted by speech therapist, reading specialist, occupational therapist; parent counseling.
7. Multiple motor-perceptual and language disabilities. Child is of normal to superior intelligence.	Psychologist, pediatrician, neurologist, speech therapist, reading specialist. (Diagnostic centers may also provide examinations by psychiatrist, ophthalmologist, and audiologist.)	Multidiscipline program, combining work by teachers, speech therapist, special tutor, physical educator; parent counseling. See Chapters 12, 13.
8. Hearing difficulty.	Pediatrician, otologist, audiologist, speech and hearing therapist.	Hearing therapist works with child and counsels parents and teachers. Early training of mothers important.
9. Cleft palate.	Physician, surgeon, orthodontist, psychologist, speech therapist (the 'cleft palate team").	Speech therapist working in conjunction with clinic; counseling of teachers and parents.
10. Voice disorders.	Speech therapist, ear, nose, and throat physician.	Speech therapist works in conjunction with physician; treatment should be reinforced by parents and teachers.
11. Language deficit in educationally deprived children, poor communicators.	Teacher, speech therapist, psychologist, social worker. Medical consultation may be necessary.	Consultant in language development and speech therapy assists teachers, parents, and volunteer helpers. See Chapter 15.

Bibliography*

ABRAMS, J. C., and BELMONT, H. S., 1965. Different approaches to the remediation of severe reading disability in children (Mimeogr.). Paper presented at the annual meeting, Amer. Orthopsychiat. Assoc. Available through The Hahnemann Medical College and Hospital of Philadelphia, 1505 Race Street, Philadelphia, Pa.

AINSWORTH, M. D., 1962. The effects of maternal deprivation: a review of findings and controversy in the context of recent research strategy. In Ainsworth, M. D., *et al.*, *Deprivation of maternal care; a reassessment of its effects*. Public Health Papers, No. 14, Geneva: World Health Organization.

ALLPORT, G. W., 1942. *The use of personal documents in psychological science.* New York: Social Science Research Council.

ALPERN, G. D., 1966. The failure of a nursery school enrichment program for culturally disadvantaged children. (Mimeogr.) Paper presented at the annual meeting, Amer. Orthopsychiat. Assoc. Available through Riley Child Guidance Clinic, 1100 West Michigan Street, Indianapolis, Indiana 46207.

AMENT, W., 1899. *Die Entwicklung vom Sprechen und Denken beim Kinde.* Leipzig: Wunderlich Verlag.

ANNELL, A. L., 1962. Die Psychopathologie der entzuendlichen Hirnschaedigung im Kindesalter. *Acta Paedopsychiatrica, 29*, Fasc. 1, 7–22. Basel/Stuttgart: Benno Schwabe & Co.

Annual Report, 1967. Neurocommunications Laboratory, Department of Psychiatry and Behavioral Sciences, The Johns Hopkins University School of Medicine. Baltimore, Maryland.

APPELT, A., 1929. *Stammering and its permanent cure.* London: Methuen & Co.

ARNOLD, G. E., undated. *Studies in Tachyphemia, an investigation of cluttering and general language disability*, Chaps. I, III. New York: Speech Rehabilitation Institute, 61 Irving Place.

ASPERGER, H., 1956. *Heilpaedagogik.* 2. Aufl., Vienna, Springer Verlag.

Auditory Discrimination Test, 1958. J. Wepman, Chicago, Ill.: Language Research Associates.

---

* For key to abbreviations see page 355.

A Visual-Motor Gestalt Test and its Clinical Use, 1938. Bender, L. New York: Amer. Ortho-psychiatric Assoc. Research Monogr. No. 3.

AYRES, A. J., 1966. Perceptual-motor dysfunction in children: a theoretical position (Mimeogr.) Position paper, annual meeting, Amer. Orthopsychiat. Assoc. Available through Dept. of Pediatrics, University of California, Los Angeles, Cal.

BAKER, S. J., 1948. Speech disturbances: a case for a wider view of paraphasias. *Psychiatry, 11,* 359–66.

———, 1951. Autonomic resistances in word association tests. *Psychoanal. Quart., 22,* 275–83.

———, 1955. The theory of silences. *J. gen. Psychol., 53,* 145–67.

BARBARA, D. A., 1954. *Stuttering: A psychodynamic approach to its understanding and treatment.* New York: The Julian Press.

BARTH, E., 1911. *Einfuehrung in die Physiologie, Pathologie und Hygiene der menschlichen Stimme.* Leipzig: Georg Thieme Verlag.

BATEMAN, B., 1964. Learning disabilities—yesterday, today, and tomorrow. *Except. Child., 31,* 4, 167–79.

———, 1965. The Illinois Test of Psycholinguistic Abilities in current research (Monogr.). Inst. for Research on Exceptional Children, University of Illinois, 43.

———, 1966. Learning disorders. *Rev. educ. Res., 36,* 1, Chap. V.

BATEMAN, W. G., 1914. A child's progress in speech. *J. educ. Psychol., 5,* 307–20.

BAX, M., and MACKEITH, R. (Eds.), 1963. *Minimal cerebral dysfunction.* London: William Heineman.

BELLAK, L., and BELLAK, S. S., 1949. Children's Apperception Test. New York: C.P.S. Co., P.O. Box 42, Gracie Station.

BENDER, L., 1938. A Visual-Motor Gestalt Test and Its Clinical Use. *Res. Monogr. No. 3.* New York: Amer. Orthopsychiatric Assoc.

———, 1957. Specific reading disability as a maturational lag. *Bull. Orton Soc., 7,* 9–18.

———, 1958. Problems in conceptualization and communication in children with develop-mental alexia. In Hoch, P., and Zubin, J. (Eds.), *Psychopathology of communication.* New York: Grune & Stratton, 155–76.

BENTON, A. L., 1962. Dyslexia in relation to form perception and directional sense. In Money, J. (Ed.), *Reading disability. Progress and research in dyslexia.* Baltimore: The Johns Hopkins Press, 81–103.

BEREITER, C., and ENGELMANN, S., 1966. *Teaching disadvantaged children in the preschool.* Englewood Cliffs, N.J.: Prentice-Hall.

BEREITER C., ENGELMANN, S., OSBORN, J., and REIDFORD, P. A., 1966. An academically oriented pre-school for culturally deprived children. In Hechinger, F. M. (Ed.), *Pre-School education today.* Garden City, New York: Doubleday & Co.

BERKO, J., 1958. The child's learning of English morphology. *Word, 14,* No. 2/3, 150–77. Reprinted in Saporta, S., and Bastian, J. R. (Eds.), *Psycholinguistics. A book of readings.* New York: Holt, Rinehart and Winston, 359–76.

BERLYNE, D. E. 1957. Recent developments in Piaget's work. *Brit. J. Educ. Psychol., 27.*

BERNSTEIN, B., 1960. Language and social class. *Brit. J. Sociol., 11,* 271–76.

———, 1961. Social class and linguistic development: a theory of social learning. In Halsey A. H., Flaud J., and Anderson, C. A. (Eds.), *Education, economy, and society.* New York: The Free Press, 288–314.

BIRCH, H. G., 1963. The problem of brain damage in children. In Birch, H. G. (Ed.), *Brain damage in children, the biological and social aspects.* Baltimore. Williams & Wilkins Co., 3–13.

BIRCH, H. G., and BELMONT, L., 1964. Auditory-visual integration in normal and retarded readers. *Amer. J. Orthopsychiat.*, *34*, 5, 852–61.

———, 1965a. Auditory-visual integration, intelligence, and reading ability in school children. *Percept. Mot. Skills*, *20*, 295–305.

———, 1965b. Auditory-visual integration in brain-damaged and normal children. *Develpm. Med., Child Neurol.*, *7*, 2, 135–44.

BIRCH, H. G., THOMAS, A., CHESS, S., and HERTZIG, M. E., 1962. Individuality in the development of children. *Develpm. Med., Child Neurol.*, *4*, 4, 370–79.

BIRNBAUM, A., 1953. *Green eyes.* New York: Capitol Publishing Co.

BLANK, M., and BRIDGER, W. H., 1964. Cross-modal transfer in nursery school children. *J. Comp. Physiol. Psychol.*, *58*, 277–82.

———, 1966. Deficiencies in verbal labeling in retarded readers. *Amer. J. Orthopsychiat.*, *36*, 5, 840–48.

BLANTON, S., and BLANTON, M. G., 1936. *For stutterers.* New York: Appleton-Century-Crofts.

BLOOM, B. S., DAVIS, A., and HESS, R., 1965. *Compensatory education for cultural deprivation.* New York: Holt, Rinehart & Winston.

BOREL-MAISONNY, S., 1951. Les troubles du langage dans les dyslexies et les dysorthographies. *Enfance*, *4*, 400–44.

BOSHES, B., and MYKLEBUST, H. R., 1964. A neurological and behavioral study of children with learning disorders. *Neurology*, *14*, 7–12.

BOSMA, J. F., TRUBY, A. J., and LIND, J. Cry motions of the newborn infant. (In press, *Acta Paediatrica.*)

BOWES, A. E., 1966. Position paper for workshop on perceptual motor dysfunction (Mimeogr.), annual meeting, Amer. Orthopsychiat. Assoc. Available through Pittsburgh Child Guidance Center.

BOWLBY, J., 1951. *Maternal care and mental health* (First Edition). Geneva, Palais des Nations: World Health Organization.

BRADLEY, J. E., 1966. Syndromes of minimal brain dysfunction in children. *Curr. Med. Dig.*, *33*, 1590–94.

BRAUN, J. S., RUBIN, E. Z., BECK, G. R., LLORENS, L. A., MOTTLEY, N., and BEALL, C. D., 1965. Cognitive-perceptual-motor functions in children—a suggested change in approach to psychological assessment. *J. Sch. Psychol.*, *3*, 3.

British Journal of Disorders of Communication, 1966, The Journal of the College of Speech Therapists, London, *1*, 1. E. & S. Livingstone, Ltd., Edinburgh & London.

BROCH, H., 1953. *Gedichte.* Zürich: Rhein Verlag.

BRODBECK, A. J., and IRWIN, O. C., 1964. *Child Develpm.*, *17*, 145.

BROWN, J. S., 1949 (Mimeogr.). A proposed program of research on psychological feedback (knowledge of results) in the performance of psycho-motor tasks. Available through University of Oregon Medical School, Portland, Ore. 97201.

BROWN, R., 1958. *Words and things.* New York: The Free Press.

BROWN, R., and BERKO, J., 1960. Word association and the acquisition of grammar, *Child Develpm.*, *31*, 1–14.

BROWN, R., and CAZDEN, C., 1965. Expansion training and the child's acquisition of grammar. Final Report to U.S. Office of Education, Project No. S-195, Contract No. OE-5-10-096. Available through Dept. of Psychology, Harvard University, Cambridge, Mass.

BROWN, R., and FRASER, C., 1964. The acquisition of syntax. In The acquisition of language. *Monogr. Soc. Res. Child Develpm.*, Serial No. *92*, *29*, 1, 43–79.

BROWN, R., FRASER, C., and BELLUGI, U., 1964. Explorations in grammar evaluation. In The acquisition of language, *Monogr. Soc. Res. Child Develpm.*, Serial No. *92, 29,* 1, 79–92.

BRYANT, N. D., 1962. Reading disability: part of a syndrome of neurological dysfunctioning. In Figurel, J. A. (Ed.), Challenge and experiment in reading, *Intl. Read. Conf. Proc.*, 7, 139–43.

———, 1964. Characteristics of dyslexia and their remedial implication. *Except. Child., 31,* 4, 195–201.

———, 1965. Some principles of remedial instruction for dyslexia. *Read. Teach., 18,* 567–72.

BUEHLER, K., 1930. *Die geistige Entwicklung des Kindes* (Sixth edition). Jena: Fischer Verlag.

BULLOWA, M., JONES, L. G., and BEVER, T. G., 1961. The development from vocal to verbal behavior in children. In Bellugi, U., and Brown, R. (Eds.), The acquisition of language. *Monogr. Soc. Res. Child Develpm., 29,* 1.

✳ BULLOWA, M., JONES, L. G., and DUCKERT, A. R., 1964. The acquisition of a word. *Language and Speech,* 7, 2, 107–11. Robert Draper, Ltd., Teddington, Middlesex, England.

BURKS, H. L., GOOD, J. A., HIGGINBOTHAM, E. S., and HOFFMAN, C. A., 1966. Treatment of language lags in a psychotherapeutic nursery school (Mimeogr.). Paper read at the annual meeting, Amer. Orthopsychiat. Assoc. Available through Division of Child Psychiatry, University of Texas, Medical Branch, Galveston, Texas.

BURLINGHAM, B. D. T., 1951. Present trends in handling the mother-child relationship during the therapeutic process. In *The psychoanalytic study of the child.* New York: International Universities Press.

BUSEMANN, A., 1927. Erregungsphasen der Jugend. *Zeitschr. f. Kinderforschung. 33.*

———, 1953. *Krisenjahre im Ablauf der menschlichen Jugend.* Ratingen Verlag.

BUXBAUM, E., 1947. Activity and aggression in children. *Amer. J. Orthopsychiat., 17.*

California Short-Form Test of Mental Maturity, S-Form, 1957. Sullivan, E. R., Clark, W. W., and Tiegs, E. W. Monterey, California.; California Test Bureau, Del Monte Research Park.

CAPLAN, G., 1955. Recent trends in preventive child psychiatry. In Caplan, G. (Ed.), *Emotional problems of early childhood.* New York: Basic Books.

———, 1959. *Concepts of mental health and consultation.* Children's Bureau, U.S. Dept. of Health, Education, and Welfare.

———, 1961. General introduction and overview. In Caplan, G. (Ed.), *Prevention of mental disorders in children.* New York: Basic Books.

CAPOBI NCO, R. J., 1964. Diagnostic methods used with learning disability cases. *Except. Child., 31,* 4, 187–95.

CASLER, L., 1961. Maternal deprivation: a critical review of the literature. *Monogr. Soc. Res. Child Develpm., 26,* 2.

✳ CAZDEN, C. B., 1966. Subcultural differences in child language: an inter-disciplinary review. *Merrill-Palmer Quart., 12,* 3, 185–221.

CHASE, R. A., 1963. Sensory feedback mechanisms and speech. *A syllabus of readings in the communications sciences* (Mimeogr.). From the Neurocommunications Unit, Clinical Neuropharmacology Research Center, National Institute of Mental Health and the Department of Psychiatry, Johns Hopkins University School of Medicine, Baltimore, Md.

CHASE, R. A., 1965a. An information model of the organization of motor activity. I: Transduction, transmission and central control of sensory information. *J. Nerv., Ment. Dis., 140,* 4, 239–51.

———, 1965b. An information model of the organization of motor activity. II: Sampling, central processing, and utilization of sensory information. *J. Nerv., Ment. Dis.*, *140*, 5, 234–350.

CHERRY, C., and SAYERS, B. MCA., 1956. Experiments upon the total inhibition of stammering by external control and some clinical results. *J. Psychosom. Res.*, *1*, 233–46.

CHESS, S., THOMAS, A., and BIRCH, H., 1959. Characteristics of the individual child's behavioral responses to the environment. *Amer. J. Orthopsychiat.*, *29*, 4, 791–802.

Children's Apperception Test. Bellak, L., and Bellak, S. S., 1949. New York: C.P.S. Co., P.O. Box 42, Gracie Station.

CLARK, A. D., and RICHARDS, C. J., 1966. Auditory discrimination among economically disadvantaged and nondisadvantaged preschool children. *Except. Child.*, *33*, 4, 259–65.

CLEMENTS, S. C., 1966. *Minimal brain dysfunction in children. Terminology and identification. Phase one of a three-phase project.* U.S. Depart. of Health, Education, and Welfare, NINDS Monogr. No. 3. Available through the Superintendent of Documents, U.S. Government Printing Office, Washington, D.C., 20402.

CLEMENTS, S. C., and PETERS, J. E., 1962. Minimal brain dysfunctions in the school age child. *Arch. Gen. Psychol.*, *6*, 181–97.

CLEMMENS, R. L., 1966. Syndromes of minimal brain dysfunction in children. *Maryland Med. J.*, *15*, 139–40.

COBB, S., 1944. *Borderlands of psychiatry.* Cambridge, Mass.: Harvard University Press.

COHN, R., 1964. The neurological study of children with learning disabilities. *Except. Child.*, *31*, 4, 179–87.

COLEMAN, R. W., KRIS, E., and PROVENCE, S., 1954. The study of variations of early parental attitudes. In *The psychoanalytic study of the child.* New York: International Universities Press.

CONNERS, C. K., 1967. The syndrome of minimal brain dysfunction: psychological aspects. *Pediatric Clinics of North America*, *14*, 4, 749–66.

CORBIN, R., and CROSBY, M., 1965. *Language programs for the disadvantaged.* The report of the NCTE Task Force on teaching English to the disadvantaged. National Council of Teachers of English, 508 South Sixth Street, Champaign, Ill. 61822.

CORIAT, I. H., 1928. *Stammering, a psychoanalytic interpretation.* New York: Nervous and Mental Diseases Publishing Co.

CRITCHLEY, M., 1964. *Developmental dyslexia.* Springfield, Ill.: Charles C. Thomas.

CRUICKSHANK, W. M., 1967. *The brain-injured child in home, school, and community.* Syracuse: Syracuse University Press.

CRUICKSHANK, W. M., BENTZEN, F. A., RATZEBURG, F. H., and TANNHAUSER, M. T., 1961. *A teaching method for brain-injured and hyperactive children.* Syracuse: Syracuse University Press.

DARLEY, F. L., 1964. *Diagnosis and appraisal of communication disorders.* Foundations of Speech Pathology Series, Englewood Cliffs, N. J.: Prentice-Hall.

DE HIRSCH, K., 1957. Tests designed to discover potential reading difficulties at the six-year-old level. *Amer. J. Orthopsychiat.*, *27*, 566–77.

——, 1961. Studies in Tachyphemia, IV. Diagnosis of developmental language disorders. *Logos*, *4*, 1, 47–54.

——, 1967. Differential diagnosis between aphasic and schizophrenic language in children. *J. Speech, Hear. Disorders*, *32*, 1, 3–11.

DE HIRSCH, K., JANSKY, J. J., and LANGFORD, W. S., 1965. The prediction of reading, spelling, and writing disabilities in children: a preliminary study (Mimeogr.). Final Report to the Health Research Council of the City of New York. Columbia University, Contract U-1270.

———, 1966. *Predicting reading failure. A preliminary study of reading, writing and spelling disabilities in children.* New York: Harper & Row.

DENES, P. B., and PINSON, E. N., 1963. *The speech chain.* Bell Telephone Laboratories.

DENHOFF, E., LAUFER, M. W., and HOLDEN, R. H., 1959. The syndromes of cerebral dysfunction. *J. Oklahoma State Med. Ass.*, June, 360–66.

DENHOFF, E., and ROBINAULT, I., 1960. *Cerebral palsy and related disorders.* New York: McGraw-Hill Book Co.

DESPERT, J., 1946. Psychosomatic study of fifty stuttering children. *Amer. J. Orthopsychiat.*, *16*, 100–113.

DEUTSCH, C. P., 1964. Auditory discrimination and learning: social factors. *Merrill-Palmer Quart.*, *10*, 3, 277–97.

DEUTSCH, M., 1963. The disadvantaged child and the learning process. In Passow, A. H., (Ed.) *Education in depressed areas.* New York: Teachers College, Columbia University, 163–80.

———, 1965. The role of social class in language development and cognition. *Amer. J. Orthopsychiat.*, *35*, 1, 78–88.

DEUTSCH, M., MALIVER, A., BROWN, B., and CHERRY, E., 1964. *Communication of information in the elementary school classroom. Summary.* Cooperative Research Project No. 908. Moravia, N. Y.: Chronicle Guidance Publications.

Developmental Articulation Test, 1955. Hejna, F., University of Connecticut, Storrs, Conn.

DOHRENWEND, B. S., and RICHARDSON, S. A., 1963. Directiveness and nondirectiveness in research interviewing. *Psychol. Bull.*, *60*, 475–86.

DREW, A. L., 1966. The clinical neurology of mental retardation. In Philips, I. (Ed.), *Prevention and treatment of mental retardation.* New York: Basic Books.

DUESS, L., 1946. Fabeltest. Trans. Despert, J. L., "Thematic Stories for Children," *Amer. J. Orthopsychiat.*, *15*, 109.

DUMKE, H. D., HEESE, G., KROKER, W., and SIEMS, L., 1963. Zur Symptomatologie des Polterns. *Folia Phoniatrica*, *15*, 2–3, 155–70.

DUNN, L. M., 1959. Peabody Picture Vocabulary Test. Nashville, Tenn.: American Guidance Service.

DURFEE, H. and WOLF K., 1933. Anstaltspflege und Entwicklung im ersten Lebensjahr. *Zeitschrift f. Kinderforschung*, *42*, 3.

EDWARDS, A. L., 1951. *Experimental design in psychological research.* New York: Rinehard & Co.

EICHORN, D., 1963. Biological correlates of behavior. *Child Psychol.* 62nd Yearbook, Part I, Chapter 1, pp. 1–61. National Society for the Study of Education, 5835 Kimbark Avenue, Chicago, Illinois.

EISENBERG, L., 1957. Psychiatric implications of brain damage in children. *Psychiat. Quart.*, *31*, 72–92.

———, 1964. Role of drugs in treating disturbed children. *Children*, II.

EISENSON, J., 1966. Perceptual disturbances in children with central nervous system dysfunctions and implications for language development. *Brit. J. Disorders of Communic.*, *1*, 1, 21–33.

EKSTEIN, R., and WALLERSTEIN, R. S., 1958. *The teaching and learning of psychotherapy.* New York: Basic Books.

ERIKSON, E. H., 1940. Problems of infancy and early childhood. In *The cyclopedia of medicine, surgery and specialties.* Philadelphia: F. S. Davis Co., 714–30.

———, 1950. *Childhood and society.* New York: W. W. Norton & Co.

ERVIN-TRIPP, S., 1966. Language development. In Hoffman, L. W., and Hoffman, M. L. (Eds.), *Review of child development research*. New York: Russell Sage Foundation, 55–107.

Exceptional Children, 1964, *31*, 4. Washington, D. C.: The Council for Exceptional Children, NEA, 1201 Sixteenth St., N.W. (Entire volume).

Fabeltest, Thematic Stories for Children, 1946. Duess, L. Translated into English by Despert, J. L. *Amer. J. Orthopsychiat., 15,* 109.

FELDMAN, S., 1964. A pre-school enrichment program for culturally deprived children. *The New Era, 45,* 3. Reprinted in Hechinger, F. M. (Ed.), 1966. *Pre-school education today*. Garden City, New York: Doubleday & Co., 97–105.

FELDMAN, SPOTNITZ, and NAGELBERG, 1953. One aspect of casework training through supervision. *Soc. Casework*, April, unnumbered. Family Service Association of America, 192 Lexington Ave., New York, N.Y. 10016

FELDMANN, H., 1965. Les bases théoriques et l'aspect clinique des troubles de la psychomotricité chez l'enfant. *Acta Paedopsychiatrica, 32,* Fasc. I, 3–11.

FELDMANN, S. C., 1965. Predicting early success (Mimeogr.) Paper read at the International Reading Assoc. conference. Available through Institute for Developmental Studies, School of Education, New York University, Washington Square, New York, N.Y.

FENICHEL, O., 1945. *The psychoanalytical theory of neurosis*. New York: W. W. Norton & Co.

FERNALD, G. M., 1943. *Remedial techniques in basic school subjects*. New York: McGraw-Hill Book Co.

FISHER, M. S., 1934. Language patterns of preschool children. *Child Develpm. Monogr., 15.*

FISKE, D. W. and MADDI, S. R., 1961. *Function of varied experience*. Homewood, Ill.: Dorsey Press.

FLOSDORF, P., 1960. Ueber das Stottern. *Jahrbuch f. Psychologie, Psychotherapie u. Medizin. Anthropologie*, 7, Jahrg., Heft 1/2, 126–74.

FOWLER, W., 1962. Cognitive learning in infancy and early childhood. *Psychol. Bull., 59,* 2, 116–62.

———, 1967. The design of early developmental learning programs for disadvantaged young children. Supplement to the *IRCD Bull., 3,* 1a, Project Beacon, Ferkauf Graduate School of Humanities and Social Sciences, Yeshiva University, 55 Fifth Ave., New York, N.Y. 10003.

FRANK, L. K., 1957. Tactile communication. *Genet. Psychol. Monogr., 56,* 209–55.

FREUD, A., and BURLINGHAM, D. T., 1943. *War and children*. New York: Medical War Books.

———, 1944. *Infants without families*. New York: International Universities Press.

FREUD, S., 1926. *Hemmung, Symptom und Angst*. Vienna: Internationaler Psychoanalytischer Verlag.

FREUND, H., 1952. Studies in the relationship between stuttering and cluttering. *Folia Phoniatrica, 4.*

FRIES, M. E., 1946. The child's ego development and the training of adults in his environment. In *The Psychoanalytic Study of the Child, 2.* New York: International Universities Press, 85–112.

FROESCHELS, E., 1925. *Lehrbuch der Sprachheilkunde*. Leipzig and Vienna: F. Deuticke.

———, 1934. Symptomatologie des Stotterns. *Monatsschrift f. Ohrenheilkunde u. Laryngo-Rhinologie, 68,* 814–32.

———, 1948. Pathology and therapy of stuttering. In *Twentieth century speech and voice correction*. New York: Philosophical Library.

FROSTIG, M., 1966. Development of psychological functions. Paper presented at the annual meeting. Amer. Orthopsychiat. Assoc. (Mimeogr.).

Frostig, (The Marianne) Developmental Test of Visual Perception, 1963 Standardization. Maslow, P., Frostig, M., and Lefever, D. W. *Percept. Mot. Skills*, Monogr. Suppl. 2, *19*, 463–99.

FROSTIG, M., and HORNE D., 1964. The Frostig Program for the Development of Visual Perception. Palo Alto, Calif.: Consulting Psychologists Press. Also, The Frostig Program for the Development of Visual Perception, Teacher's Guide. Chicago: Follett Publishing Co.

FROSTIG, M., and MASLOW, P., 1966. The Marianne Frostig Center for Educational Therapy Developmental Assessment and Training Project. Paper presented at the annual meeting, Amer. Orthopsychiat. Assoc. (Mimeogr.).

FRY, D. B., 1963. Coding and decoding in speech. In Mason, S. E. (Ed.), *Signs signals and symbols*. London: Methuen & Co., 65–83.

FULLER, G. B., and LAIRD, J. T., 1963. The Minnesota Percepto-Diagnostic Test. *J. Clin. Psychol.*, Monogr., Suppl., 1–33.

FURMANN, E., 1957. Treatment of under-fives by way of parents. In *The psychoanalytic study of the child*. New York: International Universities Press.

GALLAGHER, J. J., 1964. Learning disabilities—an introduction to selected papers. *Except. Child.*, *31*, 4, 165–67.

GARDNER, R. A., 1968a. The mutual story-telling technique in the alleviation of oedipal problems in children. *Contemporary Psychoanalysis*, *14*, 2.

GARDNER, R. A., 1968b. Mutual story-telling as a technique in child psychotherapy and psychoanalysis. Paper presented at the Meeting of the American Academy of Psychoanalysis, May 12, Boston, Massachusetts. Available through the author, 54 Forest Road, Tenafly, N.J., 07670. To be published in E. J. Masserman (Ed.), *Science and Psychoanalysis*, New York: Grune & Stratton, 1968.

GARRARD, S. D., and RICHMOND, J. B., 1963a. Factors influencing the biological substrate and early psychological development. In Ojeman, R. H. (Ed.), *Recent research on creative approaches to environmental stress*, Chap. 11. Preventive Psychiatry Committee, State University of Iowa.

———, 1963b. Psychological aspects of the management of chronic diseases and handicapping conditions in childhood. In Lief, H. I., Lief, V. F., and Lief, N. R. (Eds.). *The psychological basis of medical practice*. New York: Harper & Row, Hoeber Medical Division.

GESELL, A., 1929. *Infancy and human growth*. New York: The Macmillan Co.

GIBSON, E. J., 1963. Development of perception: discrimination of depth compared with discrimination of graphic symbols. In Wright, J. C., and Kagan, J. (Eds.), Basic cognitive processes in children. *Monogr. Soc. Res. Child Develpm.*, *28*, 5–32.

———, 1965. Learning to read. *Science*, *148*, 1066–72.

———, 1966. Perceptual learning in educational situations. Paper for Symposium on Research Approaches to the Learning of School Subjects, University of California at Berkeley, Oct. 28, 29 (Mimeogr.), Cornell University, Ithaca, N.Y.

GIBSON, E. J., OSSER, H., and PICK, A. D., 1963. A study of the development of grapheme-phoneme correspondence. *J. Verb. Learn., Verb. Behav.*, *2*, 2, 142–46.

GILLINGHAM, A., and STILLMAN, B. W., 1966, *Remedial training for children with specific disability in reading, spelling and penmanship*. Cambridge, Mass.: Educators Publishing Service (7th ed., combined with *phonetic drill cards*).

GLAUBER, P. I., 1953. Dynamic therapy for the stutterer. In Bychowski, G., and Despert, J. L. (Eds.), *Specialized techniques in psychotherapy*. New York: Basic Books.

GOLDIAMOND, I., 1964. Stuttering and fluency as manipulable operant response classes. In Krasner, L., and Ulman, L. P. (Eds.), *Research in behavior modification: new developments and their clinical implications.* New York: Holt, Rinehart and Winston.

GOLDFARB, W., 1945. Effects of psychological deprivation in infancy and subsequent stimulation. *Amer. J. Psychiat., 1–2,* 18.

GOLDMAN-EISLER, F., 1958. Speech analysis and mental processes, *Language and speech, 1,* 1, 59–75. Robert Draper, Ltd., Teddington, Middlesex, England.

———, 1961. A comparative study of two hesitation phenomena, *Language and speech, 4,* 1, 18–27. Robert Draper, Ltd., Teddington, Middlesex, England.

GOLDSTEIN, K., 1940. *Human nature in the light of psychopathology.* Cambridge, Mass.: Harvard University Press.

———, 1948. *Language disturbance.* New York: Grune and Stratton.

GOLDSTEIN, K., and SCHEERER, M. (Eds.), 1966. Abstract and concrete behavior—an experimental study with special tests (Monogr.). New York: The Psychological Corporation.

GOODENOUGH, F. L., 1954. *Measurement of Intelligence by Drawings.* New York: Harcourt, Brace, and World.

GOODMAN, L. A., 1952. Kolmogorov-Smirnov Tests for psychological research. *Psychol. Bull., 49,* 122–45.

GOODRICH, D. W., 1961. Possibilities for preventive intervention during initial personality formation. In Caplan, G. (Ed.), *Prevention of mental disorders in children.* New York: Basic Books, 249–65.

GOTKIN, L. G., CAUDLE, F. M., KUPPERSMITH, J. C., and WICH, B. S., 1964. Standard Telephone Interview. A procedure for assessing the language behavior of young children (Mimeogr.) Available through the Institute of Developmental Studies, Graduate School of Education, New York University, New York, N.Y.

GOTKIN, L. G., and FONDILLER, F., undated. Listening centers in the kindergarten (Mimeogr.). Available through the Institute for Developmental Studies, Graduate School of Education, New York University, New York, N.Y.

GRADY, P. A. E., 1963. Towards a new concept of dyslalia. In Mason, S. E. (Ed.), *Signs signals and symbols.* London: Methuen & Co., Ltd.

GRAY, S. W., and KLAUS, R. A., 1965. An experimental preschool program for culturally deprived children. *Child Develpm., 36,* 4, 887–98.

GRÉGOIRE, A., 1937. *L'apprentissage du langage: les deux premières années.* Paris: Droz.

———, 1947. *L'apprentissage du langage: II. La troisième anée et les années suivantes.* Paris: Droz.

GUBBAY, S. S., ELLIS, E., WALTON, J. N., and COURT, S. D. M., 1965. Clumsy children. A study of apraxia and agnosic defects in 21 children. *Brain, 88,* 295–312.

HALLGREN, B., 1950. *Specific dyslexia: a clinical and genetic study.* Copenhagen: Ejnar Munksgaard.

HALSEY, A. H., FLOUD, J., and ANDERSON, C. A., 1964. *Education, economy, and society.* New York: The Free Press.

HARTLEY, L. M., 1963. Analysis of the linguistic data of dyslalia. In Mason, S. E. (Ed.), *Signs signals and symbols.* London: Methuen & Co.

HEERMANN, M., 1965. *Schreibbewegungstherapie fuer entwicklungsgestoerte und neurotische Kinder und Jugendliche.* Bielefeld: Ernst und Werner Gieseking Verlag.

HEJNA, F., 1955. Developmental Articulation Test. University of Connecticut, Storrs, Conn.

HENDRICK, I., 1942. Instinct and the ego during infancy. *Psychoanal. Quart., 1,* 33–58.

———, 1951. Early development of the ego: identification in infancy. *Psychoanal. Quart., 20,* 44–61.

HESS, R. D., and SHIPMAN, V., 1965a. Early blocks to children's learning. *Children*, *12*, 189–94.
——, 1965b. Early experience and socialization of cognitive modes in children. *Child Develpm.*, *36*, 869–86.
HEWETT, F., 1964. A hierarchy of educational tasks for children with learning disorders. *Except. Child.*, *31*, 4.
HINSHELWOOD, J., 1900a. Congenital word-blindness, *Lancet*, *1*, 1506–08.
——, 1900b. *Letter-, word-, and mind-blindness.* London: Lewis.
——, 1912. The treatment of word-blindness, acquired and congenital, *Brit. med. J.*, *2*, 1033–35.
——, 1917. *Congenital word-blindness.* London: Lewis.
HUNT, J. MCV., 1961. *Intelligence and experience.* New York: Ronald Press.
——, 1964. The psychological basis for using pre-school enrichment as an antidote for cultural deprivation. *Merrill-Palmer Quart.*, *10*, 3, 209–49. Reprinted in Hechinger, F. M. (Ed.), 1966. *Pre-school education today.* New York: Doubleday & Co.
ICAA Word Blind Bulletin, Volume 1, Invalid Children's Aid Association, 4 Palace Gate, London, W.8.
Illinois Test of Psycholinguistic Abilities: experimental edition, 1961. McCarthy, J. J., and Kirk, S. A. Urbana, Ill.: University of Illinois Press.
IRWIN, O. C., 1941. Research on speech sounds for the first six months of life. *Psychol. Bull.*, *38*, 277–85.
——, 1946. Speech sound mastery during infancy. *Amer. Psychologist*, *1*, 252 (Abstract).
——, 1947. Development of speech during infancy: curve of phonemic frequencies. *J. exp. Psychol.*, *37*, 187–93.
——, 1948a. Infant speech: the effect of family occupational status of and age on use of sound types. *J. Speech Hear. Disorders*, *13*, 224–26.
——, 1948b. Infant speech: the effect of family occupational status and of age on sound frequency. *J. Speech Hear. Disorders*, *13*, 320–23.
——, 1949. Infant speech. *Scient. Amer.*, *28*, 22–24.
IRWIN, O. C., and CHEN, H. P., 1943. Speech sound elements during the first years of life: a review of the literature. *J. Speech Disorders*, *8*, 293–95.
ISAACS, S., 1937. *Social development in young children.* New York: Harcourt, Brace & World.
——, 1952. The nature and function of phantasy. In Klein, M., Heimann, P., Isaacs, S., and Riviere, J. (Eds.), *Developments in psycho-analysis.* London: The Hogarth Press, 67–122.
ISAKOWER, O., 1939. On the exceptional position of the auditive sphere. *Int. J. Psychoanal.*, *20*.
JACOBSON, E., 1946. The effect of disappointment on ego and superego formation in normal and depressive development. *Psychoanal. Rev.*, *33*, 131–45.
JACOBSON, L., 1949. Methods used in the education of mothers. In *The psychoanalytic study of the child.* New York: International Universities Press.
JAKOBSON, R., 1941. *Kindersprache, Aphasie, und allgemeine Lautgesetze.* Uppsala, Sweden: Almqvist & Wiksell.
JAKOBSON, R., and HALLE M., 1956. *Fundamentals of language.* 'S-Gravenhage Holland: Mouton & Co.
JASTAK, J., 1946. Manual, Wide Range Achievement Test. Wilmington, Del.: C. L. Story.
JOHN, V. P., 1963. The intellectual development of slum children: some preliminary findings. *Amer. J. Orthopsychiat.*, *33*, 813–22.
——, 1964. A brief survey of research on the characteristics of children from low-income backgrounds (Mimeogr.). Prepared for the U.S. Commissioner on Education.

JOHN, V. P. 1965. The relation between social experience and the acquisition of language (Mimeogr.). Lecture presented in the Orientation Conference for Professional Personnel in Child Development Centers for Project Head Start, Los Angeles, California.

JOHN, V. P., and GOLDSTEIN, L. S., 1964. The social context of language acquisition. *Merrill-Palmer Quart.*, *10*, 265–75.

JOHNSON, D. J., and MYKLEBUST, H. R., 1967. *Learning disabilities. Educational principles and practices.* New York and London: Grune & Stratton.

JOHNSON, W., 1948. *Speech handicapped school children*, New York: Harper & Row.

———, (ed.), 1955. *Stuttering in children and adults.* Minneapolis: University of Minnesota Press.

KATZ, P. A., and DEUTSCH, M., 1963. Relation of auditory-visual shifting to reading achievement. *Percept. Mot. Skills*, *17*, 323–32.

KELLER, S., 1963. The social world of the urban slum child: some early findings. *Amer. J. Orthopsychiat.*, *33*, 5, 823–32.

KEPHART, N. C., 1960. *The slow learner in the classroom.* Columbus, Ohio: C. E. Merrill.

———, 1964. Perceptual motor aspects of learning disabilities. *Except. Child.*, *31*, 201–207.

KIDD, A. H. and KIDD, R. M., 1966. The development of auditory perception in children. In Kidd, A. H., and Rivoire, J. L. (Eds.), *Perceptual development in children.* New York: International Universities Press, 113–43.

KIDD, A. H., and RIVOIRE, J. L. (Eds.), 1966. *Perceptual development in children.* New York: International Universities Press.

KIRK, S. A., 1966. The diagnosis and remediation of psycholinguistic disabilities (Mimeogr.). Institute for Research on Exceptional Children, University of Illinois.

KLEIN, D. C., and LINDEMANN, E., 1961. Preventive interventions in individual and family crisis situations. In Caplan, G. (Ed.,) *Prevention of mental disorders in children.* New York: Basic Books, 283–307.

KLEIN, D. C., and ROSS, A., 1958. Kindergarten entry, a study of role transitions. In Krugman, M. (Ed.), *Orthopsychiatry and the school.* New York: Amer. Orthopsychiat. Assoc.

KLEIN, M., 1950. A contribution to the psychogenesis of manic-depressive states. In *Contributions to psychoanalysis.* London: Hogarth Press and Institute of Psychoanalysis.

———, 1952. On the theory of anxiety and guilt. In Klein, M., Heimann, P., Isaacs, S., and Riviere, J., *Developments in psychoanalysis.* London: Hogarth Press, 271–92.

KNOBLOCH, H., and PASAMANICK, D., 1959. Syndrome of minimal cerebral damage in infancy. *J. Amer. Med. Ass.*, *106*, 1384–87.

KOCH, H., 1954. The relation of "primary mental abilities" in five- and six-year olds to sex of child and characteristics of his siblings. *Child Develpm.*, *25*, 209–23.

Kolmogorov-Smirnov Tests for Psychological Research, 1952. Goodman, L. A., *Psychol. Bull.*, *49*, 122–45.

KOPPITZ, F. M., 1964. *The Bender Gestalt Test for Young Children.* New York: Grune and Stratton.

KRIPPNER, S., 1965. Diagnostic and remedial use of the Minnesota Percepto-Diagnostic Test in a reading clinic. (Mimeogr.) Paper presented at the annual meeting, *Amer. Psychol. Assoc.* Available through Dept. of Psychiatry, Maimonides Hospital of Brooklyn, Brooklyn, N.Y.

LANGER, S. K., 1942. *Philosophy in a new key.* New York: Mentor Books.

———, 1962. *Philosophical sketches.* Baltimore: Johns Hopkins Press.

LEE, B. S., 1951. Artificial stutter. *J. Speech, Hear. Disorders*, *16*, 53–55.

LEE, L. L., 1966. Developmental sentence types: a method for comparing normal and deviant syntactic development in children's language. *J. Speech, Hear. Disorders*, November.

LETON, D. A., 1966. Perceptual–motor dysfunction in children: criterion problems (Mimeogr.). Paper presented at the annual meeting, Amer. Orthopsychiat. Assoc., Workshop #20.

LEWIS, M. M., 1951. *Infant speech: a study of the beginnings of language.* (2nd ed.) New York: Humanities Press; London: Routledge and Kegan Paul.

LIEBMANN, A., 1900. *Vorlesungen ueber Sprachstoerungen, Heft 4. Poltern (Paraphrasia praeceps).* Berlin: Oscar Coblentz Verlag.

——, 1924. *Vorlesungen ueber Sprachstoerungen, Heft. 6. Kinder, die schwer lesen, schreiben und rechnen lernen.* Berlin: Oscar Coblentz Verlag.

Lincoln-Oseretsky Motor Development Scale, 1948. Sloan, W., C. H. Stoelting.

LINDEMANN, E., 1944. Symptomatology and management of acute grief. *Amer. J. Psychiat.*, *101*, 141.

——, 1956. The meaning of crisis in individual and family living. *Teachers Coll. Rec.*, *57*, 310.

LINDNER, G., 1898. *Aus dem Naturgarten der Kindersprache. Ein Beitrag zur kindlichen Sprach-und Geistesentwicklung in den ersten vier Lebensjahren.* Leipzig: Grieben Verlag.

LOBAN, W. D., 1963. *The language of elementary school children.* A study of the use and control of language effectiveness in communication, and the relations among speaking, reading, writing, and listening. NCTE Research Report No. 1. National Council of Teachers of English, 508 South Sixth Street, Champaign, Ill. 61820.

——, 1966. *Problems in oral English. Kindergarten through grade nine.* NCTE Research Report No. 4. National Council of Teachers of English, 508 South Sixth Street, Champaign, Ill. 61820.

LOWREY, L. G., 1940. Personality distortion and early infantile care. *Amer. J. Orthopsychiat.*, *10*, 576.

LUBORSKY, L., FABIAN, M., HALL, B. H., TICHO, E., and TICHO, G. R., 1958. Treatment variables. *Bull. Menninger Clin.*, *22*, 4, 126–46.

LUCHSINGER, R., 1963. *Poltern.* Berlin-Charlottenburg: C. Marhold Verlag.

LURIA, A. R., 1961. *The role of speech in the regulation of normal and abnormal behavior.* New York, Oxford: Pergamon Press.

MACHOVER, K., 1957. Personality Projection in the Drawing of the Human Figure. Springfield, Ill.: Charles C. Thomas.

MACLAY, H., and OSGOOD, C. E., 1959. Hesitation phenomena in spontaneous English speech. *Word*, *15*, 19.

MACNAMARA, M., 1963. Helping children through their mothers. *J. Child Psychol. Psychiat.*, *4.*

MALONE, C. A., 1963. Some observations on children of disorganized families and problems of acting out. *Amer. J. Child Psychiat.*, *2*, 1, 22–41.

——, 1966. Safety first: Comments on the influence of external danger in the lives of disorganized families. *Amer. J. Orthopsychiat.*, *36*, 1, 3–13.

MANDELL, S., and SONNECK, B., 1935. Phonographische Aufnahme und Analyse der ersten Sprachäusserungen von Kindern. *Arch. ges. Psychol.*, *94*, 478–500.

MASLOW, P., FROSTIG, M., LEFEVER, D. W., and WHITTLESEY, J. R. B., 1964 The Marianne Frostig Developmental Test of Visual Perception, 1963 Standardization. Perceptual and Motor Skills. Monogr. Suppl. 2, *19*, 463–99.

MASON, S. E. (Ed.), 1963. *Signs signals and symbols.* London: Methuen & Co.

MCCARTHY, D., 1929. The vocalization of infants. *Psychol. Bull.*, *26*, 625–51.

——, 1930. The language development of the preschool child. Inst. Child Welfare (Monogr.), Ser. No. 4., Minneapolis: University of Minnesota Press.

——, 1954. Language development in children. In Carmichael, L. (Ed.), *Manual of child psychology*, 2nd ed. New York: John Wiley & Sons.

MCCARTHY, D., 1955. Discussion of Chapters 1–4. In Hoch, P. B., and Zubin, J. (Eds.), *Psychopathology of childhood*. New York: Grune & Stratton, 49–56.

———, 1959. Research in language development: retrospect and prospect. *Child Develpm. Monogr.*, *24*, 5, Serial No. 74, 3–24.

———, 1960. Language development. *Monogr. Soc. Res. Child. Develpm.*, *25*, 3 (Whole No. 77), 5–14.

MCCARTHY, J. J., and KIRK, S. A., 1961. Illinois Test of Psycholinguistic Abilities: experimental edition. Urbana, Ill.: University of Illinois Press.

MCGRAW, M. B., 1935. *Growth: a study of Johnny and Jimmy*. New York: Appleton-Century-Crofts.

MEAD, M., 1953. *Growing up in New Guinea*. New York: Mentor Books.

MEASUREMENT OF INTELLIGENCE BY DRAWINGS, 1954. Goodenough, F. L. New York: Harcourt, Brace and World.

MEDNICK, S. A., and SHAFFER, J. B. P., 1963. Mothers' retrospective reports in child rearing research. *Amer. J. Orthopsychiat.*, *23*,

MENOLASCINO, F. J., and EATON, L., 1967. Comprehensive treatment for the child with cerebral dysfunction (Mimeogr.). Paper presented at the annual meeting, Amer. Orthopsychiat. Assoc. Available through Nebraska Psychiatric Institute, University of Nebraska College of Medicine, Omaha, Nebraska.

MEREDITH, P., 1962. Psycho-physical aspects of word-blindness and kindred disorders (Mimeogr.). Available through Department of Psychology, University of Leeds, England.

———, 1964. Word-blindness: an operational approach. Excerpt from the papers read before the Health Congress of the Royal Society of Health, at Torquay, April 27 to May 1. Available through P. Meredith, Department of Psychology, University of Leeds, England.

MILLER, G. A., 1961. *Language and communication*. New York: McGraw-Hill Book Co.

MILLER, W., and ERVIN, S., 1964. The development of grammar in child language. In The acquisition of language. *Monogr. Soc. Res. Child Develpm.*, Serial No. 92, *29*, 1, 9–35.

Minnesota Percepto-Diagnostic Test. Fuller, G. B., and Laird, J. T., *J. Clin. Psychol.*, Monogr., Suppl., 1–33.

MINNIGERODE, B., 1965. Ueber die Bedeutung peripher-impressiver und zentral-sensorischer Stoerungen fuer die Entstehung der Lese-und Rechtschreibeschwaeche. *Folia Phoniatrica*, *17*, 1, 43–58.

MINUCHIN, S., CHAMBERLAIN, P., and GRAUBARD, P., 1967. A project to teach learning skills to disturbed delinquent children. *Amer. J. Orthopsychiat.*, *37*, 3, 558–68.

MONEY, J. (Ed.), 1962. *Reading disability. Progress and research needs in dyslexia*. Baltimore: The Johns Hopkins Press.

———, (Ed.), 1966. *The disabled reader: education of the dyslexic child*. Baltimore: The Johns Hopkins Press.

MONTESSORI, M., 1959. *Education for a new world*. Wheaton, Ill.: Theosophical Press.

MONTGOMERY, R. B., and COUGHLAN, S., 1953. *Sound, spell, read; the phonovisual vowel book*. Washington, D.C.: Phonovisual Products, P.O. Box 5625.

MORENCY, A. S., WEPMAN, J. M., and WEINER, P. S., 1967. Studies in speech: developmental articulation inaccuracy. *Element. Sch. J.*, *67*, 329–38.

MORLEY, M. E., 1959. Defects of articulation. *Folia Phoniatrica*, II, Nos. 1–3.

MOSES, L. B., 1952. Non-parametric statistics in psychological research. *Psychol. Bull.*, *49*, 122.

MOWRER, O. H., 1950. On the psychology of "talking birds"—a contribution to language and personality theory. In Mowrer, *Learning theory and personality dynamics*. New York: Ronald Press.

MOWRER, O. H. and VIEK, P., 1945. Language and learning: an experimental paradigm. *Harvard Educat. Rev.*, January, 35–48.

MURPHY, L. B., 1962. *The widening world of childhood*. New York: Basic Books.

MURRAY, H. A., 1953. Thematic Apperception Test. Cambridge, Mass.: Harvard University Press.

MYKLEBUST, H. R., 1954. *Auditory disorders in children: a manual for differential diagnosis*. New York: Grune & Stratton.

————, 1956, Language disorders in children. *Except. Child.*, *22*, 4, 163–66.

————, 1964. Learning disorders, psychoneurological disturbances in childhood. *Rehabilit. Liter.*, *25*, 12, 354–60. National Society for Crippled Children and Adults.

————, 1965. *Development and disorders of written language*. Volume One, Picture Story Language Test. New York: Grune & Stratton.

MYKLEBUST, H. R., and BOSHES, B., 1960. Psychoneurological learning disorders in children. *Arch. of Pediat.*, *New York*, June, 247–56.

MYKLEBUST, H. R., and JOHNSON, D., 1962. Dyslexia in children. *Except. Child.*, *29*, 1, 14–25.

NEELLY, J. M., 1961. A study of the speech behavior of stutterers and nonstutterers under normal and delayed auditory feedback. *J. Speech Hear. Disorders, Monogr. Suppl.*, No. 7.

NICE, M. M., 1917. Speech development of a child from eighteen months to six years. *Pediat. Sem.*, *25*, 204–43.

————, 1925. Length of sentences as a criterion of a child's progress in speech. *J. Educ. Psychol.*, *16*, 370–79.

NISBET, J., 1961. Family environment and intelligence. In Halsey, A. H., Floud, J., and Anderson, C. A. (Eds.), *Education, economy, and society*. New York: The Free Press, 273–87.

No-Howe (The) Speech Test for English Consonant Sounds, 1957. Smith, M. N. Distributor: College Book Store, SUNY Teachers College, Cortland, N.Y.

O'DONNELL, M., *et al.*, 1957. Alice and Jerry Books; Here we go; Skip along. *Workbook for preprimers*. New York: Harper & Row.

OLIM, B. G., HESS, R. D., SHIPMAN, V. C., 1965. Maternal language styles and the implications for children's cognitive development (Mimeogr.). Available through Urban Child Study Center, University of Chicago, Chicago, Ill.

ONG, W. J., 1967. *In the human grain. Further explorations of contemporary culture*. New York: The Macmillan Co.

ORTON, S. T., 1925. Word-blindness in school children. *Arch. neur. Psychol.*, *14*, 581–615.

————, 1928a. Specific reading disability—strephosymbolia. *J. Amer. Med. Assoc.*, *90*, 1095–99.

————, 1928b. An impediment in learning to read—a neurological explanation of the reading disability. *Sch. a. Soc.*, 286–90.

————, 1934. Some studies in language function. *Assoc. Res. Nerv. Ment. Diseases*, *13*, 614–33.

————, 1937. *Reading, writing, and speech problems in children*. New York: W. W. Norton.

————, 1943. Visual functions in strephosymbolia. *Arch. Ophth.*, *30*, 707–17.

OSTROVSKY, E., 1959. *L'influence masculine et l'enfant d'âge préscolaire*. Paris: Delachaux and Niestlé.

PAINE, R. S., 1962. Minimal chronic brain syndromes in children. *Develpm. Med. Child Neurol.*, *4*, 21–27.

PARKER, L. P., 1963. A critical investigation into the problems of dysarthria. In Mason, S. E. (Ed.), *Signs signals and symbols*, London: Methuen & Co., 183–95.

PAVENSTEDT, E., 1965. A comparison of the child-rearing environment of upper-lower and very low-lower class families. *Amer. J. Orthopsychiat.*, *35*, 1, 89–98.

Peabody Picture Vocabulary Test, 1959. Dunn, L. M. Nashville, Tenn.: American Guidance Service, Inc.

PENFIELD, W., and ROBERTS, L., 1959. *Speech and brain mechanisms*. Princeton, N. J.: Princeton University Press.

PENN, J. M., 1966. Reading disability: a neurological deficit? *Except. Child.*, *33*, 4, 243–48.

Personality Projection in the Drawing of the Human Figure 1957. Machover, K. Springfield, Ill.: Charles C. Thomas.

PIAGET, J., 1926. *The language and thought of the child*. New York: Harcourt, Brace and World; London: Routledge & Kegan Paul.

———, 1951. *Play, dreams and imitation in childhood*. New York: W. W. Norton.

———, 1954. *The construction of reality in the child*. New York: Basic Books.

POOLE, I., 1943. Genetic development of articulation of consonant sounds in speech. *Elem. English Rev.*, *11*, 159.

PREYER, W., 1893. *Die geistige Entwicklung in der ersten Kindheit*. Stuttgart: Union Verlag.

PROVENCE, S., and LIPTON, H. C., 1962. *Infants in institutions*. New York: International Universities Press.

PULVER, U., 1959. *Spannungen und Stoerungen im Verhalten des Säuglings*. Bern. u. Stuttgart: Hans Huber Verlag.

PYLES, M. K., and MACFARLAND, J. M., 1934. The consistency of reports on developmental data. *Psychol. Bull.*, *31*.

PYLES, M. K., STOLTZ, H. R., and MACFARLANE, J. W., 1935. The accuracy of mothers' reports on birth and developmental data. *Child Develpm.*, *6*, 165–76.

RABIN, A., 1965. *Growing up in the Kibbutz*. New York: Springer Publishing Co.

RABINOVITCH, M. S., 1964. *The Learning Centre* (reprint). International Copenhagen Congress on the Scientific Study of Mental Retardation.

RABINOVITCH, R. D., 1962. Dyslexia: psychiatric considerations. In Money, J. (Ed.), *Reading disability*. Baltimore: Johns Hopkins Press, 73–81.

RANSCHBURG, P., 1916. Die Leseschwaeche (Legasthenie) und Rechenschwaeche (Arithemie) der Kinder im Lichte des Experiments. *Abhand. aus d. Grenzgeb. Paed. Med.*, Berlin.

———, 1928. *Die Lese- und Schreibstörungen des Kindesalters*, Halle: Marhold Verlag.

RHEINGOLD, H. L., 1956. The modification of social responsiveness in institutional babies. *Monogr. Soc. Res. Child Develpm.*, *21*, No. 63.

RICHTER, H. E., 1963. *Eltern, Kind und Neurose*. Stuttgart: Ernst Klett Verlag.

ROACH, E. G., 1966. Evaluation of an experimental program of perceptual-motor training with slow readers. Published in the International Reading Assoc. Annual Proceedings, *Vistas in Reading*.

ROACH, E. G., and KEPHART, N. C., 1966. The Purdue Perceptual-Motor Survey. Columbus, Ohio: Charles E. Merrill Books

ROMAN, K. G., undated. *Studies in tachyphemia, an investigation of cluttering and general language disability*, Chap. VI, pp. 63–81. New York: Speech Rehabilitation Institute, 61 Irving Place.

ROSE, F. C. 1958., The occurrence of short memory span among school children referred for diagnosis of reading difficulties. *J. Educ. Res.*, *51*, 459–64.

ROUDINESCO, J., and APPELL, G., 1950. Les répercussions de la stabilization hospitalière sur le développement psycho-moteur des jeunes enfants. *Sem. Hosp. Paris, 26,* 2271.

RUBIN, E. Z., undated. Secondary emotional disorders in children with perceptual-motor dysfunction (Mimeogr.). Research report, Lafayette Clinic and Wayne State University, Detroit, Michigan.

RUBIN, E. Z., and SIMSON, C., 1960. A special class program for the emotionally disturbed child in school: a proposal. *Amer. J. Orthopsychiat., 1,* 144–53.

RUBIN, E. Z., SIMSON, C. B., and BETWEE, M. C., 1966. *Emotionally handicapped children and the elementary school.* Detroit: Wayne State University Press.

RUDERMAN, E. G. and SELESNICK, S., 1968. Multiple avenues of approach to a child with a chronic symptom: stuttering. (Mimeograph). Paper presented at the meetings of the American Academy of Psychoanalysis, May 12, Boston, Massachusetts. Available through Mrs. E. G. Ruderman, Mt. Sinai Hospital, Dept. of Child Psychiatry, 110–112 No. Hannel Road, Los Angeles, 48, California.

RUESCH, J., 1957. *Disturbed communication. The clinical assessment of normal and pathological communicative behavior.* New York: W. W. Norton.

RUSSELL, R. W., undated. A program of special classes for children with learning disability in the public schools of Glen Rock, New Jersey. New Jersey Association for Brain-Injured Children, 61 Lincoln Street, East Orange, N. J.

RUTHERFORD, W. L., 1965. Perceptual-motor training and readiness. *Reading and inquiry.* International Reading Assoc. Proceedings, *10,* Newark, Delaware, 294–96.

SANDER, L. W., 1962. Issues in early mother-child interaction. *J. Amer. Acad. Child Psychiat., 1.*

SAPIR, E., 1921. *Language, an introduction to the study of speech.* New York: Harcourt, Brace & World.

SAPORTA, S., and BASTIAN, J. R. (Eds.), 1958. *Psycholinguistics. A book of readings.* New York: Holt, Rinehart & Winston.

SARASON, S. B., DAVIDSON, K. S., and BLATT, B., 1962. *The preparation of teachers. An unstudied problem in education.* New York: John Wiley & Sons.

SARGENT, H. D., MODLIN, H. C., FARIS, M. T., and VOTH, H. M., 1958. Situational variables. *Bull. Menninger Clin., 22,* 4, 148–64.

Sceno Test (also called *Von Staabs Test*), undated. Obtainable from the author, Dr. G. von Staabs, Berlin W 15, Brandenburgische Strasse, 32, Germany.

SCHACHTEL, E. G., 1959. On memory and childhood amnesia. In Schachtel, *Metamorphosis.* New York: Basic Books, 279–322.

SCHAEFER, E. S., and FURFEY, P. H., 1966. Proposed plan: intellectual stimulation of culturally deprived infants (Mimeogr.). Application to the National Institute of Mental Health, Bethesda, Maryland.

———, 1967. Intellectual stimulation of culturally deprived infants during the period of early verbal development (Mimeogr.). Informal Progress Report to the National Institute of Mental Health, Bethesda, Maryland.

SCHNEIDER, E., 1922. *Ueber das Stottern.* Bern: A. Francke Verlag.

SCHUR, M., 1960. Discussion of Dr. John Bowlby's paper. In *The Psychoanal. Stud. of the Child, 15.* New York: International Universities Press, 63–85.

SEEMAN, M., and NOVAK, A., 1963. Ueber die Motorik bei Polterern. *Folia Phoniatrica, 15,* 2–3, 170–76.

SHANDS, H. C., 1954. Anxiety, anaclitic object, and the sign function: comments on early developments in the use of symbols. *Amer. J. Orthopsychiat., 1,* 84–97.

SHEEHAN, J. G., 1953. Theory and treatment of stuttering as an approach-avoidance conflict. *J. Psychol., 36,* 27–49.

———, 1954. An integration of psychotherapy and speech therapy through a conflict theory of stuttering. *J. Speech, Hear. Disorders, 19,* 474–82.

———, 1965. Speech therapy and recovery from stuttering. *The Voice, J. California Speech, Hear. Assoc., 14,* 3, 3–7.

———, 1966. Spontaneous recovery from stuttering. *J. Speech, Hear. Res., 9,* 1, 121–35.

SHINN, M. W., 1900. *The biography of a baby.* Boston: Houghton Mifflin.

SIGEL, I. E., 1964. The attainment of concepts. In Hoffman, M. L., and Hoffman, L. W. (Eds.), *Review of child development research.* New York: Russell Sage Foundation, 209–49.

SILVER, A. A., and HAGIN, R. A., 1964. Specific reading disability: follow-up studies. *Amer. J. Orthopsychiat., 34,* 1, 95–102.

———, 1967. Strategies of intervention in the spectrum of defects in specific reading disability (Mimeogr.). Paper read at the annual meeting, Amer. Orthopsychiat. Assoc. Available through Dept. of Psychology and Neurology, New York University Medical Center, 560 First Ave., New York, N.Y. 10016.

SILVER, A. A., HAGIN, R. A., and HERSH, M. F., 1965. Specific reading disability: teaching through stimulation of deficit perceptual areas (Mimeogr.). Paper read at the annual meeting, Amer. Orthopsychiat. Assoc. Available through Dept. of Psychology and Neurology, New York University Medical Center, 560 First Ave., New York, N.Y. 10016.

SILVER, A. A., PFEIFFER, E., and HAGIN, R. A., 1967. The therapeutic nursery as an aid in the diagnosis of delayed language development. *Amer. J. Orthopsychiat., 37,* 5, 963–70.

SILVERMAN, M., LASZLO, I. J., and CRAMER, J., 1967. Deviant preschool children: the contribution of constitutional predisposition and parental crisis (Mimeogr.). Paper read at the annual meeting. Amer. Orthopsychiat. Assoc. Available through, Meeting Street School Pre-School Program, Emma Pendleton Bradley Hospital, Riverside, R. I. 02915.

SLOAN, W., 1948. Lincoln-Oseretsky Motor Development Scale. C. H. Stoelting.

SLOBIN, D. I., 1964a. Imitation and the acquisition of syntax (Mimeogr.). Department of Psychology, University of California, Berkeley. Published under the title "Imitation and grammatical development in children." In Endler, N. S., Boulter, L. R., and Osser, H. (Eds.), *Contemporary Issues in Developmental Psychology.* Holt, Rinehart & Winston, 1967.

———, 1964b. New approaches to the study of syntactic development in children (Mimeogr.). Department of Psychology, University of California, Berkeley.

SMITH, M. E., 1926. An investigation of the development of the sentence and the extent of vocabulary in young children. *University of Iowa Studies in Child Welfare,* First Series, No. 109.

SMITH, M. N., 1957. The No-Howe Speech Test for English Consonant Sounds. Distributor: College Book Store, State University of New York, Teachers College, Cortland, N.Y.

SPITZ, R. A., 1945. Hospitalism: an inquiry into the genesis of psychiatric conditions in early childhood. In *The psychoanalytic study of the child.* New York: International Universities Press, *1,* 53–74.

SPRIGLE, H. A., 1967. Curriculum development and innovation in learning materials for early childhood education (Mimeogr.). Paper presented at the Southern Conference on Early Childhood Education, University of Georgia, March 27–29. Available through Psychological Clinic, 1939 San Marco Blvd., Jacksonville, Florida 32207.

SPRIGLE, H., and SPRIGLE, J., undated. A fresh approach to early childhood education and a study of its effectiveness. Learning to learn program (pamphlet). Available from Learning to Learn School, Inc., 1936 San Marco Blvd., Jackonsville, Florida 32207.

SRA Achievement Series, 1964. Thorpe, L. P., Lefever, D. W., and Naslund, R. A. Chicago, Ill.: Science Research Associates.

SRA Primary Mental Abilities, for ages 5 to 7, 1946. Thurstone, T. G., and Thurstone, L. L. Chicago, Ill.: Science Research Associates.

Stanford-Binet Intelligence Scale (third revision), 1960. Terman, L. M., and Merrill, M. A. Cambridge, Mass.: Houghton-Mifflin Co.

STEIN, L., 1953. Stammering as a psychosomatic disorder. *Folia Phoniatrica*, 5, 1.

STENGEL, E., 1939. On learning a new language. *Int. J. Psychoanal.*, 20, parts 3 & 4, 1–5.

STERN, C., and STERN, W., 1907. Die Kindersprache: eine psychologische und sprachtheoretische Untersuchung. *Monogr. seel. Entwickl. Kindes*, 1, Leipzig: Barth Verlag.

STEWART, G. K., and CODA, E. J., undated. An integrative multi-discipline approach to the multi-handicapped preschool child (Mimeogr.). Available through Kennedy Child Study Center, 1339 20th Street, Santa Monica, California.

STEWART, W. A., 1964. Foreign language teaching methods in quasi-foreign language situations. In Stewart, W. A. (Ed.), *Non-standard speech and the teaching of English*. Washington, D.C.: Center for Applied Linguistics, 1–15.

STONE, L. J., and CHURCH, J., 1957. *Childhood and adolescence*. New York: Random House.

STRAUSS, A. A., and LEHTINEN, L. E., 1947. *Psychopathology and education of the brain-injured child, I*. New York: Grune & Stratton.

STRAUSS, A. A., and KEPHART, N. C., 1955. *Psychopathology and education of the brain-injured child, II*. New York: Grune & Stratton.

STUART, M. F. 1963. *Neurophysiological insights into teaching*. Palo Alto, California: Pacific Books.

STUBBINGS, M. C., HAVERLY, R. L., GAYNES, W. S., and MONTGOMERY, R. B., 1953. *See, hear, say, do; the phonovisual consonant book*. Washington, D.C.: Phonovisual Products, P.O. Box 5625.

Studies in Tachyphemia, an investigation of cluttering and general language disability, undated. New York: Speech Rehabilitation Institute, 61 Irving Place.

SULLIVAN, E. R., CLARK, W. W., and TIEGS, E. W., 1957. California Short-Form Test of Mental Maturity, S-Form. Monterey, California: California Test Bureau, Del Monte Research Park.

TAYLOR, E. M., 1959. *Psychological appraisal of children with cerebral defects*. Cambridge, Mass.: Harvard University Press.

TEMPLIN, M. C., 1957. *Certain language skills in children, their development and their interrelationships*. Minneapolis: University of Minnesota Press.

TERMAN, L. M., and MERRILL, M. A., 1960. Stanford-Binet Intelligence Scale (third revision), Form L-M. Cambridge, Mass.: Houghton-Mifflin Co.

The Purdue Perceptual-Motor Survey, 1966. Roach, E. G. and Kephart, N. C. Columbus, Ohio: Charles E. Merrill Books, Inc.

Thematic Apperception Test, 1953. Murray, H. A. Cambridge, Mass.: Harvard University Press.

Thematic Stories for Children (Fabeltest), 1946. Duess, L. Trans. by Despert, J. L. *Amer. J. Orthopsychiat.*, 15, 109.

Therapeutic Play Techniques, 1955. Symposium, *Amer. J. Orthopsychiat.*, 25, 3.

THOMAS, A., BIRCH, H. G., CHESS, S., and HERTZIG, M. E., undated. The developmental dynamics of primary reaction characteristics in children. *Proceedings of the Third World Congress of Psychiatry*, 722–26.

THOMAS, D. R., 1962. Oral language, sentence structure, and vocabulary of kindergarten children living in low socio-economic urban areas. Unpublished doctoral dissertation, Wayne State University.

THORPE, L. P., LEFEVER, D. W., and NASLUND, R. A., 1964. SRA Achievement Series. Chicago, Ill.: Science Research Associates.

THURSTONE, T. G., and THURSTONE, L. L., 1946. SRA Primary Mental Abilities, for ages 5 to 7. Chicago, Ill.: Science Research Associates.

TRAVIS, L. E., 1931. *Speech pathology*. New York: Appleton-Century-Crofts.

———, 1940. The need for stuttering. *J. Speech Disorders*, 5, 193–202.

Trends in Orthopsychiatric Therapy. 1948. Symposium, *Amer. J. Orthopsychiat.*, 18, 402.

TRUBY, H. M., BOSMA, J. F., and LIND, J., in press. Infant cry sounds: a visual-acoustic analysis technique. *Acta Paediatrica*.

VAN RIPER, C., 1942. *Speech correction: principles and methods*. Englewood Cliffs, N. J.: Prentice-Hall.

VAN THAL, J. H., 1963. Evaluating nature and degree of defects and disorders of voice, speech and language. In Mason, S. E. (Ed.), *Signs signals and symbols*. London: Methuen & Co., 87–93.

VELTEN, H. V., 1943. The growth of phonemic and lexical patterns in infant language. *Language*, 19, 281–92.

VIGOTSKY, L. S., 1939. Thought and speech. *Psychiatry*, 2, 1, 29–54. Reprinted in *Thought and language*, 1962. Ed. and trans. by Hanfman, E., and Vakar, G. Cambridge, Mass.: M.I.T. Press. New York and London: John Wiley & Sons.

VON STAABS, G., *Von Staabs Test*, also called *Sceno Test*, undated. Obtainable from the author, Dr. G. von Staabs, Berlin W 15, Brandenburgische Strasse, 32, Germany.

VOSK, J. S., 1966. Study of Negro children with learning difficulties at the outset of their school careers. *Amer. J. Orthopsychiat.*, 36, 32–41.

WALDFOGEL, S., and GARDNER, G. E., 1961. Intervention in crises as a method of primary prevention. In Caplan, G. (Ed.), *Prevention of mental disorders in children*. New York: Basic Books, 307–23.

WECHSLER, D., 1940. Wechsler Intelligence Scale for Children (WISC). New York: The Psychological Corporation.

Wechsler Intelligence Scale for Children (WISC), 1940. Wechsler, D. New York: The Psychological Corporation.

WEIKART, D. P. (Ed.), undated. *Preschool intervention; preliminary report of the Perry Preschool Project*. Campus Publishers, 711 North University Ave., Ann Arbor, Michigan 48108.

WEINER, M., and FELDMANN, S., 1963. Validation studies of a Reading Prognosis Test for children of lower and middle socioeconomic status. *Educ. Psychol. Measmt.*, 23, 807–14.

WEISS, D. A., 1950. Der Zusammenhang zwischen Poltern und Stottern. *Folia Phoniatrica*, 2, 4, 252–62.

———, 1960. Therapy of cluttering. *Folia Phoniatrica*, 12, 3, 216–23.

———, 1964. *Cluttering*, Foundations of Speech Pathology Series. Englewood Cliffs, N. J.: Prentice-Hall.

WELLMAN, B., CASE, I. M., MENGERT, I. G., and BRADBURY, D. E., 1936. Speech sounds of young children. *University Iowa Stud. Child Welf.*, 5, No. 2.

WELSCH, E. E. *et al*, 1956. Qualifications for psychotherapists. Symposium, *Amer. J. Orthopsychiat.*, 25, 1, 35–65.

WENAR, C., 1963. The reliability of developmental histories. *Psychosom. Med.*, 25, 505–509.

WEPMAN, J. M., 1958. Auditory Discrimination Test. Chicago, Ill.: Language Research Associates.

WEPMAN, J. M., 1960. Auditory discrimination, speech and reading. *Element. Sch. J.*, *60*, 325–33.

——, 1964. The perceptual basis for learning. In Robinson, A. (Ed.), *Meeting educational differences in reading*. Supplementary Educational Monograph, No. 94. Chicago: University of Chicago Press.

WERNER, H., 1957. *Comparative psychology of mental development*, 2nd rev. ed. New York: International Universities Press.

WERNER, H., and KAPLAN, B., 1963. *Symbol formation*. New York: John Wiley & Sons.

WHITE, M. A., and PHILLIPS, M., 1964. Psychological predictors of school performance using group screening techniques (Mimeogr.). Paper read at annual meeting, Amer. Orthopsychiat. Assoc. Available through Teachers College, Columbia University, New York, N.Y.

WHITEMAN, M., BROWN, B. R., and DEUTSCH, M., 1966. Some effects of social class and race on children's language and intellectual abilities. *Studies in Deprivation*, Equal Opportunities Program. (In press)

Wide Range Achievement Test, Manual, 1946. Jastak, J. Wilmington, Del.: C. L. Story.

WIESENHUETTER, E., 1955. Anthropologische Deutung des Stotterns. *Zeitschr. f. Psychotherapie u. Mediz. Psychologie*.

——, 1958. Entwicklung, Reifung und Neurosen. Stuttgart: Ferdinand Enke Verlag, 34–53.

WIESENHUETTER, U., 1961. *Das Drankommen der Schueler im Unterricht*. Muenchen/Basel: Ernst Reinhardt Verlag. Erziehung und Psychologie, Heft 17.

WISCHNER, J. G., 1950. Stuttering behavior and learning: a preliminary theoretical formulation. *J. Speech, Hear. Disorders*, *15*, 324–35.

WITKIN, H. A., 1965. Heinz Werner: 1890–1964. *Child Develpm. 30*, 2, 309–28.

WITTGENSTEIN, L., 1953. *Philosophical investigations* (German and English edition). New York: The Macmillan Co.

WOOD, N. E., 1964. *Delayed speech and language development*. Foundations of Speech Pathology Series. Englewood Cliffs, N. J.: Prentice-Hall.

WYATT, G. L., 1949. Stammering and language learning in early childhood. *J. Abnorm. Soc. Psychol.*, *44*, 1, 75–84.

——, 1958a. Mother-child relationship and stuttering in children. Unpublished doctoral dissertation, Boston University Library. Microfilm copy available from University Microfilms, 313 N. First Street, Ann Arbor, Michigan. Library of Congress Number Mic 58–3130.

——, 1958b. A developmental crisis theory of stuttering. *Language and speech*, *1*. Robert Draper, Ltd., Teddington, Middlesex, England.

——, 1959. Patterns of therapy with stuttering children and their mothers (Mimeogr.). Terminal Report to the U.S. Public Health Service, National Institute of Mental Health, Small Grant M-2667-A.

——, 1961. It takes two to talk. *Parents' Magazine*, December.

——, 1963. A preventive approach to language disorders in children. In *Symposium on Going to School*. Presented by the Committee on Mental Health, Massachusetts Chapter, American Academy of Pediatrics, 9–18.

——, 1964a. Treating children with non-organic language disorders (Mimeogr.). Terminal Report to the U.S. Public Health Service, National Institute of Mental Health, Research Grant MH-4643.

——, 1964b. Review of Richter, H. E., Eltern, Kind und Neurose. *Contemp. Psychol.*, September, 337–38.

————, 1965. Speech and language disorders in pre-school children: a preventive approach. *Pediatrics*, *36*, 4, 637–47.

————, 1967. Ready for reading? *Parents' Magazine*, May.

WYATT, G. L., and HERZAN, H. M., 1962. Therapy with stuttering children and their mothers. *Amer. J. Orthopsychiat.*, *32*, 4, 645–59. Reprinted in Clark, D. H., and Lesser, G. S. (Eds.), *Emotional disturbance and school learning: a book of readings*. 1965. Chicago: Science Research Associates. 146–63.

WYATT, G. L., and COLLABORATORS, 1962. Treatment of stuttering children and their parents; report of the Wellesley research project (Mimeogr.). A series of papers presented at the 38th annual convention, Amer. Speech Hear. Assoc.

YARROW, L. J., 1961. Maternal deprivation: toward an empirical and conceptual re-evaluation. *Psychol. Bull.*, *58*, 459.

YATES, A. J., 1963a. Recent empirical and theoretical approaches to the experimental manipulation of speech in normal subjects and in stammerers. *Behav. Res. and Ther.*, *1*, 95–119, London: Pergamon Press.

————, 1963b. Delayed auditory feedback. *Psychol. Bull.*, *60*, 3, 213–32.

ZAZZO, AJURIAGUERRA, *et al.*, 1952. *L'apprentissage de la lecture et ses troubles—les dyslexies d'évolution*. Paris: Presses Universitaires de France.

ZETZEL, E. R., 1953. The depressive position. In Greenacre, P. (Ed.), *Affective disorders*. New York: International Universities Press.

ZULLIGER, H., 1953. Child psychotherapy without interpretation of unconscious content. Translated from the German by Ekstein, R., and Wallerstein, J. *Bull. of the Menninger Clin.*, *17*, 5, 180–88.

————, 1957. *Bausteine zur Kinder-Psychotherapie*. Bern und Stuttgart: Hans Huber Verlag.

————, 1959. *Heilende Kraefte im kindlichen Spiel*. Stuttgart: Ernst Klett Verlag.

Key to Abbreviations Used in Bibliography

ASSOCIATIONS AND AGENCIES

Amer. Orthopsychiat. Ass. = *American Orthopsychiatric Association*

Amer. Psychol. Ass. = *American Psychological Association*

Ass. Res. Nerv. Ment. Dis. = *Association for Research in Nervous and Mental Disease*

Inst. Child Welfare = *Institute for Child Welfare*

Inst. f. Research on Exceptional Children = *Institute for Research on Exceptional Children*

Int. Psychoanal. Library = *International Psychoanalytic Library*

NCTE = *National Council of Teachers of English*

NINDS = *National Institute of Neurological Diseases and Blindness*

JOURNALS

Abhand. aus d. Grenzgeb. Paed Med. = *Abhandlungen aus den Grenzgebieten der Paedagogie und Medizin*

Acad. Ther. Quart. = *Academic Therapy Quarterly*

Amer. J. Child Psychiat. = *American Journal of Child Psychiatry*

Amer. J. Orthopsychiat. = *American Journal of Orthopsychiatry*

Amer. J. Psychiat. = *American Journal of Psychiatry*

Arch. Gen. Psychol. = *Archives of General Psychology*

Arch. ges. Psychol. = *Archiv fuer die gesamte Psychologie*

Arch. neur. Psychol. = *Archives of Neuro-Psychology*

Arch. Ophth. = *Archives of Ophthamology*

Arch. of Pediat. = *Archives of Pediatrics*

Behav. Res. and Ther. = *Behavior Research and Therapy*

Brit. J. Disorders of Communic. = *The British Journal of Disorders of Communication*

Brit. J. educ. Psychol. = *British Journal of Educational Psychology*

Brit. J. Sociol. = *British Journal of Sociology*

Brit. Med. J. = *British Medical Journal*

Bull. Menninger Clin. = *Bulletin of the Menniger Clinic*

Bull. Orton Soc. = *Bulletin of the Orton Society*

Child Develpm. = *Child Development*

Child Develpm. Monogr. = *Child Development Monograph*

Child Psychol. = *Child Psychology*

Contemp. Psychol. = *Contemporary Psychology*

Curr. Med. Dig. = *Current Medical Digest*

Develpm. Med. Child Neurol. = *Developmental Medicine and Child Neurology*

Educ. Psychol. Measmt. = *Educational and Psychological Measurement*

Elem. English Rev. = *Elementary English Review*

Elem. Sch. J. = *Elementary School Journal*

Except. Child. = *Exceptional Children*

Genet. Psychol. Monogr. = *Genetic Psychology Monograph*

Int. J. Psychoanal. = *International Journal of Psycho-Analysis*

Int. Read. Conf. Proc. = *International Reading Conference Procedures*

Int. Read. Ass. Conf. = *International Reading Association Conference*

J. Abnorm. Soc. Psychol. = *Journal of Abnormal and Social Psychology*

J. Amer. Acad. Child Psychiat. = *Journal of the American Academy of Child Psychiatry*

J. Amer. Med. Ass. = *Journal of the American Medical Association*

J. Child Psychol. Psychiat. = *Journal o Child Psychology and Psychiatry and Allied Disciplines*

J. Clin. Psychol. = *Journal of Clinical Psychology*

J. Comp. Physiol. Psychol. = *Journal of Comparative and Physiological Psychology*

J. of Educ. = *Journal of Education*

J. Educ. Psychol. = *Journal of Educational Psychology*

J. Educ. Res. = *Journal of Ed ucational Research*

J. Exp. Psychol. = *Journal of Experimental Psychology*

J. Nerv. Ment. Dis. = *Journal of Nervous and Mental Disease*

J. Psychol. = *Journal of Psychology*

J. Psychosom. Res. = *Journal of Psychosomatic Research*

J. Oklahoma State Med. Ass. = *Journal of the Oklahoma State Medical Association*

J. Sch. Psychol. = *Journal of School Psychology*

J. Speech Disorders = *Journal of Speech Disorders*

J. Speech, Hear. Disorders = *Journal of Speech and Hearing Disorders*

J. Speech, Hear. Res. = *Journal of Speech and Hearing Research*

J. Verb. Learn., Verb. Behav. = *Journal of Verbal Learning and Verbal Behavior*

Maryland Med. J. = *Maryland Medical Journal*

Merrill-Palmer Quart. = *Merrill-Palmer Quarterly*

Monogr. seel. Entwickl. Kindes = *Monograph der seelischen Entwicklung des Kindes*

Monogr. Soc. Res. Child Develpm. = *Monograph of the Society for Research in Child Development*

Monatsschr. f. Ohrenheilk. u. Laryngo-Rhinol. *Monatsschrift fuer Ohrenheilkunde und Laryngo-Rhinologie*

Percept. Mot. Skills = *Perceptual and Motor Skills*

Psychiat. Quart. = *Psychiatric Quarterly*

Psychoanal. Quart. = *Psychoanalytical Quarterly*

Psychoanal. Rev. = *Psychoanalytical Review*

Psychol. Bull. = *Psychological Bulletin*

Read. Teach. = *Reading Teacher*

Rehabilit. Liter. = *Rehabilitation Literature*

Res. Monogr. = *Research Monograph*

Rev. Educ. Res. = *Review of Educational Research*

Sch. a. Soc. = *School and Society*

Scient. Amer. = *Scientific American*

Soc. Casework = *Social Casework*

Teachers Coll. Rec. = *Teachers College Record*

The Psychoanal. Stud. of the Child = *The Psychoanalytic Study of the Child*

The Voice, J. California Speech, Hear. Ass. = *The Voice, Journal of the California Speech and Hearing Association*

University of Iowa Stud. Child Welf. = *University of Iowa Studies in Child Welfare*

Zeitschr. f. Kinderforschung = *Zeitschrift fuer Kinderforschung*

Indexes

Index of Authors

Index of Psychological Tests

Subject Index